Hydrogen Peroxide

A HEALTH, HOMEOSTATIC and PROTECTIVE ESSENTIALITY

A scientifically verifiable, omnipresent, ubiquitous, fundamental of obligate, aerobic, carbon-based life forms

BY

Prof Randolph Michael Howes MD,PhD

Orthomolecular Scientist, Surgeon, Scholar,

Author and Biochemist

Hydrogen Peroxide

A HEALTH, HOMEOSTATIC and PROTECTIVE ESSENTIALITY

BY

PROF. HON. RANDOLPH M. HOWES, M.D., Ph.D.
Orthomolecular Scientist, Surgeon, Scholar, Author and Biochemist

Adjunct Assistant Professor of Plastic Surgery, (RET.) The Johns Hopkins Hospital, Baltimore, MD. USA

Espaldon Professor of Plastic and Reconstructive Surgery, University of Santo Tomas, Manila, Philippines

Adjunct Professor of Biological Sciences, Southeastern Louisiana University

Professor of Surgery, Biophysics and Biochemistry, Louisiana University of Medical Sciences

Dean, Louisiana University of Medical Sciences

(Also holds an Honorary Doctorate of Humanities)

DISCLOSURE AND DISCLAIMER

Prof Randolph Michael Howes MD,PhD

Notice to users:

1. User agrees not to redistribute any electronic artifacts of this resource without prior written permission from <u>Free</u> Radical Publishing Co.

2. Except as permitted under the United States Copyright Act of 1976, no part of this publication may be reproduced or distributed in any form or by any means, or stored in a data base or retrieval system, without prior written permission of the publisher.

Disclaimers:

Please note: only your personal physician or other health professional you consult can best advise you on matters of your health based on your medical history, your family medical history, your medication history, and how information from any of these databases may apply to you. Neither Dr. Howes nor any party involved in creating, producing or delivering this web site shall be liable for any damages arising out of access to or use of this material or web site, or any errors or omissions in the content thereof.

The information given herein is not intended as medical advice. Always consult with your doctor for underlying illness. Before beginning dietary investigation, consult a dietician or a physician with an interest in nutrition. Information is drawn from the scientific literature, web research, and personal enquiry; while all care is taken, information is not warranted as accurate and the author cannot be held liable for any errors and omissions.

Financial disclosure:

Dr. Howes has no financial conflicts of interest and is not involved in the sale of dietary supplements or fitness equipment. The author holds no stocks or interests in companies in the food additive or antioxidant supplement business.

Prof Randolph Michael Howes MD,PhD

Companion Books:

Howes, R. M. *U.T.O.P.I.A. - Unified Theory of Oxygen Participation in Aerobiosis.* © 2004. Free Radical Publishing Co. Kentwood, LA, available at www.iwillfindthecure.org.

Howes R. M. *The Medical and Scientific Significance of Oxygen Free Radical Metabolism.* © 2005. Free Radical Publishing Co. Kentwood, LA. USA. available at www.iwillfindthecure.org.

Howes, R. M. *Hydrogen Peroxide Monograph 1: Scientific, Medical and Biochemical Overview.* © 2006; Free Radical Publishing Co. USA. 200 pages. available at www.iwillfindthecure.org.

Howes, R. M. Monograph 2: *Antioxidant vitamins A, C & E: Equivocal Scientific Studies,* © 2006; Free Radical Publishing Co. USA. 171 pages. available at www.iwillfindthecure.org.

Howes, R. M. *Cardiovascular Disease and Oxygen Free Radical Mythology,* © 2006;

Free Radical Publishing Co. USA. 308 pages. available at www. iwillfindthecure.org.

Howes, R. M. *Diabetes and Oxygen Free Radical Sophistry,* © 2006;

Free Radical Publishing Co. USA. Free Radical Publishing Co. USA. 366 pages. available at www.iwillfindthecure.org.

Howes, R. M. *Reactive Oxygen Species Insufficiency (ROSI) as the Basis for Disease Allowance and Coexistence: Extraordinary Support for an Extraordinary Theory* Vol I, II & III. © 2008; 1564 pages. available at www.iwillfindthecure. org.
Howes, R. M. Volume I 501 pages #7 © 2008. Free Radical Publishing Co. USA.

Howes, R. M. Volume II 505 pages #8 © 2008. Free Radical Publishing Co. USA.
Howes, R. M. Volume III 562 pages #9 © 2008. Free Radical Publishing Co. USA.

Howes, R. M. *THE HOWES PAPERS*
© 2009; Free Radical Publishing Co. USA. 211 pages

Howes R.M. *"COFFEE TABLE MUSINGS of the Da Vinci in COWBOY BOOTS"*
Pithy Prose and Perspicacious Aphorisms. © 2009; 103 pages

Howes, R. M. Reactive Oxygen Species vs. Antioxidants:
"The Oxypocalypse" or
"The war that never was" © 2010; Free Radical Publishing Co. USA. 550 pages. available at www.iwillfindthecure.org.

Howes R.M. *Death in Small Doses?:*
Antioxidant Vitamins A, C & E in the 21st Century
Book One: *A Health Impact Statement For The Layman*
© 2010; Trafford Publishing. Indianapolis, USA. 90 pages

Howes R.M. *Antioxidant Vitamins are Making A Killing;*
Antioxidant Vitamins A, C & E in the 21st Century
Book Two: *A Health Impact Statement For The Medical Scientist*
© 2010; 184 pages

Howes R.M. *Antioxidant Overkill:* An antioxidant guide for the educated consumer. © 2011. CreateSpace and Free Radical Publishing Co. USA. 421 pages.

Howes R.M. *Dangers Of Excessive Antioxidants in Cancer Patients.* © 2011. CreateSpace and Free Radical Publishing Co. 524 pages.

Companion Papers:

Dr. Howes has authored over 350 medical publications in health related editorials.

Citation: R. Howes: Mythology of Antioxidant Vitamins?. *The Journal of Evidence-Based Alternative and Complimentary Medicine.* April, 2011. 16(2): 149-189.

Citation: R. Howes: Cancer Therapy: A Review with Scientific Validation for the Role of Electronically Modified Oxygen Derivatives in Oncologic Treatment Modalities. *The Internet Journal of Alternative Medicine.* 2010 Volume 8 Number 1.

Citation: R. Howes: Hydrogen Peroxide: A review of a scientifically verifiable omnipresent ubiquitous essentiality of obligate, aerobic, carbon-based life forms. *The Internet Journal of Plastic Surgery.* 2010 Volume 7 Number 1.

Howes M.D., PhD., R. (2009). Dangers of Antioxidants in Cancer Patients: A Review. *PHILICA.COM Article number 153.* Published 7th February, 2009. (20 pages)

Howes M.D., PhD., R. (2008). Aging and anti-aging claims: a review on antioxidant vitamins A, C & E. *PHILICA.COM Article number 116.* Published on 12th January, 2008. (16 pages)

Howes M.D., PhD., R. (2007). Sleep: An original "radical" proposal. *PHILICA.COM Observation number 42.* Published on 5th October, 2007. (1 page)

Howes M.D., PhD., R. (2007). Antioxidant Vitamins A, C & E; Death in Small Doses and Legal Liability? *PHILICA.COM Article number 89.* Published on 5th April, 2007. (23 pages)

Howes M.D., PhD., R. (2007). Cancer, Apoptosis and Reactive Oxygen Species: A New Paradigm. *PHILICA.COM Article number 86.* Published on 26th February, 2007. (11 pages)

Howes M.D., PhD., R. (2007). Antioxidant Vitamins A, C and E: Assessing Potential for Harm. *PHILICA.COM Article number 83.* Published on 15th February, 2007. (14 pages)

Howes M.D., PhD., R. (2007). The Consequent Downfall of the Free Radical Theory. *PHILICA.COM Article number 75.* Published on 22nd January, 2007. (9 pages)

Howes, R.M.: "The Free Radical Fantasy," The Annals of New York Academy of Sciences, 2006, Vol. 1067, pp. 22-26.

(Howes, 2005) (Howes, R.M. Tumoricidal Activity of An Injectable Singlet Oxygen System Generated From Physiological Agents: The Howes Singlet Oxygen Cancer Therapy System). In The Medical and Scientific Significance of Oxygen Free Radical Metabolism. © 2005. Free Radical Publishing Co. Kentwood, LA. pp. 893-912).

(Howes, Farber, 2005) (Howes, R.M. and Farber, G. Tumoricidal Activity of the Howes Singlet Oxygen Delivery System in Human Basal Cell Carcinoma. In The Medical and Scientific Significance of Oxygen Free Radical Metabolism. © 2005. Free Radical Publishing Co. Kentwood, LA. pp. 883-892).

(Howes et al, 1977) (Howes, R.M., Steele, R.H. and Hoopes, J.E., The role of Electronic excitation states in collagen biosynthesis, Persp. In Biol. And Med., Summer 1977, 20; 4:539-544).

(Howes, Steele, 1976) (Howes, R.M., Steele, R.H. and Hoopes, J.E., Peroxide induced Chemiluminescence in an in vitro proline hydroxylation system, 1976, 8; 1:77-84).

(Howes et al, 1976) (Howes, R. M., Allen, R.C., Su, C.T. and Hoopes, J.E., Altered polymorphonuclear leukocyte bioenergetics in patients with thermal injury, the Surgical Forum, 1976, 27:558-560).

(Howes, Steele, 1972) (Howes, R.M. and Steele, R.H., Microsomal chemiluminescence induced by NADPH and its relation to aryl-hydroxylations, Res Commun. Chem. Path. Pharmacol., March 1972, 3; 2:349-357).

(Howes, Steele, 1971) (Howes, R. M. and Steele, R. H., Microsomal chemiluminescence induced by NADPH and its relation to lipid peroxidation, Res. Commun. Chem. Path. Pharmacol., July-Sept. 1971, 2; 4 & 5:619-626).

**I despise precious time wasted,
for it alone, is the unfinished canvas
displaying the portrait of my life.**
R. M. Howes, M.D., Ph.D.
9/7/09

"We are what we repeatedly do. Excellence then, is not an act, but a habit." ~Aristotle

OTHER BOOKS PUBLISHED:
Partial list.

The Fire Eaters, Molding your own destiny more easily, Carnivore Press, © 1982

Uplift, The Answer Book to your plastic and cosmetic

surgery questions, Carnivore Press, © 1986

The Pundit Speaks, vol. I. An Anthology of Neoclassical Poetic

Philosophy, Carnivore Press, © 1990

The Pundit Speaks, Volume II, An Anthology of Neoclassical

Poetic Philosophy, Free Radical Press, © 1994

The Pundit Speaks, Volume III, An Anthology of Neoclassical

Poetic Philosophy, Free Radical Press, © 1996

The Pundit Speaks, Volume IV, An Anthology of Neoclassical

Poetic Philosophy, Free Radical Press, © 2000

The Fable of the Chocolate Covered Strawberry Coloring

Book, Free Radical Press, © 2001

The Pundit Speaks, Volume IV, An Anthology of Neoclassical

Poetic Philosophy, Free Radical Press, © 2003

The Pundit Speaks, Volume V, An Anthology of Neoclassical

Poetic Philosophy, Trafford Publishing, © 2009

Coffee Table Musings of The DaVinci In Cowboy Boots, Trafford

Publishing, © 2010

Death In Small Doses? Trafford Publishing, © 2010

Antioxidant Overkill, CreateSpace and Free Radical Publishing, © 2011

Da in Cancer Patients, CreateSpace and Free Radical Publishing, © 2011

Heart Disease and Antioxidant Failures, CreateSpace and Free

Radical Publishing, © 2011

Antioxidant Failures and Dangers, CreateSpace and Free Radical

Publishing, © 2011

Anti-Aging Anti-oxidant Scams, CreateSpace and Free Radical

Publishing, © 2011

Sports, Athletes, Exercise Facts and Antioxidant Myths, CreateSpace and Free Radical Publishing, © 2011

Alzheimer's Disease: Forget Antioxidants and Supplements, CreateSpace and Free Radical Publishing, © 2012

Antioxidants Linked To Deadly Unintended Consequences, CreateSpace and Free Radical Publishing, © 2012

Sex, Performance, Reproduction, Naked Radicals and Antioxidants, CreateSpace and Free Radical Publishing, © 2012

U.T.O.P.I.A.: Unified Theory of Oxygen Participation In Aerobiosis, CreateSpace and Free Radical Publishing, © 2013

Diabetes and Oxygen Free Radical Sophistry, CreateSpace and Free Radical Publishing, © 2014, revised

Available at: www.philica.com

www.medi.philica.com
www.iwillfindthecure.org
www.amazon.com

Prof Randolph Michael Howes MD,PhD

**If you believe the implausible,
you will accept the indefensible and
not recognize the inexcusable.**
R. M. Howes, M.D., Ph.D.
6/5/11

DOC
R _x **ANDOLPH**
HOWES

RAD!CAL

ABOUT THE AUTHOR

Dr. Randolph M. Howes M.D., Ph.D.
Biographical sketch:

As a champion of the people, Dr. Howes anticipates and hopes for the active involvement of all connected parties (patients, caregivers, healthcare professionals, etc.) as an integral approach to educating consumers and the public about the potential dangers of excessive antioxidant-containing supplements and "antioxidant stacking."

Some people are born with a silver spoon in their mouth but Dr. Howes had to earn his. Even as a child, Dr. Howes could think with adult clarity. He could envision his future but it would require "decades of dedication" to make it a reality.

From childhood, Dr. Howes was motivated to become a medical doctor and scientist. Assuredly, having been born on a small strawberry farm in rural Louisiana, his journey to the top has proved to be arduous and demanding.

However, he was fortunate to acquire the confidence of Sister Elizabeth at St. Joseph's school and went on to gain the support of his high school speech teacher, Mrs. Iris Brann, who also had strong beliefs in his abilities and potential. Ultimately, with the help of his guitar and his singing ability, he defeated the star quarter back of the high school football team to become the president of the student body.

With the aid of a $25 dollar legislative scholarship, he went on to Southeastern Louisiana College (SLC). At SLC, he was selected for honors chemistry, made the Dean's list, worked at the Psychology Research Lab forty hours a week, maintained a premed study load, and was elected president of the Junior Class and the Interfraternity Council.

Prof Randolph Michael Howes MD, PhD

To earn badly needed funds, he played music on weekends in a small combo, The Three Blind Mice. Next, he matriculated to Tulane University School of Medicine.

His initial dream was to try to combine both medicine and science. In that regard, he began work as a technician with Dr. Andrew Schally at the Endocrine Polypeptide Lab in the isolation of thyrotropin releasing factor. This work led to a Nobel Prize for Dr. Schally.

Dr. Howes had been highly impressed with the enthusiasm of biochemist, Dr. Richard H. Steele, who accepted him as a doctoral candidate under his tutelage. Dr. Howes graduated in the top 10 of his class, won the Louisiana Pathology Association Award, was elected to the Sigma Xi honor fraternity and was the first in the history of Tulane to become a Doctor of Medicine and a Ph.D. in biochemistry concurrently.

Next, he was selected to pursue a career in surgery at the prestigious Johns Hopkins Hospital.

Unbelievably, at Dr. Howes' urging, he was allowed to operate his own research lab during his surgical internship and residency training while at Johns Hopkins Hospital. He worked hand in hand with the greats in American medicine and surgery.

Independently, he garnered grants, trained lab techs, wrote papers, slept on the cold floor, proudly served as a Captain in the U.S. Army Reserves Medical Corp and finished with board eligibility in both general and plastic surgery in an unheard of six year period.

In another first, he was appointed as an Adjunct Assistant Professor of Plastic Surgery at Johns Hopkins Hospital.

For decades, Dr. Howes gave unselfishly to pro bono medical missions in the Philippines and he holds the Ernesto Espaldon Chair as Professor of Plastic Surgery at the University of Santo Tomas.

Upon retirement from a career in cosmetic plastic surgery, he is living his dream of trying to revolutionize the treatment of cancer, heart disease, HIV/AIDS and malaria, with his in depth knowledge of the arcane biochemistry of oxygen metabolism. He is a work in progress! Dedicated and passionate, he is on a mission for mankind.

Dr. Howes invented the triple lumen venous catheter, which has been credited with helping save the lives of over 20 million critically ill patients worldwide. His catheter became the number one venous catheter in the world and his name is well recognized in over 100 countries. He has been recognized as a humanitarian, visionary, entrepreneur, singer, songwriter, inventor and author.

He received the Harper Award for innovative research from the American College for Advancement in Medicine, served as their keynote speaker and his peers refer to him as "a walking encyclopedia on oxygen metabolism."

He is a Dr. Norman Vincent Peale Unsung Hero award winner, which recognized his awesome versatility. Additionally, even though he is humble and does not like talking about it, he is a self made multi-millionaire.

He is currently doing extensive research on cures for cancer and heart disease and development of revolutionary treatment modalities. He has written 16 books over the past 8 years on the subject of oxygen metabolism, as it relates to protection from cancer, heart disease, diabetes, malaria, HIV/AIDS, Alzheimer's disease, aging and arthritis. He has written many scientific and medical papers and has lectured nationally and internationally.

His research has shown that currently common antioxidant vitamins, such as vitamins A & E, (and vitamin C to a lesser extent) can be harmful and that oxygen free radicals protect us from bacterial, fungal and viral infections and they help to control cancer growth.

He has developed an effective, inexpensive singlet oxygen generating system, from orthomolecular agents, for the treatment of cancer and heart disease. He is passionate about his research and hopes to have his discoveries at the patient's bedside in his lifetime. Admittedly, this is an extremely ambitious goal.

There are over 8,000 pages in his magnum opus and at the Howes World Selective Library on Oxygen Metabolism. **Over 3,000 pages of his opus are available online in a searchable format www.iwillfindthecure.org** © by R.M. Howes

NOTE: An avid researcher, Dr. Howes has authored more than 350 original publications, including over 30 medical and scientific books, such as Death In Small Doses (Antioxidant vitamins A, C & E in the 21st Century), Antioxidant Overkill and Dangers of Excessive Antioxidants In Cancer Patients. He has written numerous articles for medical and consumer publications, including The Journal of American Academy of Cosmetic Surgery, Annals of the New York Academy of Science, The Journal of Evidence Based Complementary And Alternative Medicine, The Baton Rouge Advocate, and The Houma Courier. He has a weekly science/medicine column in the Hammond Daily Star and The Ponchatoula Times. His research interests include truthful reporting of antioxidant dangers, adverse effects of vitamins A, C & E, other antioxidant's deadly unintended consequences, free radicals, oxygen metabolism, and cancer and heart disease treatment and prevention, global health care policy, and oxidative means to revolutionize treating and preventing HIV/AIDS and malaria.

Dr. Howes is also an active and well-known speaker and media personality, having been featured on PBS's The American Health

Journal, WWL-TV New Orleans and WDSU-TV New Orleans, Sirius/XM satellite radio, as well as many other national talk and news shows across America.

In 2013, he received from the American College for Advancement In Medicine the first Charles Farr Award for "excellence in oxidative medicine."

After reading Dr. Howes' book, *Dangers of Excessive Antioxidants In Cancer Patients,* Robert C. Allen, M.D., Ph.D., Chairman of the Department of Pathology at Creighton Medical School in Omaha, Nebraska, described Dr. Howes this way,
"During my forty-five-year association with Dr. Randolph M. Howes, I've been consistently impressed, and sometimes exhausted, by his brilliance, energy and intensity. Over the past several years his attention has been focused on debunking the meme that oxidants are "bad" and antioxidants are "good". We should all appreciate that oxidation provides the energy that drives all complex life forms. *Dangers of Excessive Antioxidants in Cancer Patients* presents convincing arguments with supporting evidence that simplistically assuming antioxidants are somehow "good" is not valid. Dr. Howes is *The Scientific Voyager* poetically described herein, and this book is the product of his voyage."

Dr. Allen answered the question, "If you or a loved one had cancer, would you now take or recommend antioxidants?" He answered, "If I had cancer and was undergoing chemotherapy, I certainly would not be taking BHT, vitamins A and E, or any "antioxidant" formulation, nor would I recommend antioxidants to my family, loved ones, or anyone else." His support of Dr. Howes' work is clear and undeniable.

Following the same scenario, Dr. Robert Muller, M.D. (Ob-Gyn) answered this way: "Dr Howes book shows the extensive research done on antioxidants, BUT the difficulty lies in overcoming the social norms established by the brainwashing of the public by the pharmaceutical industry. If common sense prevails, the choice becomes very clear—antioxidants are worthless in the prevention and treatment of cancer (and CVD)." Robert Muller, M.D. 5-12-11

These are just two examples of highly qualified, medically-involved, individuals who recognize the innovative brilliance of Dr. Howes' new approach to disease prevention, causation and coexistence.

Dr. Howes' origin from a small Louisiana farming community imbedded in him a unique level of morality, ethical behavior and common sense. He feels that common sense is "commonly missing" in the world of medical science today. True, one must be trained to deal with the arcane biological and physiological sciences but one must also be open-minded and willing to rely on common sense, especially when certain scientific theories go against or fly in the face of inductive/deductive reasoning and clear thinking.

**If you can not see what is illogical,
you can not fix the irreconcilable.
If you can not sense flawed logic,
you will never taste truth.**
R. M. Howes, M.D., Ph.D.
6/5/11

Dr. Howes spent over a quarter of a century in educational training to prepare himself for the challenging world of medical science. He is fulfilling his dreams of making significant contributions to the prevention and cure of some of mankind's most deadly diseases, such as cancer, heart disease, malaria and HIV/AIDS.

He feels strongly that he must place his innovative ideas onto the public forum, utilizing printed media and the world wide web. Thus, others can evaluate the validity of his contributions and continue in the pursuit of his dreams.

DEDICATION

To a couple of special friends:
dr. paul manson, dr. robert allen and
dr. robert rowen

Monograph I: HYDROGEN PEROXIDE

TABLE OF CONTENTS:

The U.T.O.P.I.A. Institute and Free Radical Publishing Co.

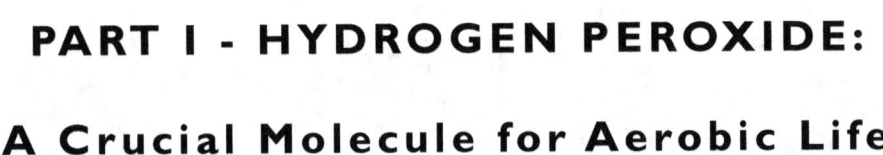

PART I - HYDROGEN PEROXIDE:

A Crucial Molecule for Aerobic Life

1.0 INTRODUCTION

Oxygen is constantly being metabolized, from the moment of conception until the moment of death, in every aerobic cell in our body. Consequently, reactive oxygen species or electronically modified oxygen derivatives (EMODs) and oxygen excited states are constantly being generated in every aerobic cell in our body. Healthy tissue maintains a steady state of $[H_2O_2]$ of 10^{-9} to 10^{-7} (Physiological Reviews 1979, 59: 564).

We derive our energy from oxidation, which requires, at least, slightly prooxidant conditions. (Halliwell)

Humans consume about 250 grams of oxygen every day, and of this, approximately 3-5% is converted to superoxide anion (O_2^{-}) and other modifications of oxygen (Rice-Evans, C A and Burdon, R H. Free radical damage and its control. Amsterdam: Elsevier, 1994; p. 25-27). **That calculates out to 12.5 grams of superoxide per person per day.** These are overwhelming quantities of **superoxide, which are likely rapidly converted to hydrogen peroxide.**

"We can look at oxygen deficiency or oxygen starvation as the single greatest cause of all disease." (Stephen Levin, Ph.D., entitled, Oxygen and Life: Original Hypothesis concerning Oxygen Deficiency as a Cause of Disease States). **I agree with the importance of ground state oxygen but I believe that the electronically modified oxygen derivates (free radical oxygen modifications and excitation states, i.e., (EMODs) are of far greater importance for fighting pathogens and neoplasia. Additionally, one could have adequate levels of ground state oxygen and yet, not be able to generate adequate levels of EMODs, such as in the case of chronic granulomatous disease.**

The roles of these reactive species in host defense and antimicrobial activity are well documented as impaired EMOD (ROS or RNS) production results in susceptibility to bacterial (Babior BM, Lambeth JD, and Nauseef W. The neutrophil NADPH oxidase. *Arch Biochem Biophys* 397: 342–344, 2002) **or parasitic infection** (Murray HW and Nathan CF. Macrophage microbicidal mechanisms in vivo: reactive nitrogen versus oxygen intermediates in the killing of intracellular visceral *Leishmania donovani. J Exp Med* 189: 741–746, 1999).

The Term ROS (EMODs)

The term **ROS (EMODs) encompasses** many species including:

- **singlet oxygen**
- **the superoxide anion radical**
- **H_2O_2**
- **lipid peroxides**
- **nitric oxide (NO)**
- **peroxynitrite (ONOO)**
- **the thiyl peroxyl radical (RSOO·)**
- **the ferryl radical (FeO^{2+})**
- **and the hydroxyl radical (OH·)**

Hydrogen peroxide biochemistry has had a history of controversy, conflict and perceived paradoxes. I believe that many of the paradoxes are due to the nigh carte-blanche, unquestioning acceptance and application of the erroneous principles taught by the free radical theory, as they related to the biochemistry of aerobic cells (Howes, R. M. 2004. Revised 2014, U.T.O.P.I.A. - Unified Theory of Oxygen Participation in Aerobiosis. (767 page text) Free Radical Publishing Co. Kentwood, LA) (Howes, R.M. 2005. The Medical and Scientific Significance of Oxygen Free Radical Metabolism. (931 page text) Free Radical Publishing Co. Kentwood, LA).

I hereby present the scientific basis for prooxidant protection and oxidative self-healing. I make the case that hydrogen peroxide is a major player in maintaining healthy homeostasis and occupies on unparalleled role as a secondary cellular messenger. Without steady state levels of hydrogen peroxide, our very existence would be in jeopardy, just as it is in patients with chronic granulomatous disease or in patients with absence of myeloperoxidase.

1.1 Oxidative-Cure and the Peroxide-Spike

Aging increases the risk for many diseases and disorders. In general, elderly people have an increased rate of chronic disorders, arteriosclerosis, infections, autoimmune disorders and cancer. Most of these disorders are gradually progressive and do not show symptoms for many years.

And additional factor for the increased risk of disease in the elderly is the decline in the immune system. **It seeks out and destroys bacteria, viruses, fungi and cancerous cells before they can damage the body. These are the same pathogens which are destroyed by EMODs and a deadly oxidative event (DOA). This is a most important finding.** It has memory and learns to distinguish between "self" and "non-self" particles.

This system of self-cure is primarily a system of "oxidative-cure" and is responsible for the killing of bacteria, viruses, fungi, protozoa and tumor cells. **Oxidation serves as the first line of our defense and occurs with the respiratory burst, which should more properly be referred to as the "peroxide spike", secondary to spontaneous or enzymatic dismutation of superoxide.** Ergo, our lives are sustained by an innate "oxidative-cure" and during times of need, to fight invaders or tumors, we rely on the **"peroxide-spike" or ("Vis medicatrix naturae":** The Healing Power of Nature).

Prof Randolph Michael Howes MD,PhD

Disruption of the delicate balance between pro-oxidants and antioxidants has been implicated in the pathophysiology of many chronic diseases, such as atherosclerosis (Halliwell B. Oxidants and human disease: some concepts. *FASEB J.* 1987;1:358–364).

Short sighted investigators suggest that anything which serves as an antioxidant is good and anything which oxidizes something else is bad. That is just not true. All antioxidants can serve as prooxidants. The synthesis of thyroxine depends on the actions of H_2O_2 and thyroid peroxidase. Further, H_2O_2 is now well recognized as an important and widespread second messenger for all aerobic cells. To imply or give the false impression that the presence of H_2O_2 is a bad thing is more nonscience/ nonsense.

Many molecules are designed to accept and receive electrons (with no wear and tear) as a natural part of their reactivity, especially the transitions metals and the heme proteins.

The flawed free radical has created a **paradox** whereby strong oxidizing agents have been used by many physicians for alleviating symptoms of syndromes that are purported to be evidently caused by accelerated oxidative molecular injury. **I believe that this paradox exists only because we have erroneously been led to accept the free radi-crap theory.** Evidently, these diseases are not caused by oxidative molecular injury and can, in fact, be controlled or cured by EMODs (i.e., H_2O_2, ozone, hyperbaric oxygen, singlet oxygen, etc.). H_2O_2 should no longer be vilified and should be recognized as a ubiquitous and naturally occurring substance which has extremely important modulatory cellular functions. **Oxygen, in its varying electronic configurations and states, is the primary reason that we do not have an infection or a tumor to appear at any and all times in our lives, from conception to birth.**

Oxygen is fundamental for life and its concentration and those of electronically modified oxygen derivatives (EMODs) are an important signal for virtually all cellular processes. Oxygen is an important signal in all major aspects of stem cell biology including proliferation and tumorigenesis, cell death and differentiation, self-renewal, and migration. (Oxygen in the Cultivation of Stem Cells. Marie Csete. *Ann. N.Y. Acad. Sci.* 1049: 1–8 (2005).

1.2   The Breath of Life

**"Aerobic life is choreographed by its oxygen in-structor to
perform the dance of the electron."**
R. M. Howes, M.D., Ph.D.
2/25/04

The breath of life is filled with oxygen, which serves as the primary adjunct to aerobic metabolism and as fuel for our bodies. **I believe that if you analyze the contents of that breath of life, you will find that it is because of the presence of its 21% oxygen content, which makes it is the breath of life.**

I quote, "And the Lord God formed man of the dust of the ground, and breathed into his nostrils the breath of life; and man became a living soul. Genesis 2:7."

Some say that 10^{12} O_2 molecules are consumed everyday.

Emergency procedures emphasize the importance of establishing an airway and an adequate supply of oxygen. **Aerobic exercises are based on oxygen metabolism to aid the immune system, improve overall health and disease prevention.**

The importance of oxygen could not be more readily apparent. It is the essential sustaining and driving force for all aerobic cellular metabolism. The primary thing which stands between us and constant or perpetual infections or manifestations of neoplasia, is our ability to generate oxidative events in the form of RONS/excytomers (EMODs).

It is unheard of to attempt to resuscitate a patient with a large dose of β-carotene, melatonin or lipoic acid or any other antioxidant. To the contrary, based on experience we know that they need oxygen and oxidative help and healing.

There are a growing number of studies which fail to implicate oxygen free radical reactions as being causative of specific diseases.

Attempts, with antioxidants, to prevent cancer have failed.
" " " " diabetes have failed.
" " " " atherosclerosis have failed.
" " " " strokes have failed.
" " " " amyloidosis have failed.
" " " " Alzheimer's disease have failed.
" " " " Parkinson's disease have failed.
" " " " arthritis have failed.

This pattern has repeated itself over and over again in attempts to prevent any and all diseases and to stop the aging process. Attempts to extend the normal lifetime expectancy have been very disappointing and inconclusive.

To the contrary, diseases of EMOD deficiency states, such as chronic granulomatous disease, clearly demonstrate the crucial need for EMOD generation.

Anaerobic metabolism is favorable to many pathogenic organisms and hypoxia is the predominant condition within cancerous cells.

Hypoxia has been closely associated with pathological processes. (Hypoxia Promotes Lymph Node Metastasis in Human Melanoma Xenografts by Up-Regulating the Urokinase-Type Plasminogen Activator Receptor. Einar K. Rofstad, Heidi Rasmussen, Kanthi Galappathi, Berit Mathiesen, Kristin Nilsen and Bjørn A. Graff. Cancer Research 62, 1847-1853, March 15, 2002).

Further, **I believe that the decreasing levels of EMODs are associated with the overall decline that we see in the aging process, which results in decreased O$_2$ intake, O$_2$ utilization, lowered EMODs and allowance of arteriosclerosis, diabetes, cancer, cataracts, etc. This is specifically the reason that antioxidants have failed to curtail or prevent these diseases.**

Investigators, who apply the free radical theory, have based conclusions on loose associations, in vitro studies and counter-intuitive observations. I believe that we now have adequate data to make more reasonable conclusions regarding this amazing and crucial molecule (H$_2$O$_2$) of human metabolism. The cell is a dynamic entity of incomprehensible complexity, in which all biochemical pathways are inter-related. These interrelationships have to be considered, especially as they apply to the redox status of the cell and to organismal homeostasis.

In the case of **"redox signaling" this is achieved by discrete, localized redox circuitry rather than generalized "oxidative stress"** (Go YM, Gipp JJ, Mulcahy RT, and Jones DP. H$_2$O$_2$-dependent activation of GCLC-ARE4 reporter occurs by mitogen-activated protein kinase pathways without oxidation of cellular glutathione or thioredoxin-1. *J Biol Chem* 279: 5837–5845, 2004). This realization represents a significant departure from traditional views that ROS (EMODs) are simply a by-product of normal oxidative metabolism or a tool through which phagocytes accomplish antimicrobial action. With this paradigm shift comes the challenge of understanding how ROS production is regulated and localized within cells in both normal and pathological circumstances. **Current evidence would support a role for EMODs as a generalized "injury" response in tissues. This is exactly what I have been saying for years. For EMODs to mediate signaling, one would assume that some specific protein modification would be involved.** Available evidence supports a role **for protein thiol groups in this process as they represent a well-known target for reactive species.** Recently, **a number of proteins have been identified as targets for ROS-mediated signal transduction.**

The biochemistry of H_2O_2 is also the biochemistry of the superoxide anion. Superoxide anion converts rapidly to H_2O_2 either spontaneously or with the help of the superoxide dismutase enzyme. Since many of the electronically modified oxygen derivatives (EMODs) are rapidly converted and/or transformed into other EMOD species, it is also the story of all EMODs.

Chance, et al., have reviewed the metabolism of H_2O_2 in mammalian systems (Chance, B., Sies, H. and Boveris, A. Hydrogen peroxide metabolism in mammalian organs. Physiol Rev 1979; 59: 527). H_2O_2 may be produced directly as a product of biological oxidations, or it may be produced by the dismutation of superoxide. Their relative **estimates of subcellular sources of H_2O_2 are as follows:**

Estimates of subcellular sources of H_2O_2 are as follows:

- **Endoplasmic reticulum (mixed function oxidations)**   **45%**
- **Peroxisomes (metal-catalyzed oxidations)**   **35%**
- **Mitochondria (oxidative phosphorylation)**   **15%**
- **Cytosol (xanthine oxidation)**   **5%**

These **EMODs are formed continuously** in all aerobic cells, either via oxygen energy metabolism, through reactions with drugs or toxins or via metabolism of fatty acids.

In 1999, Juan and Buettner calculated the steady state levels to be as follows:

> **$[H_2O_2]$ss in red cells is 10^{-10} M**
> **$[H_2O_2]$ss in mitochondrial membrane is 10^{-8} M**
> **$[H_2O_2]$ss in liver cells is 10^{-8} M**
> **$[O_2]$ss is 10^{-5} M, much higher than $[H_2O_2]$**
> **$[O_2^{\cdot-}]$ss in cells is 10^{-10} M**

Naturally, we will have to consider an in depth study of small molecular weight antioxidants, and antioxidant enzymatic systems involved in the production and removal of H_2O_2, such as NADPH oxidase, myeloperoxidase, catalase, superoxide dismutase, glutathione peroxidase, cytochrome P450s, vitamins C & E, β-carotene, α-tocopherol, glutathione, melatonin, etc. Many of these agents influence the redox status of the cell.

1.3 H_2O_2, the Most Common Oxidant In Vivo

Virtually all mammalian cells produce EMODs. It was generally believed that these were by-products of cellular respiration and metabolism, and that they exerted dastardly toxic effects, including DNA damage and lipid oxidation. Recent evidence has demonstrated that this concept is wrong and that **EMODs are produced in a controlled fashion and likely have critical signaling functions.** Likewise, antioxidant defenses play a role in modulating the ambient steady-state levels of reactive oxygen species. Actually, **I believe that the antioxidants are there as co-metabolic factors and not just there for the purpose of countering "dangerous" EMODs.** Biological or pharmacological manipulation of endogenous antioxidants can have a profound effect on cellular function.

Hydrogen peroxide (H_2O_2) plays a particularly important role in signal transduction. H_2O_2 is uncharged and is freely diffusible within and between cells. Compared with other reactive oxygen species, it is also quite stable.

One major source of H_2O_2 is a membrane-bound NADH/NADPH oxidase, the activity of which is regulated by **hormones, growth factors, and physical forces**. The primary product of this enzyme system is superoxide ($O_2\ ^{\cdot-}$), which is rapidly dismutated to H_2O_2 by the superoxide dismutases. Removal of H_2O_2 is regulated by two important enzymes, catalase and glutathione peroxidase. Reaction products of H_2O_2, including lipid hydroperoxides, are also biologically active, as is the regenerated oxygen.

Given the fact that the molecule is diffusible and stable and that its production and removal are highly regulated, **H_2O_2 is an obvious candidate as a second messenger**. Indeed, **many studies have demonstrated that H_2O_2 mediates intracellular responses to extracellular stimuli.**

Non-destructive and reversible oxidative modifications may be achieved by H_2O_2 and other hydroperoxides with or without the aid of redox mediators such as GSH or thioredoxin. **The most common oxidant in vivo is H_2O_2 that, in inflammatory conditions, is amply formed by dismutation of $O_2\ ^{\cdot-}$ released from activated phagocytes** (Babior, B.M. NADPH oxidase: An update. Blood 1999; 93: 1464-1476), but physiologically also by intracellular NADPH oxidases (Bayraktutan, U., Blayney, L. and Shah, A.M. Molecular characterization and localization of the NADPH oxidase components gp91-phox and p22-phox in endothelia cells. Arterioscler Thromb Vasc Biol 2000; 20: 1903-1911), and other enzymatic systems. Although some H_2O_2 appears to be produced constitutively, receptor-mediated H_2O_2 formation appears to be more common. Typical examples **are TNFα-induced mitochondrial $O_2\ ^{\cdot-}$ formation** (Goossens, V., Grooten, J.,

DeVos, K. and Fiers. W. Direct evidence for tumor necrosis factor-induced mitochondrial reactive oxygen intermediates and their involvement in cytotoxicity. Proc Natl Acad Sci USA 1995; 92: 8115-8119), or **cytoplasmic increase of H_2O_2 upon growth factor receptor stimulation** (Finkel, T. Redox-dependent signal transduction. FEBS Lett 2000; 476: 52-54).

Nonetheless, **H_2O_2 is the most common oxidant in vivo**.

Nearly every disease process responds favorably to any therapy that effectively increases cellular oxygen content (Thomas Levy MD).

The primary reactive oxygen metabolites EMODs are O_2^{-} and H_2O_2. All other oxygen radicals (.OH, RO., ROO.) are produced via secondary reactions of these initially formed metabolites.

(O_2^{-}), is the stoichiometric precursor of H_2O_2. The amount of H_2O_2 produced by brain mitochondria is up to 5% of the amount of O_2 consumed. However, some H_2O_2 is produced directly and not via the superoxide anion.

H_2O_2 is also generated by:
    Arachidonic acid-metabolizing enzymes
    Xanthine oxidase
    Nitric oxide synthase
    Cytochrome P450
    as well as in the cellular response to ultraviolet radiation.

Halliwell states that H_2O_2 is widely regarded as a cytotoxic agent, whose levels must be minimized by the action of antioxidant defense enzymes. Actually, **H_2O_2 is poorly reactive in the absence of transition metal ions and exposure to certain human tissues to H_2O_2 may be greater than is commonly supposed.** Cell culture is frequently used for studies on "physiological" processes such as **signal transduction and regulation of gene expression** and chemical reactions involving the **culture media need to be considered because they may lead to the generation of substantial amounts of H$_2$O$_2$** in vitro. Some or all other reported effects of ascorbic and polyphenolics compounds (e.g., quercetin, catechins, epigallocatechin, epigallocatechin gallate) on cells in culture may be due to H$_2$O$_2$ generation by interaction of these compounds with cell culture media (Halliwell, B., Clement, M.V., Ramalingam, J. and Long, L.H. Hydrogen peroxide. Ubiquitous in cell culture and in vivo? IUBMB Life. 2000. Oct-Nov;50(4-5):251-257). In other words, investigators should be constantly aware of artifacts during the measurements of H$_2$O$_2$ in culture media.

Others have found that **mammalian cells are not killed by H$_2$O$_2$-generated .OH radicals** (Ward JF, Blakey WF, Joner EL. Mammalian cells are not killed by DNA single-strand breaks caused by hydroxyl radicals from hydrogen peroxide endothelial cells against oxidant damage. Biochem Biophys Res Commun 1985;127-270-276).

**The unanswerable mysteries
of being alive
are surpassed only by
the incomprehensible mysteries
of being dead.**
R. M. Howes, M.D., Ph.D.
10/30/11

2.0 UBIQUITOUS HYDROGEN PEROXIDE (A PRODUCT OF NATURAL METABOLISM)

H_2O_2 is now recognized as a ubiquitous intracellular messenger under subtoxic conditions.

Gaseous H_2O_2 is recognized to be a key component and product of the earth's lower atmospheric photochemical reactions. **Surface water concentrations of H_2O_2 have been found to vary between 51-231 mg/L, increasing both with exposure to sunlight and the presence of dissolved organic matter. H_2O_2 has been detected in the human breath at levels ranging from 1.0 ug/L to 0.34 ug/L (IARC, 1985), and even in the breath of babies. H_2O_2 is a naturally occurring substance. H_2O_2 has been detected in serum and in intact liver** (IARC, 1985). (IARC. 1985. International Agency for Research on Cancer. Hydrogen Peroxide. In: IARC Monographs on the Evaluation of Carcinogenic Risk if Chemicals to Humans: Allyl compounds, Aldehydes, Epoxides and Peroxides, Vol. 36. IARC, Lyon, pp. 285-314).

H_2O_2 as a human food additive is generally regarded as safe and may be used as a component of articles for use in packaging, handling, transporting or holding food in n accordance with prescribed conditions [FDA 21 CFR 175.105 (4/1/93)].

H_2O_2 has been used on fresh fruits and vegetables for decades. It has been used in dentistry and oral hygiene for decade upon decade. It has been used on wounds, as an antiseptic and debriding agent, for three quarters of a century on millions and millions of human wounds. **All of these umpteen examples of H_2O_2 application and ingestion have nearly been essentially without adverse effects.**

3.0 NATURAL CELLULAR H_2O_2 SOURCES

3.1 All Aerobic Cells and H_2O_2

According to the director of the Linus Pauling Institute, Dr. Frei Balz, **under normal metabolic conditions, each cell in our body is exposed to about 10^{10} molecules of superoxide each day.** For a person weighing 150 pounds, this amounts to about 4 pounds of superoxide per year, a substantial amount! Once formed, superoxide is converted to other **EMODs**. For a 200 pound man this equates to formation of 5.3 pounds of O_2^- per year. That means that in 37.7 years, this person would have formed an amount of O_2^- equal to his body weight and **at 75 years of age, he would have formed 2 times his body weight of O_2^-.** Please remember that O_2^- is immediately converted into H_2O_2 and **one would have a corresponding amount of H_2O_2 formed in the same time frame** (Dr. Balz Frei at lpi@oregonstate.edu**).

Any mitochondrial substrate incorporated in the respiratory chain through NADH or ubiquinone, will generate H_2O_2. Thus, H_2O_2 generation is a physiologic event under aerobic conditions.

Basically, all cells continuously form O_2^- and submitochondrial particles generate O_2^- at a rate of 4-7 nmol/min^{-1}/mg protein^{-1} (Chance, B., Sies, H. and Boveris, A. Hydroperoxide metabolism in mammalian organs. Physiol Rev 59: 527-605, 1979).

I look at the production of **superoxide anion as an innate pathway for hydrogen peroxide production.**

Prof Randolph Michael Howes MD,PhD

Cells, other than neutrophils, which generate EMODs include:

> **colonic epithelia**
> **smooth muscle**
> **fibroblasts**
> **osteocytes**
> **endothelial cells**
> **keratinocytes**
> **chondrocytes**
> **adipocytes**

and **a variety of cancer cells** (Burdon, R. Superoxide and hydrogen peroxide in relation to mammalian cell proliferation. Free Radic Biol Med 1995; 18: 775-794). Thus, **get out of your head the concept that EMODs are some cellular assassinating radical products generated only by angry PMNs. EMODs are intentionally generated salutary cellular products intended to help regulate critical metabolic and reproductive mechanisms. (Signal Transduction by reactive Oxygen and Nitrogen Species: Pathways and Chemical Principles. Edited by H.J. Forman, J. Fukuto and M. Torres, Kluwer Academic Publishers, 2003.)**

H_2O_2 and O_2^{-} Enzymatic Production

Enzyme	Tissue	Location
Monoamine oxidase	liver	mitochondrial outer membrane
D-amino acid oxidase	kidney	peroxisome
Glycolate oxidase	liver	peroxisome
Fatty acyl-CoA oxidase	liver	peroxisome
L-Gulonolactone oxidase	liver	microsomal
Pyridoxamine-5'-phosphate	liver	cytosol
Diamine oxidase	placenta	
Thiol oxidase	kidney	plasma
Urate oxidase	liver	peroxisome

Xanthine oxidase   milk
Sulfite oxidase   liver mitochondria
Xanthine oxidase   neutrophil   specific granules
Aldehyde oxidase

Superoxide and H_2O_2 are Produced Enzymatically By

- NADPH oxidases (phagocytosis)
- Mitochondrial cytochrome c oxidase (cell respiration)
- Liver Cytochrome P 450 (oxidation of xenobiotics)
- Xanthine oxidase (ischemic reperfusion)
- Prostaglandin synthetase
- Lipoxygenase
- Aldehyde oxidase
- Amino acid oxidase
- Myeloperoxidase (uses H_2O_2 to oxidize chloride ions to form HOCl)

Frequently, **EMODs are generated in response to signals such as:**
     growth factors (Platelet Derived Growth Factor)
     cytokines (Tumor Necrosis Factor,
     Interferon-gamma)

In addition to mitochondrial sources of **EMODs**, O_2^- and/or H_2O_2, can be derived from:

-cyclooxygenase
-lipoxygenase
-NO synthase
-heme oxygenases
-peroxidases (in addition to myeloperoxidase)
-hemoproteins such as heme and hematin
-and NAD(P)H oxidases (also in non-phagocytic cells)

Several investigators have known that these latter enzymes, **the membrane-associated NAD(P)H oxidase(s), are the** primary physiological producers of EMODs in vascular tissue. Of importance, the activity of these enzymes can be modulated by vasoactive hormones and the low-molecular-weight G protein rac-1, providing a critical characteristic of any second messenger: "regulation of its production." Metabolism of these EMODs is also tightly controlled. Dismutation of O_2^{-} by superoxide dismutase (SOD) produces the more stable EMOD, H_2O_2.

Cells deficient in heme oxygenase-1 are hypersensitive to oxidants like H_2O_2 (Poss KD and Tonegawa S. Reduced stress defense in heme oxygenase 1-deficient cells. *Proc Natl Acad Sci USA* 94: 10925–10930, 1997), and experiments modulating cellular enzyme activity demonstrate that heme oxygenase-1 can mediate protection against oxygen toxicity, although protection is seen only over a narrow range of enzyme expression.

3.2 The Red Blood Cell

"The Oxygen Paradox," Eds. K.J.A. Davies and F. Ursini. Cleup University Press, 1995. A Tribute of Paul Hochstein. K.J.A. Davies, J.M.S. Davies, E. Cadenas, L. Packer, A Sevanian, H.J. Forman, T.M. Chan, J.R. Landolph and F. Ursini. Page 3.

Dr. Hochstein studies were subsequently on the H_2O_2 production and H_2O_2 steady-state levels in red cells (Guilivi, C., Hochstein, P. and Davies, K.J.A. Hydrogen peroxide production by red blood cells. Free Radical Biol Med 1994; 16: 123-129).

Red blood cells are believed to be constantly under oxidative stress due to high oxygen tension and generation of EMODs by autoxidation of oxyhemoglobin.

The concept of oxidative stress was developed primarily by Sies, with synonymous terms such as "oxidant stress" and "pro-oxidant stress," or the related term "reductive stress" receiving comparatively less emphasis. **Sies described oxidative stress as a "disturbance in the pro-oxidant/antioxidant balance in favor of the former"** (Sies H. Oxidative stress: introductory remarks. In: *Oxidative Stress*, edited by Sies H. New York: Academic, 1985, p. 1–8). This original denotation has been modified since to the **more refined definition of "imbalance between oxidants and antioxidants in favor of the oxidants, potentially leading to damage." This is basically an unnecessary and confusing concept.**

3.3 Vascular Cells

Virtually all types of vascular cells produce O_2^-. and H_2O_2 (Griendling, K. K., Sorescu, D. and Ushio-Fukai, M. NAD(P)H oxidase: role in cardiovascular biology and disease. Cir Res 2000: 86; 494-501).

The production of **reactive oxygen species in the blood vessel wall is enhanced in experimental models of hypercholesterolemia, hypertension, diabetes, and balloon injury to the coronary arteries**. Moreover, in angiotensin II–induced hypertension, excess **free radical production was predominantly localized to the media. All layers of the vascular wall produce EMODs.**

The smooth muscle cell response to growth factors is now known to be dependent on the intracellular generation of H_2O_2 (Bae YS, Kang SW, Seo MS, Baines IC, Tekle E, Chock PB, and Rhee SG. Epidermal growth factor (EGF)-induced generation of hydrogen peroxide. Role in EGF receptor-mediated tyrosine phosphorylation. *J Biol Chem* 272: 217–221, 1997) (Sundaresan M, Yu ZX, Ferrans VJ, Irani K, and Finkel T. Requirement for generation of H_2O_2 for platelet-derived growth factor signal transduction. *Science* 270: 296–299, 1995).

Among 2e-oxidants produced in vivo, H_2O_2 is perhaps the most abundant. It freely diffuses through cell membranes and may travel several cell diameters before reacting with **targets such as thiols and heme. Diseased vessels produce increased levels of H_2O_2 (**Griendling KK, Sorescu D, and Ushio-Fukai M. NAD(P)H oxidase: role in cardiovascular biology and disease. *Circ Res* 86: 494–501, 2000**), and activated neutrophils at normal circulating concentrations can produce 200–400 μM H_2O_2 over a 60-min period** (Liu X and Zweier JL. A real-time electrochemical technique for measurement of cellular hydrogen peroxide generation and consumption: evaluation in human polymorphonuclear leukocytes. *Free Radic Biol Med* 31: 894–901, 2001). **I believe that this is a protective mechanism of the body to protect itself from accumulation of microaggregates and plaque formation.**

H_2O_2 **may be involved in modulating •NO bioactivity. Although H_2O_2 does not react with •NO, it does produce arterial relaxation in an endothelium- and eNOS-dependent manner** (Thomas SR, Chen K, and Keaney JF Jr. Hydrogen peroxide activates endothelial nitric-oxide synthase through coordinated phosphorylation and dephosphorylation via a phosphoinositide 3-kinase-dependent signaling pathway. *J Biol Chem* 277: 6017–6024, 2002).

Hydrogen peroxide treatment also promotes chronic increases in eNOS activity by upregulating transcription and enhancing mRNA stability (Drummond GR, Cai H, Davis ME, Ramasamy S, and Harrison DG. Transcriptional and posttranscriptional regulation of endothelial nitric oxide synthase expression by hydrogen peroxide. *Circ Res* 86: 347–354, 2000) via a mechanism that involves activation of Ca^{2+}/calmodulin kinase II and janus kinase 2 signaling pathways. Therefore, H_2O_2 **may promote both acute and chronic increases in eNOS activity that could serve as a compensatory response to oxidative stress. This supports my view that H_2O_2 is protective for the vascular wall.**

Paradoxically, although treatment of endothelial cells with H_2O_2 promotes eNOS activity above basal levels, ambient levels of H_2O_2 can inhibit agonist-stimulated NO bioactivity. For example, **in cerebral arterioles, H_2O_2 impairs NO-mediated arterial relaxation in response to acetylcholine or authentic NO, an effect that appears to involve O_2^- · as it is reversed by SOD.** I believe that this argues that more H_2O_2 will not impair NO-mediated arterial relaxation, but, in fact, corrects it.

Mice with a defect in H_2O_2 detoxification due to cellular glutathione peroxidase deficiency have impaired endothelium-dependent vasodilator function (Forgione MA, Weiss N, Heydrick S, Cap A, Klings ES, Bierl C, Eberhardt RT, Farber HW, and Loscalzo J. Cellular glutathione peroxidase deficiency and endothelial dysfunction. *Am J Physiol Heart Circ Physiol* 282: H1255–H1261, 2002).

H_2O_2 increases smooth muscle cell gelatinase activity and $ONOO^-$ activates matrix metalloproteinase-9 to generate collagenase activity (Rajagopalan S, Meng XP, Ramasamy S, Harrison DG, and Galis ZS. Reactive oxygen species produced by macrophage-derived foam cells regulate the activity of vascular matrix metalloproteinases in vitro. Implications for atherosclerotic plaque stability. *J Clin Invest* 98: 2572–2579, 1996).

A number of smooth muscle cell mitogens actually require H_2O_2 production for a proliferative response (Sundaresan M, Yu ZX, Ferrans VJ, Irani K, and Finkel T. Requirement for generation of H_2O_2 for platelet-derived growth factor signal transduction. *Science* 270: 296–299, 1995). However, **higher concentrations of H_2O_2 are associated with smooth muscle cell apoptosis and necrosis** (Deshpande NN, Sorescu D, Seshiah P, Ushio-Fukai M, Akers M, Yin Q, and Griendling KK. Mechanism of hydrogen peroxide-induced cell cycle arrest in vascular smooth muscle. *Antioxid Redox Signal* 4: 845–854, 2002),

Blood vessels exposed to H_2O_2 exhibit relaxation that is blocked by methylene blue, an inhibitor of soluble guanylyl cyclase (Burke TM and Wolin MS. Hydrogen peroxide elicits pulmonary arterial soluble relaxation and guanylate cyclase activation. *Am J Physiol Heart Circ Physiol* 252: H721–H732, 1987). **The activity of H_2O_2 to increase smooth muscle cell cGMP is dependent on catalase and is temporally related to the formation of compound I. Emerging evidence that H_2O_2 also acts as an endothelium-derived hyperpolarizing factor suggests that the mechanism outlined above is relevant for the control of vascular tone** (Matoba T, Shimokawa H, Nakashima M, Hirakawa Y, Mukai Y, Hirano K, Kanaide H, and Takeshita A. Hydrogen peroxide is an endothelium-derived hyperpolarizing factor in mice. *J Clin Invest* 106: 1521–1530, 2000).

The molecular mechanisms whereby H_2O_2 prevents vascular smooth muscle cells from becoming apoptotic remain to be determined. While the findings of some studies indicate that H_2O_2 stimulates smooth muscle cell proliferation, reports by other groups indicate that H_2O_2 can also induce apoptosis and/or promote vascular smooth muscle cell death. These studies collectively suggest that under certain conditions, H_2O_2 can promote either vascular smooth muscle cell proliferation or cell death, **a paradox** that underscores the importance of this reactive oxygen species to smooth muscle cell function. **I believe that this is not a paradox but is an illustration of the modulatory capabilities of EMODs, especially H_2O_2, even in the vascular wall. This is no paradox if one considers the secondary messenger activity of H_2O_2.**

Shingu, et al, showed that **endothelial cells and smooth muscle cells have very low levels of catalase activity** and therefore are more susceptible to damage by H_2O_2 (Shingu M, Yoshioka K, Nobunaga M, Yoshida K. Human vascular smooth muscle cells and endothelial cells lack catalase activity and are susceptible to hydrogen peroxide. Inflammation. 1985;9:309–320). However, **I believe that this is excellent evidence which shows that the** endothelium and the vascular wall needs high levels of H_2O_2 to protect itself from atherosclerotic particle aggregation. If the endothelium does not need high levels of H_2O_2 then I ask, "Why has it not evolved high levels of catalase to deal with the EMODs and H_2O_2, which are produced by all three layers of the vascular wall?"

The pivotal role of GSH-Px in vascular antioxidant protection is further pointed out by the findings **that catalase activity is lacking in human vascular cells** (Shingu M, Yoshioka K, Nobunaga M, Yoshida K. Human vascular smooth muscle cells and endothelial cells lack catalase activity and are susceptible to hydrogen peroxide. Inflammation. 1985;9:309–320). **I believe that a most important question is, "If antioxidant protection is so important in preventing atherosclerosis, then, why is catalase missing from human vascular cells?" I believe the answer is that the prooxidative protective activity is much more important in preventing plaque aggregation and allowance of plaque formation.**

Other agonists and mechanical forces have also been shown to increase **EMOD** production in vascular cells. **PDGF, thrombin, TNF-*a*. and lactosylceramide activate NAD(P)H oxidase dependent $O_2^{\cdot-}$ production in SMCs.**

In endothelial cells, mechanical forces, including cyclic stretch and laminar and oscillatory shear stress, stimulate NAD(P)H oxidase activity (De Keulenaer, G. W., Chappell, D. C., Ishizaka, N., Nerem, R. M., Alexander, R. W. and Griendling, K. K. Oscillatory and steady laminar shear stress differentially affect human endothelial redox state. Circ Res. 1998; 82; 1094-1101).

Macrophages, platelets, fibroblasts, and tumor cells themselves are a major source of angiogenic factors such as basic fibroblast growth factor, vascular endothelial growth factor, inflammatory cytokines (e.g., tumor necrosis factor

[TNF]-alpha, interleukin [IL]-1-beta, IL-6, chemokines (e.g., IL-8, GRO-alpha), prostaglandins-1 and -2, and nitric oxide (Jackson, J.R., Seed, M.P., Kircher, C.H., et al: The codependence of angiogenesis and chronic inflammation. FASEB J 11:457-465, 1997).

Antiangiogenic therapy was the rage in the 1990s for eradicating cancers in mice but subsequent **clinical studies were failures**. It appeared that the drug's ability to block formation of new blood vessels to bring oxygen and nutrients to tumors was not enough to stop established tumors. **Antiangiogenic drugs kill the very blood vessels needed to deliver oxygen and drugs to the tumor and oxygen is required for effective radiation therapy to be successful.** Too high of a dose of antiangiogenic drugs can kill too many vessels and cause adverse effects such as stroke and myocardial infarction.

In SMCs, H_2O_2 **induces tyrosine phosphorylation** of the EGF-r and stimulates it association with Shc (src homology complex)-Grb2 (growth factor receptor-bound protein 2)-Sos (son-of-sevenless) complex to activate subsequent signaling cascades (Rao, G. N. Hydrogen peroxide induces complex formation of SHC-Grb2-SOS with receptor tyrosine kinase and activates ras and extracellular signal-regulated protein kinases group of mitogen activated protein kinases. Oncogene. 1996; 13; 713-719).

A weak glutathione-related enzymatic antioxidant shield is present in human atherosclerotic plaques. **I believe that a specific antioxidant/prooxidant imbalance, operative in the vascular wall may be involved in atherogenic processes in humans and that balance is shifted in the antioxidant direction, as evidenced by the presence of a high content ascorbate, vitamin E, and urate.**

An emerging consensus also underscores the importance in vascular disease of oxidative events in addition to LDL oxidation. These include the production of reactive oxygen and nitrogen species by vascular cells, as well as oxidative modifications contributing to important clinical manifestations of coronary artery disease such as endothelial dysfunction and plaque disruption.

Despite this abundant data however, fundamental problems remain with implicating oxidative modification as a (requisite) pathophysiologically important cause for atherosclerosis. These include the poor performance of antioxidant strategies in limiting either atherosclerosis or cardiovascular events from atherosclerosis, and observations in animals that suggest dissociation between atherosclerosis and lipoprotein oxidation.

Indeed, **it remains to be established that oxidative events are a cause rather than an injurious response to atherogenesis.**

In this context, inflammation needs to be considered as a primary process of atherosclerosis, and oxidative stress as a secondary event. To address this issue, Stocker and Keaney have proposed an "oxidative response to inflammation" model as a means of reconciling the response-to-injury and oxidative modification hypotheses of atherosclerosis. **But any way you look at it, antioxidants fail to protect, reverse or stop the atherosclerotic plaque development in humans.**

At the molecular level, signaling in response to pro-atherogenic agents requires as well as causes generation of **EMODs**. Proatherogenic agents comprise a large variety of molecules. It has been identified that **cytokines, including tumor necrosis factor-γ (TNF-γ), interferon-γ (IFN-γ), interleukin-1,-6 (IL-1, IL-6), and angiotensin II (Ang II) stimulate intracellular generation of EMODs. High levels of low-density lipoprotein (LDL), especially in the form of oxidized low-density lipoprotein (ox-LDL), have also been shown to increase intracellular EMODs generation.**

Actually, hyperlipidemia drugs (e.g., ciprofibrate and elofibrate) results in the proliferation of peroxisomes, an increase in the activity of oxidases and the excessive production of H_2O_2. (RMH Note: this argues that hydrogen peroxide acts to help cure arteriosclerosis).

3.4　The Lung

Type II pneumocytes, alveolar macrophages and endothelial cells produce H_2O_2.

Exposure of lung cells, subcellular organelles and tissue to hyperoxia (100% O_2) increases mitochondrial H_2O_2 production 10- to 15-fold (Turrens, JF, Freeman BA, Crapo JD. Hyperoxia increases H_2O_2 release by lung mitochondria and microsomes. Arch Biochem Biophys 217:411-421, 1982). Thus, it appears to me that both hypoxemia and hyperoxia can result in increased production of **EMODs**.

Asbestos fibers can induce the formation of **EMODs**, as can silica and coal mine dust. Both **chrysotile and crocidolite stimulate in vitro production of $O_2^{.-}$** by human alveolar macrophages.

3.5　The Liver

One rat liver mitochondrion produces 3×10^7 superoxide radicals per day.
　　　　(Figures vary according to the reference cited.)

The hepatocytes steady state H_2O_2 concentration can be up to 25 uM.

The major source of oxygen-derived radicals ($O_2^{.-}$) is the electron transport chain located in the inner membrane of mitochondria and from flavin-linked enzymes in the endoplasmic reticulum of liver and kidney. Any compound

with quinone-type structure is suspect as a source of superoxide radical anion.

Several studies indicate that **xanthine oxidase** is released from the liver and the intestine into the circulation and it binds to pulmonary epithelium, where it serves as a locus for **the intense production of EMODs** (Weinboum, A, Nielsen, VG, Tan S, Gelman S, Matalon S, et al. Liver ischemia-reperfusion increases pulmonary permeability in rat: role of circulating xanthine oxidase. Am J Physiol 268:G988-G996, 1995).

3.6   The Neutrophil

Activated phagocytic cells, such as monocytes, neutrophils, eosinophils and macrophages generate O_2^{-}.

The major role of the neutrophil is to protect the body against infectious organisms and, in my opinion and that of many others, against cancer. The killing event is thought to occur with the participation of both oxidative and non-oxidative mechanisms. Metchnikoff described the process of phagocytosis, in which the neutrophil engulfs the foreign agent and forms a phagosome, wherein fusion of intracellular azurophilic granules and specific granules occur. Specific granules activate the complement cascade and contain collagenase and gelatinase.

The heme-containing protein complex, NADPH oxidase, can produce large amounts of O_2^{-} and its derivative upon activation. **In an inflammatory environment, H_2O_2 is produced by activated** macrophages at an estimated rate of 2-6 X 10^{-14} mol/h^{-1}/cell^{-1} and **can reach as high as 10-100 μM** in the vicinity of these cells

Generation of superoxide anions (O_2^{-}) by NADPH oxidase complex of PMN is indispensable to the host defense response, as it is essential for killing of invading microorganisms. Superoxide rapidly leads to the formation of hydrogen peroxide and singlet oxygen.

200 μM H_2O_2 which is a level seen during activation of phagocytes in vitro.

Oxidative mechanisms, producing bacterial cell death, usually follow a massive increase in the consumption of oxygen by the neutrophil and are referred to as the **respiratory burst.** The respiratory burst is a sequence of four metabolic events which consists of (1) a massive, **10-15X increase in oxygen consumption,** (2) formation of the superoxide anion by a one electron reduction, (3) formation of **hydrogen peroxide** by another one electron reduction and (4) activation of the hexose monophosphate shunt, which is used to regenerate NADPH. NADPH is nicotinamide adenine dinucleotide phosphate, and NADP+ is the oxidized form of NADPH.

NADPH is provided primarily by the oxidative pentose phosphate pathway (Chance B, Sies H, and Boveris A. Hydroperoxide metabolism in mammalian organs. *Physiol Rev* 59: 527–605, 1979) that is initiated by **glucose-6-phosphate dehydrogenase and that maintains the cellular redox couple NADPH/NADP$^+$** in balance. **In this context, glucose-6-phosphate dehydrogenase can be considered an antioxidant.** For example, overexpression of glucose-6-phosphate dehydrogenase in endothelial cells decreases oxidative stress and increases the bioavailability of ·NO.

Hydrogen peroxide is utilized in myeloperoxidase-dependent bacterial killing, where it combines with chloride (Cl-) to form **hypochlorous acid (HOCl)** or with bromide (Br-) to form hypobromous acid. **These oxidized halogens are potent antimicrobial agents.** These reactive oxygen species can recombine or be converted to other species such as **singlet oxygen (which is bactericidal, fungicidal, virucidal, parasiticidal and tumoricidal)** or the hydroxyl radical.

Phagocytic cells attack and destroy invading organisms and cancer cells by consuming large amounts of oxygen in a process called **the** "respiratory burst." Of the oxygen consumed, 70-90% is converted into the superoxide anion, which readily forms H_2O_2.

This respiratory burst is initiated by the activation of NADPH-oxidase by exposure to: immunoglobulin-coated bacteria,
>immune complexes,
>complement 5a,
>or leukotrienes.

Activated phagocytes can produce as much as 47 nmol of $H_2O_2/10^6$ cells within 30 minutes corresponding to a concentration of 47 μM H_2O_2 in a diluted volume of 1 ml.

200 μM H_2O_2 is a level seen during activation of phagocytes in vitro.

PMNs plasma membrane contains NADPH oxidase bound to the extracellular surface, which faces the lumen of the phagosome after phagocytosis of bacteria, and catalyzes formation of RONS (superoxide, hydrogen peroxide, hypochlorous acid), within the phagosome of neutrophils.

Eosinophils produce free radicals (HOBr) facilitating access of EMODs (e.g., superoxide, and hydrogen peroxide) to kill parasites.

Once activated, phagocytes produce large quantities of superoxide, on the order of 10 nmol·min-1·10^6 neuutrophils-1 during the oxidative burst (Babior, B.M., NADPH oxidase: an update. Blood 1999; 93: 1464-1476).

White cells deliberately generate O_2^- to kill invading pathogens. An enzyme, NADPH oxidase, is found on the surfaces of macrophages and neutrophils and is stimulated by invading pathogens to produce $O_2^{\cdot-}$. The neutrophil also contains myeloperoxidase which reacts with H_2O_2 and salt (chloride ions) to produce $^1O_2$. **Myeloperoxidase** is in such high concentrations in neutrophils that it gives a **greenish color** to phlegm during times in which our bodies are fighting respiratory infections.

The rate of superoxide production in vascular cells is thought to be ~1-10% of that in leukocytes (Hohler, B.; Holzapfel, B., and Kummer W. NADPH oxidase submits and superoxide production in porcine pulmonary artery endothelial cells. Histochem Cell Biol 2000; 114: 29-37) (Rueckschloss, U. Galle, J., Zerkowski H. R. and Morawietz, H. Induction of NAD(P) H oxidase by oxidized low-density lipoprotein in human endothelial cells: antioxidative potential of hydroxymethylglutaryl coenzyme A reductase inhibitor therapy. Circulation 2001; 104: 1767-1772), as confirmed recently using highly specific electron spin resonance (ESR) methods. **In contrast to the cytotoxic amounts of superoxide generated by phagocytes, most nonphagocytic cells produce low amounts of EMODs** that stimulate numerous transcription factors as well as signaling cascades via activation of kinases and inhibition of tyrosine phosphatases.

It should be noted here that in physiological conditions, the intracellular production of **EMODs** does not alter the **redox state of cells which have large reserves of reducing agents,** notably reduced glutathione, as well as extremely effective antioxidant defense mechanisms, such as SOD, catalase, and peroxidases. **This reducing intracellular environment (RMH Note: I do not fully accept this view of a continuous reducing intracellular environment. In fact, I believe that a continuous oxidative status is necessary for prooxidant protection) actually allows agonist-induced increases in EMODs to function as second messengers by limiting their effecting time and space in a manner similar to other well-known intracellular signals,** such as calcium ion. Thus, because of their confinement, it is possible for **EMODs** to promote cell proliferation despite the fact that transition from a differentiated to a proliferating phenotype is marked by a shift toward a more reduced overall cellular state (Schafer, F. Q. and Buettner, G. R. Redox environment of the cell as viewed through the redox state of the glutathione disulfide/glutathione couple. Free Radic Biol Med 2001; 30: 1191-1212). **Therefore, in physiological conditions, EMODs production is not accompanied by oxidative stress, but rather provides a means of finely regulating signaling in vascular cells. This is a very important view.**

3.7   Fibroblasts

Fibroblasts exhibit increased NADH- or NADPH-driven O_2 production in response to TNF-a, IL-1, and platelet-activating factor (Meiser, B. Regulation of the superoxide releasing system in human fibroblasts. Adv Exp Med Biol. 1996; 387; 113-116).

3.8   The Brain and H_2O_2

H_2O_2 and the Central Nervous System

Post mitotic neurons (brain cells cannot regenerate), **the brain is prone to oxidation because:** 1) it has high amounts of easily peroxidizable 20:4 and 22:6 fatty acids; 2) it is not particularly enriched with antioxidant enzymes or with vitamin E; 3) certain regions of the brain (especially in humans), contain lots of Fe (iron). Brain homogenates rapidly peroxidize at 37 degrees but it is blocked by an iron ligate or dopamine. **Thus, the brain should peroxidize rapidly, but it does not.**

EMODs have recently been implicated in a variety of redox-based signaling mechanisms that can mediate changes in neural plasticity including:

> **activation of oxidative stress-responsive transcription factors**
> **modulation of LTP induction**

and mediation of nonsynaptic communication between neurons and glia.

Concentrations of up to 250 μM H_2O_2 could be generated every minute within the brain neutrophil. The rate of O_2 consumption is roughly 10-fold higher in neurons than in glia.

Concentrations of up to 250 mM H_2O_2 could be generated every minute within brain neutrophil. The rate of O_2 consumption is roughly 10-fold higher in neurons than in glia.

In brain tissue, H_2O_2 levels are regulated largely by the intracellular enzyme, glutathione (GSH) peroxidase, and by endogenous catalase in peroxisomes.

The amount of H_2O_2 produced by brain mitochondria is up to 5% of the amount of O_2 consumed.

($O_2^{\cdot-}$), is the stoichiometric precursor of H_2O_2. The amount of H_2O_2 produced by brain mitochondria is up to 5% of the amount of O_2 consumed.

Given that the rate of O_2 consumption in gray matter is 2-5 μmol/g tissue wet weight per minute; or 2-5mM (assuming 1 g = 1 mL), this would mean that **concentrations of up to 250 μM H_2O_2 could be generated every minute within brain neutrophils**. Because **the rate of O_2 consumption is roughly 10-fold higher in neurons than in glia**, however, this H_2O_2 would be produced predominantly in the neuronal compartment, which could lead to higher, intra-neuronal concentrations. Moreover, the presence of mitochondria within 250 nm of the synapse in **DA (dopamine)** terminals suggests that even higher levels could be reached in the restricted, intracellular compartment of a synaptic terminal. It is relevant to note, however, that such local increases are likely to be transient because H_2O_2 is membrane permeable and thus can readily leave the compartment in which it is produced. DA is involved in epinephrine synthesis.

In addition to mitochondrial sources, H_2O_2 will also be produced in DA terminals by **monoamine oxidase (MAO),** which is a metabolizing enzyme for DA. Importantly, **MAO is localized on the outer membrane of mitochondria,** which would further enhance H_2O_2 concentrations near DA synapses. DA transmits nerve impulses.

In brain tissue, H_2O_2 levels are regulated largely by the intracellular enzyme, glutathione (GSH-Px) peroxidase, and by endogenous catalase in peroxisomes. Catalase is present in trace quantities in brain and is localized in peroxisomes, which in the brain are referred to as "microperoxisomes." **In contrast to glutathione peroxidase and catalase, which exhibit relatively low enzymatic activity in brain, superoxide dismutase is relatively abundant** (Sies, H. Oxidative Stress. Academic Press 1985; 388). This indicates **to me that high levels of hydrogen peroxide are generated and needed within the brain.**

High levels of EMODs and low levels of antioxidant enzymes are the normal conditions in the brain from early age through adulthood and should result in early onset of Alzheimer's disease or other neurodegenerative diseases (Huntington's, ALS and prion disorders), but it does not. The two factors of high levels of EMODs and low levels of antioxidant enzymes argues that the brain should be dramatically effected, in a damaging and harmful way, in all individuals. However, that is not the case and many, if not most, individuals live to old ages, while still free of any of the above neurological diseases. In my opinion, this clears EMODs of the harmful effects of the doom and gloom crowd. Furthermore, these are post-mitotic cells.

Chageaux noted that **once a nerve cell has become differentiated it does not divide anymore. A single nucleus, with the same DNA, must serve an entire lifetime for the formation and maintenance of tens of thousands of synapses.**

I believe that this is remarkable for brain cells which use very high amounts of O_2, have high levels of lipids (over 50% by dry weight), have high levels of nonheme iron, produce high amounts of EMODs and have low levels of antioxidant enzymes. To me, it does not make sense that such a vulnerable, post-mitotic cellular system could survive for a life time, if it was under the constant attack of harmful and damaging EMODs. Ergo, I ask, "How toxic are EMODs?" Thus, I conclude that EMODs are not very harmful to brain cells and in fact, I submit that they are needed by neurons for normal physiological and biochemical functioning.

Additionally, I ask, "Isn't it curious that three crucial organs of the body (heart, brain and lungs), which use extremely high levels of oxygen, have evolved such that they have innately low levels of antioxidant enzymes?" If there is any credence to the Free Radi-Crap theory of oxidative stress and aging, a further complication, in our evolutionary ascent to the top of the phylogenetic tree, is the fact that we do not synthesize many of the low molecular weight antioxidants and they must be ingested in the diet. I ask, "How could natural selection have been so faulted during its last 2.3-2.5 million years of evolution?" Many bugs, birds and other mammals can do this. Thus, I ask, "How could man's evolutionary process be so lacking and incomplete?"

The fact that the antioxidant enzymes in the brain do not completely deplete H_2O_2 levels is again evidence of the need for these RONS for normal brain function.

According to the Free Radi-Crap theory, leaving steady state levels of H_2O_2 and extremely dangerous RONS would have disastrous consequences, especially a chain reaction involving lipid peroxidation, but ....that does not happen.

Please keep asking yourself, "Just how toxic are EMODs?" Many individuals produce exponential numbers of EMODs, from exponential numbers of cells, and appear to do so for a life time without untoward effects.

3.9 H_2O_2 from the Cornea

Hydrogen peroxide (H_2O_2) is produced by the cornea and neighboring tissues. Aqueous humor itself generates H_2O_2 with reported maximum levels of approximately **0.09 mM H_2O_2 in bovine aqueous** (Spector A, Ma W, Wang RR. The aqueous humor is capable of generating and degrading H_2O_2. Invest Ophthalmol Vis Sci 1998;39:1188–97).

High intraocular concentrations of reactive oxygen species such as H_2O_2 have been found in inflammatory disorders of the eye and are associated with tissue damage (Rose RC, Richer SP, Bode AM. Ocular oxidants and antioxidant protection. Proc Soc Exp Biol Med 1998;217:397–407) (Green K. Free radicals and aging of anterior segment tissues of the eye: a hypothesis. Ophthalmic Res 1995;27:143–9).

Based on the fact that corneal cells do not divide and that they are constantly exposed to EMODs, e.g., H_2O_2, I ask, "How can some people live a full and long life and not develop cataracts, if EMODs are the causative agent?"

The age of onset of cataracts links them to the decreasing levels of oxygen consumption and oxygen utilization of oxygen by the cells.

3.10 The Peroxisome

Peroxisomes produce H_2O_2, but not O_2^- under physiological conditions **(Chance et al. 1979). Peroxisomes are now found to be present in virtually all eukaryotic cells (except mature red blood cells).**

Microsomes are responsible for 80% of the H_2O_2 produced in vivo at 100% hyperoxia sites. Peroxisomes are primarily in the liver but other organs contain them. **Peroxisomal oxidation of fatty acids has been recognized as an important source of H_2O_2 with prolonged starvation. This may be involved in increased longevity with caloric restriction.**

(Signal Transduction by reactive Oxygen and Nitrogen Species: Pathways and Chemical Principles. Edited by H.J. Forman, J. Fukuto and M. Torres, Kluwer Academic Publishers, 2003. Page 292). **Peroxisomes account for a large fraction of total cellular H_2O_2 production** (Boveris, A., Oshino, N. and Chance, B. The cellular production of hydrogen peroxide. Biochem J 1972; 128: 617-630).

Peroxisomes contain **H_2O_2-generating enzymes including:**

> **glycollate oxidase**
> **D-amino acid oxidase**
> **urate oxidase**
> **L-a-hydroxylases oxidase**
> **and fatty acyl-CoA oxidase.**

Peroxisomal catalase utilizes H_2O_2 produced by these oxidases to oxidize a variety of substrates in "eradicative" reactions. I believe that this is a good thing.

In liver and kidney cells, peroxisomes detoxify a variety of toxic molecules, including ethanol, that enter the circulation.

Oxidative reactions in peroxisomes also mediate β-oxidation of fatty acids. Due to high concentrations of peroxisomal catalase, minimal amounts of H_2O_2 are capable of escaping from these intracellular organelles.

Interestingly, **many of the effects of peroxidized fatty acids and H_2O_2 can be mimicked** by **hydroxy derivatives of fatty acids, such as hydroxy linoleic acids (HODEs) and hydroxy arachidonic acids (HETEs).** Gordon and associates found that **peroxidized arachidonic acids are degraded in cellular peroxisomes** (Gordon JA, Heller SK, Kaduce TL, Spector AA. Formation and release of a peroxisome-dependent arachidonic acid metabolite by human skin fibroblasts. J Biol Chem. 1994;269:4103–4109).

Peroxisomal degradation of fatty acids, in contrast to their mitochondrial degradation, generates H_2O_2 (Mannaerts GP, Van Veldhoven PP. Metabolic pathways in mammalian peroxisomes. Biochimie. 1993;75:147–158. Review). Investigators measured the resistance of these cells to cytotoxicity induced not only by the addition of H_2O_2 but also by the addition of **13-hydroperxyoctadecadienoic acid (13-HPODE).**

The novel results demonstrated that **the cells enriched in catalase are resistant to the damaging effects of an oxidized lipid. Oxidized lipids and H_2O_2 profoundly affect cellular properties.** A number of different cell types respond to these agents. Cell proliferation, activation of the synthesis and secretion of specific gene products, expression of cell adhesion molecules, and a number of other effects have been described for both oxidized lipids and H_2O_2. **Redox metals** could use H_2O_2 and peroxidized lipids to generate hydroxyl and lipid peroxy radicals, which could propagate oxidation (Girotti AW. Mechanisms of lipid peroxidation. J Free Radic Biol Med. 1985;1:87–95. Review).

The Santanam study is the first to generate a stable cell line that overexpressed the enzyme to demonstrate that the **overexpression of catalase** indeed affords protection against H_2O_2-induced cytotoxicity. **Surprisingly, since CAT is only supposed to break down hydrogen peroxide, these cells were also resistant to the effects of 13-HPODE, a peroxidized fatty acid**.

Pioneering studies by Gordon and coworkers have demonstrated that oxidized arachidonic acid derivatives are targets of peroxisomal degradation. **Degradation of fatty acids in the peroxisomes would result in the generation of H_2O_2.**

These results go on to create or explain a **puzzling paradox**. How do the hydroxy fatty acids such as the HODEs and HETEs affect cells and why would antioxidants prevent their effects? **These lipids do not propagate oxidation even in the presence of metal ions**.

These results also suggest that cellular peroxisomes are an important target for gene induction and the prevention of metabolic toxicity.

3.11 Hydrogen Peroxide in Breath Condensates

There **is no correlation between the levels of exhaled H_2O_2 and age, sex, or lung function in healthy children** (Jöbsis Q, Raatgeep HC, Schellekens SL, Hop WCJ, Hermans PWM, de Jongste JC. Hydrogen peroxide in exhaled air of healthy children: reference values. Eur Respir J 1998; 12: 483-485).

However, **exhaled H_2O_2 concentration is related to the number of sputum eosinophils and airway hyper-responsiveness in asthma of different severity, and it is elevated in patients with severe unstable asthma**, although exhaled **NO is significantly reduced by treatment with**

corticosteroids. This may be related to the fact **that neutrophils, prevalent in severe asthma, generate higher amounts of superoxide radicals and therefore H_2O_2** (Antczak A, Nowak D, Bialasiewicz P, Kasielski M. Hydrogen peroxide in expired air condensate correlates positively with early steps of peripheral neutrophil activation in asthmatic patients. Arch Immunol Ther Exp (Warsz) 1999;47:119-126).

Asthmatic patients also exhale significantly higher levels of thiobarbituric acid-reactive products (TBARs), which indirectly reflect increased oxidative stress (Antczak A, Nowak D, Shariati B, Krol M, Piasecka G, Kurmanowska Z. Increased hydrogen peroxide and thiobarbituric acid-reactive products in expired breath condensate of asthmatic patients. Eur Respir J 1997; 10: 1235-1241).

Cigarette smoking causes an influx of neutrophils and other inflammatory cells into the lower airways, and fivefold higher levels of H_2O_2 have been found in exhaled breath condensate of smokers than in nonsmokers (Nowak D, Antczak A, Krol M, Pietras T, Shariati B, Bialasiewicz P, Jeczkowski K, Kula P. Increased content of hydrogen peroxide in the expired breath of cigarette smokers. Eur Respir J 1996; 9: 652-657).

Levels of **exhaled H_2O_2 are increased** compared with those in normal subjects in patients with stable COPD and are further increased during exacerbations (Dekhuijzen PN, Aben KK, Dekker I, Aarts LP, Wielders PL, van Herwaarden CL, HC, Bast A. Increased exhalation of hydrogen peroxide in patients with stable and unstable chronic obstructive pulmonary disease. Am J Respir Crit Care Med 1996;154:813-816).

Cigarette smoking is by far the commonest cause of COPD, but only 10 to 20% of smokers develop symptomatic COPD. **No significant differences have been found between H_2O_2 levels in current smokers with COPD and subjects with COPD who have never smoked, and there is no correlation**

between expired H_2O_2 concentration and daily cigarette consumption (Nowak D, Kasielski M, Pietras T, Bialasiewicz P, Antczak A. Cigarette smoking does not increase hydrogen peroxide levels in expired breath condensate of patients with stable COPD. Monaldi Arch Chest Dis 1998; 53: 268-273). Thus, oxidative stress is a characteristic feature of COPD and presumably related to airway inflammation, and it cannot be explained entirely by the oxidants present in tobacco smoke.

I believe that the increased H_2O_2 levels represent the body's response to perceived injury, such as an irritant, cigarette smoke, etc.

Increased levels of free fatty acids, including linoleic and arachidonic acids, have been measured in exhaled condensate and sweat in children and in adults with acute pneumonia and lung edema. In contrast, **the level of lipid peroxidation in patients with cancer was significantly reduced compare with that in healthy control subjects** (Khyshiktyev BS, Khyshiktueva NA, Ivanov VN, Darenskaia SD, Novikov SV. Diagnostic value of investigating exhaled air condensate in lung cancer. Vopr Onkol 1994; 40: 161-164).

I believe that the lower level of lipid peroxidation in the cancer patients is indicative of low EMOD levels, which allows for the cancer development.

3.12 Hydrogen Peroxide in the Breath

Activation of inflammatory cells, including neutrophils, macrophages, and eosinophils, result in an increased production of O_2^-, which by undergoing spontaneous or enzyme-catalyzed dismutation lead to formation of H_2O_2. As **H_2O_2 is less reactive than other reactive oxygen species, it has the propensity to cross biologic membranes and enter other compartments** (Freeman BA, Crapo JD. Biology of disease: free radicals and tissue injury. Lab Invest 1982; 47: 412-426).

Because it is soluble, increased H_2O_2 in the airway equilibrates with air (Dohlman AW, Black HR, Royall JA. Expired breath hydrogen peroxide is a marker of acute airway inflammation in pediatric patients with asthma. Am Rev Respir Dis 1993; 148: 955-960). Compared with the cellular antioxidant scavenging systems, the extracellular space and airways have significantly less ability to scavenge reactive oxygen species (356, 357). **Catalase is the major enzyme involved in removing H_2O_2 and is preset in low concentrations in the respiratory tract. I believe that this is another example, in which, an area of the body which is constantly exposed to extremely high levels of EMODs, has low levels of catalase. This does not make teleological sense that such would be the occurrence, if EMODs are so harmful.** Thus, again I ask, **"How toxic are EMODs?"** Exhaled H_2O_2 has potential as a marker of oxidative stress in the lungs.

In summary, I can say that in the three areas of high ROS or EMOD generation of the body (e.g., brain, heart and the lungs), we normally have low levels of antioxidant enzymes. Additionally, we do not synthesize any of the traditional low molecular weight antioxidants and we must get them by the dietary route. Thus, I ask, "How toxic are EMODs?" How could the evolutionary process make such glaring errors and egregious mistakes in not protecting humans as equally well as much lower phylogenetic species? **These observations lead me to believe that EMODs are not nearly as toxic as they have been accused of being. In fact, I believe that they are naturally and normally beneficial to health.**

3.13 The Electron Transport Chain

One out of every 20 of the O_2 molecules or 5% of the O_2 passing along the electron transport chain is converted into $O_2^{.-}$ and this occurs when one of the electron carriers, called Coenzyme Q, passes the electron to O_2 instead of the next electron carrier.

Considering the inhibition of cytochrome c oxidase as a mechanism to generate H_2O_2 implies that the production of this molecule is coupled to ATP production.

The main sites for H_2O_2 and O_2^- production are the:

1) NADH-ubiquinone-reductase (complex I)
2) ubiquinol-cytochrome c-reductase (complex III)
Both have ubiquinone as a common component, and act **as prooxidants**.

(Signal Transduction by reactive Oxygen and Nitrogen Species: Pathways and Chemical Principles. Edited by H.J. Forman, J. Fukuto and M. Torres, Kluwer Academic Publishers, 2003. **H_2O_2 as Intracellular Messenger**. C. Giulivi and M.J. Oursler. Page 313).

All mitochondria exhibit lower (or negligible) rates of hydrogen peroxide production in State 3 (active ATP production), whereas, is maximum in State 4 (resting, nonphosphorylating mitochondria). Hyperbaric oxygen and hyperoxia exposure results in a marked increase in for hydrogen peroxide production by isolated heart and liver mitochondria.

Focusing on isolated mitochondria, and considering the succinate dehydrogenase-ubiquinone segment as the most important source of EMODs (60-80%), then the rate of EMOD production is modulated by the steady-state concentrations of ubisemiquinone and oxygen (assuming that superoxide anion is the chemical precursor of hydrogen peroxide) for the production of hydrogen peroxide is formulated as non-enzymatic oxidation of ubisemiquinone (UQ^-) by oxygen. Thus, **this is a major source of H_2O_2.**

As a consequence, several metabolic conditions that result in an increased level of ubiquinone include:

> **fasting**
> **chronic treatment with dinitrophenol**
> **cortisone treatment**
> **or higher availability of oxygen (e.g., hyperoxia) are**
expected to have increased rates of EMODs.

This may shed light on caloric restriction.

Antimycin A (a site 2 inhibitor) increases H_2O_2 generation and utilizes almost all O_2 consumed to produce H_2O_2; whereas, rotenone (a site 1 inhibitor) reduces H_2O_2 production.

Any electron transport chain operating in the presence of O_2 "leaks" some of the electrons, passing them directly onto O_2. Cytochrome oxidase keeps the partially reduced intermediates on the pathway to water tightly bound to its active site; they do not escape into free solution. **The rate at which $O_2^{\cdot-}$ is produced rises as the concentration of O_2 in the system is raised** (Freeman, BA, Crapo JD: Hyperoxia increases oxygen radical production in rat lungs and lung mitochondria. J Biol Chem 256: 10986-10992, 1981). A number of compounds slowly become oxidized on exposure to O_2 and $O_2^{\cdot-}$ is generated; these include adrenalin, tetrahydrofolate, reduced FMN and oxyhemoglobin.

3.14 Aging Deficiencies and Exercise

I believe that aging is, in part, a disease of EMOD deficiencies.

Aging is directly associated with an increase in overall disease occurrence, which I believe is related to an overall decrease in oxygen metabolism. William E. Roundtree writes in the Hughston Health

Alert, that a decline in our physical abilities starts around age 30, continues throughout our life, and reaches a plateau between ages 60 and 70. After the plateau, a slower decline follows. **Maximum breathing capacity decreases approximately 40% during this period and individuals with chronic lung diseases, such as emphysema, suffer a more significant decline. Cardiovascular function declines approximately one half of one percent each year starting around age 30** and it is no coincidence that world-class and endurance athletes begin gradually leaving their sport after this age. **There is a 40-50% decline in muscle mass and a similar decline in bone mass, along with a simultaneous increase in body fat in both men and women. The metabolic rate also declines with age and is primarily affected by muscle mass.** Periods of extreme starvation can produce as much as a 45% decline in the metabolic system and is believed to be the reason for increased life span with caloric restriction. Sadly, there is no corresponding decline in the appetite with aging. In fact, **after 25 years of age, we tend to gain one pound per year as we age.**

These decreases in the breathing capacity and the cardiovascular function, fit well with my **Unified theory**, and could well explain the increased incidence of diseases associated with aging as it relates to decreased levels of oxygen intake and utilization and thus allows for diseases to occur or to manifest themselves.

It appears to me that aging is a disease of attrition and deficiencies, with deficits of the following:

Oxygen (superoxide anion, hydrogen peroxide and singlet oxygen)
Hormones (DHEA, testosterone, estrogen, etc.) (the equivalent of castration)
Muscle mass
Thymus activity
Immunologic responsiveness
Oxygen consumption

Cellular oxygen utilization
Compliance of the chest wall
Decreased heart function
Decreased cardiac output
Decreased coronary artery blood flow
Decreased brain blood flow
Decreases number of neurons
Decreased oxygen in the skin
Decreased collagen cross linking
Decreased red blood cells (anemia)

According to Dr. Michael Olpin, there are considerable benefits of **aerobic conditioning** with exercise. **I believe that the most common denominator for the body's responses to exercise, are an increase in oxygen consumption and oxygen utilization, both of which result in increased levels of EMODs.** Olpin's list is as follows:

Cardiovascular benefits

> Increase in the diameter of blood vessels
> Allows blood to move through the blood vessels more easily
> Increase in cardiac output
>> **Gets more oxygen and nutrients into the cells throughout the body**
> Increase in the number of red blood cells
>> This provides more oxygen carrying capacity to cells
> Increase in capillarization characterized by a decrease in surface area within capillaries
> **Increases the blood hemoglobin levels for oxygen transport**
> Increases total blood volume (up to 25%)
> Decreases existing plaque buildup along the wall of arteries
> Increases the amount of blood that goes to the brain
> **Increases mitochondrial "reticulum"**
> **Increases in size and number of the mitochondria**

Allows more oxygen to be absorbed into muscle cells

Helps reduce the amount of insulin required to control blood sugar levels

Decreases risk of type II diabetes

Increases tissue responsiveness to the actions of insulin

Increases the number of enzymes involved in aerobic activity

Increases activity of Kreb's cycle

Increases the diffusion of oxygen capacity of the lungs

Enhances the exchange of oxygen from the lungs to the blood

Increase in surface area of alveoli

Increases oxygen getting to the cells where they can generate more RONS

Increase amount of oxygen circulating through the blood stream

Increases air intake

Increases A-V O_2 difference (means more O_2 being taken from the blood)

Decreases risk of the following cancers (cancer development – normal ratio 1:3, athletes 1:7). Due to increased levels of interleukin-1 and interferon and increased numbers of natural killer cells, circulating lymphocytes, granulocytes and other protective bodies

> **Colon, Breast, (shown to decrease breast cancer in women by 60%), Prostate, Uterus, Ovaries, Cervix, Vagina**

Helps body resist upper respiratory tract infections

Reduces risk of endometriosis

Slows some of the physical impairment of Alzheimer's disease (JAMA Oct. 15, 2003)

Increases longevity (2-4 years)

Increases function of the immune system

With the decreasing pulmonary and cardiovascular function associated with aging and with the increasing accumulation of fats (lipids) seen in obesity, it appears to me that the development of disease is a direct consequence of progressively decreasing O_2 levels, O_2 consumption and O_2 delivery to the tissue and cells. The accumulating fats are responsible for trapping more and more of the EMODs and $^1O_2$ generated. To me, **this is the reason for the changes seen with aging and with the appearance of diseases, such as cancer, arteriosclerosis, diabetes, arthritis and cataracts.**

In 1954, Rebeca Gerschman and her colleagues were the first to introduce the idea that free radicals are toxic agents and Dr. Harman, in 1956, developed the free radical theory of aging. The free radical theory of aging simply argues that aging results from the damage generated by **EMODs**. Most experimental evidence in favor of the free radical theory of aging has been based on studies of invertebrates. **Transgenic fruit flies, Drosophila melanogaster, overexpressing the cytoplasmic form of SOD, called Cu/ZnSOD or SOD1, and catalase have a 34% increase in average longevity and a delayed aging process** and in Drosophila, **expression of SOD1 in motor neurons increases longevity by 40%.** Additionally, certain long-lived strains of both Drosophila and the nematode worm Caenorhabditis elegans also have increased levels of antioxidant enzymes. **I believe that this is likely due to H_2O_2 generation by SOD.**

Further, I believe that the increased stores of body fat (obesity) serve as a "sink" for EMODs and thereby decrease their availability to fight diseases and aging.

Physical activity has a major role in reducing the risk for cardiovascular diseases, including coronary artery disease, stroke, hypertension, obesity and diabetes. The prevalence of obesity in the United States has increased dramatically in the past 20 years, especially in Mexican American men and women and black women, and diabetes is increasing at alarming rates. **Type 2 diabetes is beginning to appear in children** and adolescents, **just as is arteriosclerosis** (Flegal, K.M., Carroll M.D., Ogden, C.L., et al: Prevalence and trends in obesity among US adults, 1999-2000. JAMA 2002;288(14):1723-1727) (Ogden, C.L., Flegal, K.M., Carroll, M.D., et al: Prevalence and trends in overweight among US children and adolescents, 1999-2000. JAMA 2002;288(14):1728-1732). **I believe that the fats accumulated in young obese patients serve as a trap for EMODs and this "allows" for the development of diabetes and atherosclerosis.**

Risk reduction for chronic degenerative diseases can occur with low levels of **exercise** as was made clear in consensus statements published by the Centers for Disease Control and Prevention and the ACSM (Pate, R.R., Pratt, M., Blair, S.N., et al: Physical activity and public health: a recommendation from the Centers for Disease Control and Prevention and the American College of Sports Medicine. JAMA 1995;273(5):402-407) (Physical activity and cardiovascular health. NIH Consensus Development Panel on physical activity and cardiovascular health. JAMA 1996; 276(3):241-246). **I do not believe that the affects of aging are the result of accumulated oxidative products, as taught by the free radical theory. To me, it makes more sense that the appearance of the myriad diseases associated with aging are the result of the deficiencies of aging, especially H_2O_2 and EMODs.**

It has often been stated that physical activity has only a limited influence on changing body composition, and that even exercise of a vigorous nature results in the expenditure of too few calories to lead to substantial reductions in body fat. What was once referred to as "oxygen debt" is now called post-exercise oxygen consumption (EPOC) and it is felt to be responsible for additional caloric expenditure following exercise. **I believe that** the important aspect of this observation is the increased oxygen consumption, which has the associated noted salutary effects and not the additional caloric expenditure.

3.15 Breast Cancer and Exercise

Evidence from both animal and human studies indicates that **exercise may reduce the risk of breast cancer. Among eleven human studies that took into account many of the established risk factors for breast cancer, eight reported a decrease in the risk of breast cancer** in pre-menopausal, post-menopausal or all women with high levels of physical activity compared to women with low levels of activity (Cornell University Program on Breast Cancer and Environmental risk Factors. January 1999, Fact Sheet #19).

According to several large studies of occupational (work-related) activity, women who reported a high level of physical at work had an **18% to 52% reduction in their risk of developing breast cancer** compared to women with low levels of activity at work. In studies of recreational activity, women who exercised during their leisure time were reported to have a **12% to 60% reduction in their risk of developing breast cancer.** However, there is some inconsistency in all of these studies.

3.15.1 EMODs and Breast Tumors

Breast tumors are frequently infiltrated by large numbers of macrophages. Tumor-associated **macrophages have been shown to deliver a sublethal oxidative stress to murine mammary tumor cells** (Kundu N, Zhang S, Fulton AM. Sublethal oxidative stress inhibits tumor cell adhesion and enhances experimental metastasis of murine mammary carcinoma. Clin Exp Metastasis 1995;13:16–22). This may be due to oxygen radical production by the macrophages. In addition, tumour necrosis factor-α is secreted by tumour-associated macrophages, and is known to induce cellular oxidative stress. **This is exactly as I have said, "If the body could generate more of an oxidative assault, it could kill the cancer."**

The chemotherapeutic agents doxorubicin, mitomycin C, etoposide and cisplatin are superoxide generating agents (Yokomizo A, Ono M, Nanri H, Makino Y, Ohga T, Wada M, Okamoto T, Yodoi J, Kuwano M, Kohno K. Cellular levels of thioredoxin associated with drug sensitivity to cisplatin, mitomycin C, doxorubicin, and etoposide. Cancer Res 1995;55:4293–4296).

Radiotherapy and photodynamic therapy generate oxygen radicals within the carcinoma cell.

The **anti-estrogen tamoxifen, increasingly used alongside other breast cancer therapies, has also been shown to induce oxidative stress within carcinoma cells** *in vitro* (Ferlini C, Scambia G, Marone M, Distefano M, Gaggini C, Ferrandina G, Fattorossi A, Isola G, Benedetti Panici P, Mancuso S. Tamoxifen induces oxidative stress and apoptosis in estrogen receptor-negative human cancer cell lines. Br J Cancer 1999;79:257–263).

A breast tumor rapidly outgrows its blood supply, leading to glucose deprivation and **hypoxia.** Glucose deprivation rapidly induces cellular oxidative stress within the MCF-7 breast carcinoma cell line, although it does not cause oxidative stress in non-transformed cell lines. This may be because glucose deprivation depletes intracellular pyruvate within the breast carcinoma cell, preventing the decomposition of endogenous oxygen radicals. Breast carcinomas usually support their growth by stimulating blood vessel development (angiogenesis). **Blood flow within these new vessels is often chaotic, causing periods of hypoxia followed by reperfusion. Reperfusion** after myocardial infarction or cerebral ischemia is known to cause the generation of EMODs.

Sublethal oxidative stress promotes cell proliferation *in vitro*, with both superoxide and hydrogen peroxide stimulating growth (Burdon RH. Superoxide and hydrogen peroxide in relation to mammalian cell proliferation. Free Radic Biol Med 1995;18:775–794). Proliferation in response to hydrogen peroxide may be due to the activation of mitogen-activated protein kinases (MAPKs). HeLa cells treated with hydrogen peroxide undergo a sustained activation of all three MAPK pathways: extracellular signal related protein kinase; c-Jun amino-terminal kinase/stress-activated protein kinase; and p38.

Severe oxidative stress leads to apoptosis. Conversely, persistent oxidative stress at sublethal levels may cause resistance to apoptosis. The induction of programmed cell death by EMODs is dependent on p53 in both mouse and human cell lines (Yin Y, Solomon G, Deng C, Barrett JC. Differential regulation of p21 by p53 and Rb in cellular response to oxidative stress. Mol Carcinog 1999;24:15–24).

The antioxidant thiols thioredoxin and metallothionein are rapidly upregulated in response to EMODs, and the antioxidants malondialdehyde, superoxide dismutase, glutathione peroxidase and catalase show increased expression or activity in breast tumor tissue as compared with normal controls. An upregulation of anti-ROS defenses in cancer cells may explain why tumor cell lines *in vitro* are extremely resistant to cytolysis by hydrogen peroxide (O'Donnell-Tormey J, DeBoer CJ, Nathan CF. Resistance of human tumor cells in vitro to oxidative cytolysis. J Clin Invest 1985;76:80–86). In addition, antiapoptotic Akt (protein kinase B) is activated by hydrogen peroxide (Shaw M, Cohen P, Alessi DR. The activation of protein kinase B by H_2O_2 or heat shock is mediated by phosphoinositide 3-kinase and not by mitogen-activated protein kinase-activated protein kinase-2. Biochem J 1998;336:241–246).

EMODs increase tumor cell production of the angiogenic factors IL-8 and vascular endothelial growth factor (VEGF). Tumour cell **EMODs** also promotes secretion of the matrix metalloproteinase-1 (MMP-1), a collagenase that aids vessel growth within the tumour microenvironment (Brown NS, Jones A, Fujiyama C, Harris AL, Bicknell R. Thymidine phosphorylase induces carcinoma cell oxidative stress and promotes secretion of angiogenic factors. Cancer Res 2000;60:6298–6302). **Hydrogen peroxide induces inducible nitric oxide synthase (NOS)** in cytokine stimulated rat pleural mesothelial cells (Milligan SA, Owens MW, Grisham MB. Augmentation of cytokine-induced nitric oxide synthesis by hydrogen peroxide. Am J Physiol 1996;271:L114–L120). The nitric oxide produced would activate cGMP within nearby smooth muscle cells, leading to vasodilatation. Vasodilatation could also be triggered by carbon monoxide, because oxidative stress powerfully induces heme oxygenase-1, which degrades heme to biliverdin and carbon monoxide. Carbon monoxide, like nitric oxide, activates cGMP.

Rac1 can activate the NADPH-oxidase in tumour cells, causing superoxide production. **EMODs have been shown to mediate the role of Rac1 in actin cytoskeleton reorganization** (Moldovan L, Irani K, Moldovan NI, Finkel T, Goldschmidt-Clermont PJ. The actin cytoskeleton reorganization induced by Rac1 requires the production of superoxide. Antiox Redox Signal 1999;1:29–43).

3.15.2 H_2O_2 Is Not a Mutagen but Rather an Epigenetic Toxicant

H_2O_2 may act as a "genotoxicant" or "epigenetic" agent in its role as a promoting agent. However, although it can cause DNA damage, **peroxide is at best a very weak mutagen in mammalian cells** (Takeuchi, T., Matsugo, S. and Morimoto, K. (1997) Mutagenicity of oxidative DNA damage in Chinese hamster V79 cells. Carcinogenesis, 18, 2051-2055). This is in contrast to the work of others who state **that $O_2^{\cdot-}$ and H_2O_2 do not react with DNA bases at all** (Dizdaroglu, M. (1993) In DNA and Free Radicals (Halliwell, B., and Aruoma, O.I. eds.), pp. 19-39, Ellis Horwood, Chichester.) OH· generates a variety of products from all four DNA bases and this pattern is used as a **diagnostic "fingerprint" of OH· attack** (Halliwell, B. and Aruoma, O.I. (1991) FEBS Lett. 281, 9-19). **Singlet oxygen** selectively attacks guanine to produce the **8-hydroxyguanine (8-OHG)**, which is also used as an index of oxidative damage to DNA and it can be measured as the nucleoside, **8-hydroxydeoxyguanosine (8-OHdG).**

In vitro, H_2O_2 can induce single-strand breaks in cellular DNA, oxidation of DNA bases, chromosomal aberrations and DNA-protein crosslinks. This indicates that RONS are involved in the redox state of the cell and are important mediators for many cellular functions. In spite of the long speculation on the involvement of H_2O_2 in the tumor promotion process, **current knowledge concerning the mechanism by which H_2O_2 promotes tumor formation is still scarce** (Huang, et al, Tumor promotion by hydrogen peroxide in rat liver epithelial cells. Carcinogenesis, Vol. 20, No. 3, pp. 485-492, 1999).

It has been postulated that tumor promotion by H_2O_2 is likely operating via "epigenetic" rather than "genotoxic" mechanisms. **I believe that this again indicates that it is not known where peroxide has an impact on tumor growth and it must be kept in mind that these studies were carried out using non-physiological levels of H_2O_2, which are known to have cytotoxic activity.**

Otto Warburg was the first scientist to implicate oxygen in cancer (Warburg, O. On the origin of cancer cells. Science 1956; 123: 309-314). Organic and hydrogen peroxides have been shown to act as tumor promoters and not as initiators, indicating that these oxidants are **not mutagens** but rather **epigenetic toxicants**. In the past decade, much research has shifted to the understanding of how **EMODs** can reversibly control the expression of genes at noncytotoxic doses (Allen, R.G. and Tresini, M. Oxidative stress and gene regulation. Free Rad Biol Med 2000; 28: 463-499). In this regard, **at least 127 genes and signal transducing proteins have been reported to be sensitive to reductive and oxidative (redox) states in the cell** (Allen, R.G. and Tresini, M. Oxidative stress and gene regulation. Free Rad Biol Med 2000; 28: 463-499).

The metabolism of glutathione by **membrane gamma-glutamyl transpeptidase (GGT) has been recently recognized as a basal source of H_2O_2 in the extracellular space**. Significant levels of GGT activity are expressed by malignant tumors and in **melanoma** cell lines they were found to correlate with the malignant behavior (J Cell Sci. Vol 113, Issue 15 2671-2678).

A study on synergism between tumor necrosis factor-alpha and H_2O_2, levels of cellular toxicity were found. With PC12 tumor cells, TNF alpha **toxicity was seen at >50 ng/ml**, and that of H_2O_2 **at > 150 microM**, however, when together, **sub-lethal levels (25 ng/ml TNF alpha and 30 microM H_2O_2)** induced toxicity (Trembovler, V., Abu-Raya, S. and Shohami, E. Synergism between tumor necrosis factor-alpha and H_2O_2 enhances cell damage in rat PC12 cells. Neurosci Lett. 2003 Dec 19; 353(2):115-118).

Many human cancer cells overproduce hydrogen peroxide. High levels (up to 0.5 nmol/hr/10^4 cells) of hydrogen peroxide are constitutively released from a wide range of human tumor cells. I believe that this makes the tumor cell more vulnerable to increases in EMODs and creates selectivity for PDT and cancer therapy.

Clearly, this illustrates the great importance of H_2O_2 and EMODs in the regulation of cellular homeostasis and redox status.

3.15.3 Gap Junction Communications and EMODs

Cell to cell communication via gap junctions is essential for the maintenance of the homeostatic balance in multicellular organisms (Yamasaki, H. and Naus, C.C.G. (1996) Role of connexin genes in growth control. *Carcinogenesis*, 17, 1199–1213). Accumulated evidence suggests an important role of GJC in tumor promotion (Trosko, J.E., Chang, C.C. and Madhukar, B.V. (1994) The role of modulated gap junctional intercellular communication in epigenetic toxicology. *Risk Anal.*, 14, 303–312). This stems from several findings, including: (i) many tumor promoting agents inhibit GJC; (ii) GJC is usually down-regulated in tumors; (iii) on the other hand, up-regulation of GJC is associated with prevention of carcinogenesis (Schmidt, J.N., Traenckner, E.B., Meier, B. and Baeuerle, P.A. (1995) Induction of oxidative stress by okadaic acid is required for activation of transcription factor NF-kappa B. *J. Biol. Chem.*, 270, 27136–27142) (Lau, A.F., Kanemitsu, M.Y., Kurata, W.E., Danesh, S. and Boynton, A.L. (1992) Epidermal growth factor disrupts gap-junctional communication and induces phosphorylation of connexin43 on serine. *Mol. Biol. Cell*, 3, 865–874).

Recently Trosko's group reported that H_2O_2 inhibits GJC in WB-F344 rat liver epithelial cells with an I_{50} value of 200 µM, but it seems that this effect does not involve oxidative stress because the antioxidants they used did not block the effect of H_2O_2 on the disruption of GJC (Upham, B.L., Kang, K.S., Cho, H.Y. and Trosko, J.E. (1997) Hydrogen peroxide inhibits gap junctional intercellular communication in glutathione sufficient but not glutathione deficient cells. *Carcinogenesis*, 18, 37–42). Again, this illustrates that attempts to verify the Free Radi-Crap theory falls flat on its face. This is because the theory is wrong....good data.....wrong theory.

Nonetheless, many investigators refer to the possibility of EMOD damage to DNA and infer that it can induce neoplastic changes. From the knowledge that 8-OH-dG is only one of many oxidized products formed and that about 6.4×10^{10} oxygen radicals are estimated to be produced per rat cell each day, they calculated that one oxidized DNA residue is produced for every 7.6×10^5 oxygen radicals generated, or about 9×10^4 oxidized DNA bases are formed per cell per day.

The involvement of reactive oxygen species (**EMODs**), particularly H_2O_2, in the tumor promotion process is supported by both *in vivo* and *in vitro* studies. **(RMH Note: these studies use non-physiological levels of peroxide).** H_2O_2 is capable of promoting neoplastic transformation in several two-stage transformation systems, including rat urothelial cells, murine myeloid progenitor cells, mouse epidermal cells and mouse embryo fibroblast.
In vivo studies also suggest that H_2O_2 is a mouse skin tumor promoter (Mitchel, R.E., Morrison, D.P. and Gragtmans, N.J. (1987) Tumorigenesis and carcinogenesis in mouse skin treated with hyperthermia during stage I or stage II of tumor promotion. *Carcinogenesis*, **8**, 1875–1879). **The production of EMODs and H_2O_2 is a common feature of tumor promoters such as TPA, TCDD, UV, OA, peroxisome proliferators, steroidal estrogens, phenobarbital, chlordane and aroclor.**

Disruption of functional gap junctions is evident in tumor promotion and carcinogenesis. H_2O_2 treatment, especially at a concentration of 200 μM, rapidly and transiently disrupts GJC in T51B cells. Collectively, these data indicate that the actions of H_2O_2 on tumor promotion, IE gene expression and GJC interruption are dependent on oxidative stress and antioxidants may be useful in chemoprevention. Remember, **antioxidants have been shown not to prevent cancer.** The mechanisms responsible for tumor promotion by H_2O_2 still remain unclear. H_2O_2 may act as a `genotoxicant' or `epigenetic' agent in its role as a promoting agent.

I repeat, although H$_2$O$_2$ can cause DNA damage, it is, at best, a very weak mutagen in mammalian cells (Takeuchi, T., Matsugo, S. and Morimoto, K. (1997) Mutagenicity of oxidative DNA damage in Chinese hamster V79 cells. *Carcinogenesis*, **18**, 2051–2055).

Chronic infection/inflammation is implicated in the pathogenesis of several forms of cancer, including hepatoma. It is well known that during inflammation, cells release reactive oxygen species, particularly H$_2$O$_2$. However, **the role of H$_2$O$_2$ in the development of cancer and the underlying mechanisms are not well defined. It is also well known that inflammation is associated with hypoxia.**

4.0 H$_2$O$_2$ AS INTRACELLULAR MESSENGER

Different from O$_2$$^-$ that is charged, hardly permeable, and extremely short-lived, **H$_2$O$_2$** produced either intracellularly, within mitochondria, or at extracellular space is uncharged, relatively longer-lived, and freely diffusible. As with NO, **this property makes H$_2$O$_2$ an ideal signaling molecule.**

There is evidence that diffusable reactive oxygen intermediates such as nitric oxide (NO) and **hydrogen peroxide (H$_2$O$_2$) (EMODs) can modulate cellular functions through altering signal transduction in many cell types, including endothelial cells (ECs), vascular smooth muscle cells (VSMC), and T cells** (Los, M., W. Droege, K. Stricker, P. A. Baeuerle, K. Schulze-Osthoff. 1995. Hydrogen peroxide as a potent activator of T lymphocyte functions. Eur. J. Immunol. 25:159) (Harlan, J. M., K. S. Callahan. 1984. Role of hydrogen peroxide in the neutrophil-mediated release of prostacyclin from cultured endothelial cells. J. Clin. Invest. 74:442) (Lewis, M. S., R. E. Whatley, P. Cain, T. M. McIntyre, S. M. Prescott, G. A. Zimmerman. 1988. Hydrogen peroxide stimulates the synthesis of platelet-activating factor by endothelium and induces endothelial cell-dependent neutrophil adhesion. J. Clin. Invest. 82:2045) (Sundaresan, M., Z-X. Yu, V. J. Ferrans, K. Irony, T. Finkel. 1995. Requirement for generation of H$_2$O$_2$ for platelet-derived growth factor signal transduction. Science 270:296) (Rao, G. N., B. C. Berk. 1992. Active oxygen species stimulate vascular smooth muscle cell growth and proto-oncogene expression. Circ. Res. 70:593)

H$_2$O$_2$ is known to:

> **induce transcription factor activation**
> **modulate K$^+$ channels expressed in Xenopus oocytes**
> **regulate Ca^{2+} signaling**

induce Ca^{2+} influx by directly activating Ca^{2+} channels on the plasma membrane
stimulate protein phosphorylation

It has recently been shown that H_2O_2:

increases intracellular Ca^{2+}
decreases the ATP/ADP ratio
and inhibits glucose-stimulated insulin secretion from isolated mouse islets

Many investigators have shown that **calcium is essential for production of EMODs** and believe that elevated calcium levels are responsible for activation of **EMOD**-generating enzymes and formation of free radicals by the mitochondrial respiratory chain. Conversely, **an increase in intracellular calcium concentration may be stimulated by EMODs** and H_2O_2 has been recently shown to accelerate the overall channel opening process in voltage-dependent calcium channels in plant and animal cells. Data support the speculation that **Ca^{2+} and RONS are two cross-talking messengers in various cellular processes** (Gordeeva, A.V., Zvyagilskaya, R.A. and Labas, Y.A. Cross-talk between reactive oxygen species and calcium in living cells. Biochemistry (Moscow), Oct. 2003, vol. 68, no. 10, pp. 1077-1080.). Please keep in mind that many investigators believe that Ca^{2+} overload is considered to be the final pathway leading to cell death under pathological conditions. I believe that this is related to RONS induced apoptosis.

RONS have recently been implicated in a variety of redox-based signaling mechanisms that can mediate changes in neural plasticity including:

activation of oxidative stress-responsive transcription factors
modulation of LTP induction

and mediation of nonsynaptic communication between neurons and glia.

(Signal Transduction by reactive Oxygen and Nitrogen Species: Pathways and Chemical Principles. Edited by H.J. Forman, J. Fukuto and M. Torres, Kluwer Academic Publishers, 2003. **H_2O_2 as Intracellular Messenger** (S.O. Rhee, S. Lee, K. Yang, J. Kwon and S.W. Kang Page 167).

Hydrogen peroxide is also generated by:

> **arachidonic acid-metabolizing enzymes**
> **xanthine oxidase**
> **nitric oxide synthase**
> **cytochrome P450**
> **as well as in the cellular response to ultraviolet radiation.**

Many cells types produce H_2O_2 in response to a variety of extracellular stimuli including:

> **cytokines**
> **neurotransmitters**
> **peptide growth factors**
> **hormones**
> **and phorbol myristate acetate (PMA).**

H_2O_2 thus produced in response to receptor stimulation is known to mediate the activation of such crucial protein kinases as the members of:

> **MAPK family**
> **Src family**
> **receptor protein tyrosine kinase family**
> **and PKC family.**

The addition of exogenous H_2O_2 or the intracellular production in response to receptor stimulation, affect the function of various proteins including:

> **transcription factors**
> **phospholipases**
> **protein phosphates**
> **ion channels**
> **and G proteins.**

H_2O_2 is the mediator of the eNOS up-regulation.

Accordingly, H_2O_2 **is now recognized as a ubiquitous intracellular messenger, under subtoxic conditions** (Rhee, S.G. Redox signaling: Hydrogen peroxide as intracellular messenger. Exp Mol Med 1999; 31: 53-59), (Finkel, T. Oxygen radicals and signaling. Curr Opin Cell Biol 1998; 10: 248-253), (Suzuki, Y.J. and Ford, G.D. Redox regulation of signal transduction in cardiac and smooth muscle. J Mol Cell Cardiol 1999; 31: 345-353), (Thannickal, V.J. Fanburg, B.L. Reactive oxygen species in cell signaling. Am J Physiol Lung Cell Mol Physiol 2000; 279: L1005-1028), (Griendling, K.K. and Ushio-Fukai, M. Reactive oxygen species as mediators of angiotensin II signaling. Regul Pept 2000; 91: 21-27), (Patel, R.P., Moellering, D., Murphy-Uhrich, J., Jo., H., Beckman, S. and Darley-Usmar, V.M. Cell signaling by reactive nitrogen and oxygen species in atherosclerosis. Free Radic Biol Med 2000; 28: 1780-1794), (Forman, H.J. and Torres, M. Signaling by the respiratory burst in macrophages. IUBMB Life 2001; 51: 365-371).

H_2O_2 levels are increased within the cell in response to growth factors and **act as an intracellular messenger** (Rhee, S.G., et al Hydrogen peroxide: a key messenger that modulates protein phosphorylation through cysteine oxidation. Signal Transduct. Knowl. Environ. 53: 1-6, 2000). Low levels of H_2O_2 produced by the mitochondria regulate physiological processes, including **cell proliferation**, while high levels of H_2O_2 are toxic to the cell and cause apoptosis.

Recent evidence that specific **inhibition of H_2O_2 generation results in a complete blockage of signaling by:**

PDGF
EGF
and angiotensin II is a strong indication that H_2O_2 serves in a messenger role. However, the mechanism by which H_2O_2 mediates receptor signaling has not been well characterized. This reinforces the point that **it is time to discard the outdated and erroneous Free Radi-Crap Theory of Aging and oxidative stress.**

The limited reactivity with many biological molecules and the low intracellular concentrations of O_2^- and H_2O_2 (10 pM and 1-100 nM, respectively) have raised questions about their toxicity per se in vivo. I have repeatedly questioned their reputed toxicity throughout my research.

-H_2O_2 production is 8.1% total O_2 consumed (liver cell) mitochondria.
-H_2O_2 production is 5.3% total O_2 consumed (liver cell) peroxisomes.
-Thus, a total of 13.4% H_2O_2 production in liver cell (Oxygen Paradox, page 93).

Peroxisomal oxidation of fatty acids has been recognized as an important source of H_2O_2

with prolonged starvation. **This may be related to the affects of caloric restriction and aging.**

Ceramide Signaling. T. Goldkorn, T. Ravid and E.A. Medina. Page 194

Under basal conditions, human cells produce about 2 billion $O_2.-$ and H_2O_2 molecules per cell per day (Hoidal, J.R. Reactive oxygen species and cell signaling. Am J Respir Cell Mol Biol 2001; 25: 661-663). **EMODs were once considered as only waste byproducts of aerobic metabolism or molecules of defense produced by host inflammatory cells against invading organism.** Now, **EMODs are recognized as controlling key steps in cellular signal transduction cascades** (Schreck, R., Rieber, P. and Baeuerle, P.A. Reactive oxygen intermediates as apparently widely needed messengers in the activation of the NK-k B transcription factor and HIV-1. Embo J 1991; 10: 2247-2258), (Sen, C.K. and Packer, L. Antioxidant and redox regulation of gene transcription. Faseb J 1996; 10: 709-720).

Treatment of airway epithelial cells with **exogenous H_2O_2, the agent commonly produced during lung inflammatory processes, has been shown to activate EGF receptor tyrosine kinase** but not the receptor's trafficking. This presents a mechanism by which **RONS directly mediate transduction of mitogenic signals to the nucleus.** Our laboratory has also examined the role of ROS in another key physiologic process, apoptosis.

Goldkorn found that **H_2O_2 at physiological concentrations [50-250 nmoles/mg protein], induces epithelial apoptosis via the ceramide signal transduction pathway.** This work provides **a direct link between two important aspects of mammalian stress responses: the generation of RONS and activation of the sphingomyelin/ceramide cycle leading to apoptosis.**

Importantly, **several agonists increase H_2O_2 generation by epithelial cells, including:**

> **`cytokines (TNFa, IL1 and Fas ligand)**
> **cytotoxic agents**
> **ionizing radiation**
> **and infections (e.g., HIV or bacteria).**

Gene Regulation by EMODs ("The Oxygen Paradox," Eds. K.J.A. Davies and F. Ursini. Cleup University Press, 1995. A. Eisenstark, A. Ivanova and C. Miller Page 573). **About 30 proteins are induced when a low, non-lethal, dose of hydrogen peroxide is added to cells.** In addition, **cells become resistant to doses of H_2O_2 that would be toxic to non-induced cells.** Nine of these proteins are under regulation of the product of **the oxyR gene.** An interesting aspect of its regulatory mechanism is that **it activates transcription from the nine promoters only when the protein is oxidized. When a reductant is added to a culture, transcription is turned off.** Indeed, mutations within the oxyR gene may prohibit this oxidation, resulting in highly increased synthesis of the known proteins under its regulation (Storz, G., Tartaglia, L.A. and Ames, B.N. Transcriptional regulator of oxidative stress-inducible genes: Direct activation by oxidation. Science 1990; 248: 189-194). **This illustrates the point that interference with or blocking of EMOD signaling, with reducing agents or antioxidants, has potentially harmful effects.**

Environmental oxidants that increase EMOD production are:

> **ultraviolet**
> **ionizing radiation**
> **heavy metals**
> **redox active chemicals**
> **anoxia**
> **and hyperoxia.**

Monoamine oxidase (MOA), located on the cytoplasmic face of the outer mitochondrial membrane, represents another source of H_2O_2 that can lead to apoptosis.

H_2O_2 itself is a mild oxidant and is relatively inert to most biomolecules.

In an inflammatory environment, H_2O_2 is produced by activated macrophages at an estimated rate of $2\text{-}6 \times 10^{-14}$ mol/h^{-1}/cell^{-1} and can reach as high as 10-100 μM in the vicinity of these cells.

5 μM H_2O_2 is non-toxic (O_2 Paradox, page 574).

(Mitochondrial ROS/RNS Signaling. C. Giulivi and M.J. Oursler. Page 312). **Both NAD- and FAD-linked substrates support rates of hydrogen peroxide production (0.2-0.8 nmol hydrogen peroxide/min mg protein) modulated by** various **metabolic states** (Boveris, A. and Chance, B. The mitochondrial generation of hydrogen peroxide: General properties and effect of hyperbaric oxygen. Biochem J 1973; 134: 707-716), (Loschen, G., Assim, A. and Richter, C. Superoxide radicals as precursors of mitochondrial hydrogen peroxide. FEBS Lett 1973; 33: 84-88).

Possible H_2O_2 consequences:

   1) hexose monophosphate shunt activation
   2) glutathione redox cycle activation
   3) oxidation of intracellular sulfhydryls
   4) decreased intracellular ATP
   5) possible DNA damage (unlikely)
   6) loss of NAD$^+$
   7) Poly (ADP-ribose) polymerase activation
   8) increased free Ca^{++}
   9) cytoskeleton alterations
   10) plasma membrane alterations
   11) inhibition of glycolysis

EMODs modulate fibroblast proliferation and collagen synthesis, and are involved not only in MMP activation but also increased MMP expression. **EMODs influence extracellular matrix remodeling through the activation of matrix metalloproteinases (MMPs). EMODs can modulate the activity of diverse intracellular**

signaling pathways and the activity of diverse intracellular signaling pathways and molecules (a mechanism commonly termed 'redox signaling').

Many cells types produce H_2O_2 in response to a variety of extracellular stimuli including:

> **Cytokines**
> **Neurotransmitters**
> **Peptide growth factors**
> **Hormones**
> **and phorbol myristate acetate (PMA).**

Cytochrome P450 and *b*5 enzymes oxidize unsaturated fatty acids and xenobiotics and, in the process, generate O_2^- and/or H_2O_2.

Other cytoplasmic sources of oxidants include:

> **soluble enzymes such as xanthine oxidase**
> **aldehyde oxidase**
> **and lipoprotein dehydrogenase that can generate**
> **RONS during catalytic cycling.**

Cytochrome p450 and *b*5 enzymes oxidize unsaturated fatty acids and xenobiotics and, in the process, generate $O_2 \cdot^-$ and/or H_2O_2. I might add that, based on my past work and that of Japanese investigators, Cyt P450 also generates $^1O_2$.

Stimulation of rat vascular smooth muscle cells (VSMCs) by PDGF transiently increased the intracellular concentration of H_2O_2.

4.1 Mitogen-Activated Protein Kinases (MAP Kinases)

The MAPKs are a family of serine/threonine kinases that control cellular responses to growth, apoptosis, and stress signals.

There are 4 main MAPKs including:

-extracellular signal-regulated kinases (ERK1/2)
-c-Jun N-terminal kinases (JNKs, also termed SAPKs
-p38 MAPKs
-and big MAPK-1.

These proteins are the best studied in terms of their redox sensitivity. In SMCs, **H_2O_2, has been shown to activate p38 MAPK, JNK and big MAPK-1.** Its effects on ERK1/2 are controversial, with some reports showing inhibition and others demonstrating stimulation.

In endothelial cells, H_2O_2 activates p38 MAPK and its downstream target, MAPK-activated protein (MAPKAP) kinase 2/3, leading to phosphorylation of heat-shock protein 27 (Hsp27). ERK1/2 activation also seems to be redox sensitive in this cell type, based of the observation that shear stress-**induced ERK1/2 phosphorylation is inhibited by anti-oxidants** and dominant-negative Rac-1. In neonatal rat ventricular myocytes, **all 3 MAPKs (ERK1/2, p38 MAPK, and JNK) have been demonstrated to be activated by H_2O_2.** Thus, regulation of MAPK activity by RONS varies not only among family members but also among cells.

The recently identified serine/threonine kinase Akt/protein kinase B has been shown to play a key role in many cellular processes, including cell survival and protein synthesis (Coffer, P. J. and Woodgett, JR, Jim J. Protein kinase B (c-Akt): a multifunctional mediator of phosphatidylimositol 3-kinase activation. Biochem J. 1998;335; 1-13). **Similar to p38 MAPK, both exogenous H_2O_2 and Ang II activate Akt in SMCs.**

Most likely, only a glimpse of the cadre of oxidant-sensitive signaling pathways have been seen. Many proteins, including phospholipase D, Fyn, proline-rich tyrosine kinase (Pyk) 2, JAK2, and signal transducer and activator of transcription (STAT) 1, appear to be redox sensitive, based on their activation by addition of exogenous EMODs. **H$_2$O$_2$ and lipid hydroperoxides activate phospholipase D in endothelial cells. In mouse fibroblasts, H$_2$O$_2$, activate JAK2 via Fyn Kinase**, resulting in the stimulation of Ras activity (Abe, J.I. and Berk, B.C. Fyn and JAK2 mediate ras activation by reactive oxygen species. J Biol Chem. 1999; 274; 21003-21010).

EMODs regulate several general classes of genes including:

-adhesion molecules and chemotactic factors
-antioxidant enzymes
-and vasoactive substances.

4.2   EMOD Response to Injury

Proof that balloon angioplasty increases oxidant stress has been provided in 2 studies.

Please keep in mind the fact that the reaction to injury is quite different from the reaction to hypercholesterolemia. **It appears to me that the body reacts to the injury of angioplasty, the cardiac by-pass pump and hemodialysis by triggering the oxidative self-healing system.** (Maher ET, Wickens DG, Griffin JFA, Kyl P, Curtis JR, Dormandy TL. Increased free radicals during hemodialysis. Nephrol Dial Transplant 1988; 2: 169-71) (Market M, Heirly C, Kuwahara T, Frei J, Wauters JP. Dialyzed polymorphonuclear neutrophil oxidative metabolism during hemodialysis. A comparative study with 5 new and reused membranes. Clin Nephrol 1988; 3: 129-36) (Himmelfarb J, Lazarus JM, Hakim R. Reactive oxygen species production by monocyte and polymorphonuclear leukocytes during dialysis. Am J Kidney Dis 1991; 17: 271-6) (Rosenkranz AR, Templ E, Traindl O, Hinzl H, Zlabinger GJ. Reactive oxygen product formation by human neutrophils as an early marker for biocompatibility of dialysis membranes. Clin Exp Immunol 1994; 98: 300-5). **Thus, we** need to figure a way to do these procedures, such that we do not induce such a strong oxidative reaction to these procedures, even though the oxidative response may fight any potential infections.

Cellular antioxidant regulation does not completely remove endogenously generated H_2O_2. Rather these processes appear to permit levels of H_2O_2 that are sufficient to exert modulatory actions.

EMODs, including H_2O_2, play roles including:

> Hypoxic signaling
> Physiological redox signaling
> Adaptive signaling
> Apoptotic signaling
> and ultimately necrosis

5.0 INTRACELLULAR KILLING AND DIGESTION OF PATHOGENS

Several minutes after phagolysosome formation, **the first detectable effect on the microorganism is the loss of the ability to reproduce**. Inhibition of macromolecular synthesis occurs sometime later and many **pathogenic and non-pathogenic bacteria are dead 10 to 30 minutes after ingestion.** The mechanisms phagocytes use to carry out this killing are diverse and complex, consisting of both metabolic products and lysosomal constituents. Each type of phagocyte (neutrophils, monocytes or macrophages) will have a slightly different mix of killing methods. **The killing mechanisms that phagocytes use can be organized into two broad groups: oxygen-dependent and oxygen-independent mechanisms.**

5.1   Oxygen-Dependent Mechanisms

Binding of Fc receptors on neutrophils, monocytes and macrophages and mannose receptors on macrophages causes an increase in oxygen uptake by the phagocyte called **the respiratory burst**. This influx of oxygen is used in a variety of mechanisms to cause damage to microbes inside the phagolysosome, but the common theme is the creation of highly reactive small molecules that damage the biomolecules of the pathogen. Binding of these receptors activates an NADPH oxidase that reduces O_2 to O_2^- (superoxide). Superoxide can further decay to hydroxide radical ($OH\cdot$) or be converted into hydrogen peroxide (H_2O_2) by the enzyme superoxide dismutase. In neutrophils, these oxygen species can act in concert with the enzyme myeloperoxidase to form hypochlorous acid (HOCl) and H_2O_2. **HOCl then reacts with a second molecule of H_2O_2 to form singlet oxygen ($^1O_2$),** another reactive oxygen species. Macrophages in some mammalian species catalyze the production of nitric oxide (NO) by the enzyme nitric oxide synthase. NO is toxic to bacteria and directly inhibits viral replication. It may also combine with other oxygen species to form highly reactive peroxynitrate radicals. All of **these pathogen-toxic oxygen species are potent oxidizers and will attack many targets in the pathogen.** At high enough levels, **reactive oxygen species overwhelm the protective mechanisms of the microbe, leading to its death.**

Superoxide in aqueous media undergoes a spontaneous second order reaction with itself, a dismutation reaction that yields one molecule each of H_2O_2 and oxygen in a relatively slow reaction at pH 7.4 (the second order rate constant is of the order of 10 to the 4.5[th] power), when compared with the rate at which superoxide or HO_2.- can abstract an H-atom from such key biological targets as catecholamines or the allylic CH in lipid where the second order rate constant exceeds 10^7. Theoretically, in vivo, the presence of highly active **SOD enzymes will lead to an increase in the local concentration of H_2O_2.**

Although the dismutation would be spontaneous at physiological pH at high superoxide concentrations, **the concentration of superoxide approaches 10 μM (physiological)** as the self reaction slows down considerably and its lifetime becomes extended by many seconds. **Nature has evolved a class of superoxide dismutase (SOD2) enzymes to accelerate H_2O_2 production from superoxide anion. These enzymes can react rapidly with superoxide (rates approaching or exceeding 10^9 power) and dismutate the radical to the nonradical products, O_2 and H_2O_2, faster than superoxide can react with other potential biological targets.** The short half-life should not be misinterpreted as mitigating the potential reactivity of O_2^- because the half-life is actually quite long in relation to the **phenomenal diffusion coefficient of the radical.** Given that superoxide can interact with a variety of biological target molecules, the reaction with the enzyme literally can shunt the superoxide production into H_2O_2 and oxygen.

Proteolysis (protein breakdown) is enhanced by 20-400 μM H_2O_2, whereas millimolar concentrations inhibit proteolysis. As usual, **the effects of H_2O_2 are concentration dependent.**

Phagocytes are a key feature of defense against microorganisms (The Jeremiah Metzger Lecture. Microbial defenses against killing by phagocytes. Mandell GL, Frank MO. Trans Am Clin Climatol Assoc. 1992;103:199-209).

Hydrogen peroxide generated in mononuclear phagocytes and polymorphonuclear cells is of pivotal importance in the intracellular killing of several pathogens (Babior BM. Oxygen-dependent microbial killing by phagocytes (second of two parts). N Engl J Med. 1978 Mar 30;**298**(13):721–725).

Intracellular hydrogen peroxide may also mediate, in part, the antineoplastic activity of macrophages (Nathan C, Cohn Z. Role of oxygen-dependent mechanisms in antibody-induced lysis of tumor cells by activated macrophages. J Exp Med. 1980 Jul; **152**(1):198–208) (Nathan CF, Cohn ZA. Antitumor effects of hydrogen peroxide in vivo. J Exp Med. 1981 Nov 1;**154**(5):1539–1553).

Reports have suggested that **hydrogen peroxide released by mononuclear phagocytes and neutrophils may extend the antimicrobial, antitumor,** and oxidant-injury activities of these cells to adjacent tissues (Nathan CF, Brukner LH, Silverstein SC, Cohn ZA. Extracellular cytolysis by activated macrophages and granulocytes. I. Pharmacologic triggering of effector cells and the release of hydrogen peroxide. J Exp Med. 1979 Jan 1;**149**(1):84–99) (Nathan CF, Silverstein SC, Brukner LH, Cohn ZA. Extracellular cytolysis by activated macrophages and granulocytes. II. Hydrogen peroxide as a mediator of cytotoxicity. J Exp Med. 1979 Jan 1;**149**(1):100–113).

In 1976, the highly respected Dr. Klebanoff stated that H_2O_2 is one of the most important antimicrobial and antitumor weapons of polymorphonuclear leukocytes (Klebanoff SJ. Phagocytic cells: products of oxygen metabolism. In: Gallin JI, Goldstein IM, Snyderman R, eds. Inflammation: basic principles and clinical correlates, 1 ed. New York: Raven Press Ltd, 1988).

The bactericidal and cytotoxic actions of phagocytes and particularly neutrophils have been attributed mainly to O_2-dependent systems that depend on the accumulation of chemically reactive derivatives toxic to the bacteria (A reevaluation of the roles of the O_2-dependent and O_2-independent microbicidal systems of phagocytes. Elsbach P, Weiss J. Rev Infect Dis. 1983 Sep-Oct;5(5):843-53). However, it is concluded that effective antimicrobial activity rests on the coexistence of O_2-independent bactericidal proteins that are highly specific for certain microbial species and O_2-requiring systems that nonspecifically attack all cells.

The respiratory burst oxidase is an activatable, membrane-bound flavo(?hemo) protein that catalyzes the NADPH-dependent reduction of oxygen to superoxide (O_2-) in stimulated phagocytes. Chronic granulomatous disease (CGD), a group of disorders in which phagocytes cannot manufacture O_2-, is caused by a biochemical lesion involving this oxidase or its activating system (The respiratory burst oxidase. Babior BM. Hematol Oncol Clin North Am. 1988 Jun;2(2):201-12).

The products of oxygen reduction (superoxide anion, hydrogen peroxide, hydroxyl radicals) and excitation (singlet oxygen) have been implicated in the toxic properties of phagocytes (neutrophils, eosinophils, and mononuclear phagocytes). Enzymes that potentiate (such as peroxidase) or limit (such as catalase, superoxide dismutase) the toxicity of these agents contribute to the complexity of the oxygen-dependent antimicrobial systems of phagocytes. These toxic systems are dormant when the phagocyte is at rest but are activated when the need arises and directed to the destruction of invading microorganisms and other foreign cells (Oxygen metabolism and the toxic properties of phagocytes. Klebanoff SJ. Ann Intern Med. 1980 Sep;93(3):480-9).

Both nonlethal *Plasmodium yoelii* and lethal *Plasmodium berghei* **(malaria) were killed in vitro by hydrogen peroxide at concentrations as low as 10^{-5} M. Higher concentrations** were required in the presence of added normal erythrocytes. Injection of hydrogen peroxide in vivo significantly reduced *P. yoelii* parasitemia but had less effect on *P. berghei* (Dockrell, Hazel M.; Playfair, John H L. Killing of Blood-Stage Murine Malaria Parasites by Hydrogen Peroxide. Infect Immun. 1983 Jan;**39**(1):456–459).

These observations, together with reports of successful infusions of hydrogen peroxide into patients (Mallams JT, Finney JW, Balla GA. The use of hydrogen peroxide as a source of oxygen in a regional intra-arterial infusion system. South Med J. 1962 Mar;**55**:230–232) (Oliver, T.H., and D.V. Murphy. 1920. Influenzal pneumonia: the intravenous injection of hydrogen peroxide. Lancet 1:432-433) (Balla GA, Finney JW, Aronoff BL, et al: Use of Intra-arterial Hydrogen Peroxide to Promote Wound Healing. Am J Surg 1964; 108: 621-629), **suggest that exogenous hydrogen peroxide might be effective in the therapy of selected infectious and neoplastic diseases.**

Providing additional support for a potential therapeutic role for parenterally administered hydrogen peroxide, (Dockrell, HJ. M., and J. H. L. Playfair. 1983. Killing of blood-stage murine malaria parasites by hydrogen peroxide. Infect. Immun. 16:75-80) reported that **murine Plasmodium yoelii parasitemia was reduced after the intravenous administration of hydrogen peroxide.**

Oxidizing agents such as ozone, hydrogen peroxide, sodium hypochlorite and UV light oxidative mechanisms kill pathogens on the outside of the body and likewise, they kill them on the inside of the body.

5.2   Oxygen-independent Killing

Oxygen-independent mechanisms also play a part in bacterial killing in anaerobic conditions. Some of these non-oxidative agents are acids, lysozyme, lactoferrin, defensins, BPI, azurocidin, serine proteinases, elastase, cathepsin G, and proteinase 3.

6.0 H_2O_2 PRODUCTION

H_2O_2 is involved in any metabolic pathway which utilizes oxidases, peroxidases, cyclo-oxygenases, lipoxygenases, myeloperoxidase, catalase, etc. In some it is generated and in others, it is altered or removed.

The most important sources of **EMOD** generation are:

-endoplasmic reticulum (cytochrome P450)
-peroxisomes (fatty acid oxidation)
-mitochondrial electron transport system (univalent reduction of molecular oxygen NADH dehydrogenase complex)
-endothelial cells (xanthine oxidase reaction)
-inflammatory cells (myeloperoxidase, NADPH oxidase)
-catecholamine oxidation
-and metabolism of arachidonic acid (Toufektsian MC, Boucher FR, Tanguy S, Morel S, de Leiris JG. Cardiac toxicity of singlet oxygen: implication in reperfusion injury. Antioxid Redox Signal. 2001 Feb;3(1):63-9).

NORMAL METABOLISM UTILIZES OXYGEN AND PRODUCES HYDROGEN PEROXIDE. **All aerobic organisms, including humans, derive most of their metabolic energy from the reduction of oxygen and, consequently, produce significant amounts of O_2^- and H_2O_2 that are generated during the metabolism of oxygen.** (Genetic Contributions to Plasma Total Antioxidant Activity. Xing Li Wang; David L. Rainwater; Jane F. VandeBerg; Braxton D. Mitchell; Michael C. Mahaney. *Arteriosclerosis, Thrombosis, and Vascular Biology.* 2001;21:1190.)

H_2O_2 is a normal product of metabolism and is continually produced in the human body. **I believe that one of the most compelling arguments for the harmless nature of H_2O_2 in the human body is the fact that individuals, who lack one of the primary enzymes to break down H_2O_2 (acatalasemia),** their peroxide levels do not cause them harm. Patients lacking catalase (the primary enzyme for breaking down hydrogen peroxide) appear to live relatively normal lives and the Swiss type acatalasaemic patients show no signs of oxidative damage (Goth, L and Pay, A. Genetic heterogeneity in acatalasemia. (1992) Electrophoresis 17: 1302-1303).

Activated phagocytes can produce as much as 47 nmol of $H_2O_2/10^6$ cells within 30 minutes corresponding to a concentration of 47 μM H_2O_2 in a diluted volume of 1 ml.

The rapid dismutation of O_2^{-} to H_2O_2 is (spontaneous, 10^5 $[mol/L]^{-1} \cdot s^{-1}$, SOD-catalyzed, $10^9 [mol/L]^{-1} \times s^{-1}$).

Chance et al. estimate that rat liver microsomes produce:

> 6 to 15 nmol H_2O_2
> and 2 to 10 nmol O_2^{-} per min/mg protein, primarily from autooxidation of reduced cytochromes c and P-450.

Hyperoxia and hyperbaric oxygen enhance hydrogen peroxide generation at the subcellular and cellular levels at different extents (60 to 200%).

Catalase does not appear to be nearly so important as SOD, judging from the weak phenotypes of cells that lack it (Imlay, J. A., and Linn, S. (1988) *Science* **240**, 1302-1309) and persons with acatalasemia (Eaton, J. W., and Ma, M. (1995) in *The Metabolic and Molecular Bases of Inherited Disease* (Scriver, C. R., Beaudet, A. L., Sly, W. S., and Valle, D., eds), 7th Ed., pp. 2371-2383, McGraw-Hill, Inc., New York).

In mammalian cells catalase is largely contained in peroxisomes and to a lesser extent it is secreted.

Mycobacterium tuberculosis can survive and grow inside macrophages, likely due to production of cell wall glycolysis that remove EMODs (**some bacteria have catalase to break down hydrogen peroxide**) and these types of organisms that survive inside phagocytes produce persistent diseases.

Mitochondrial respiration is an important proximal component of the signaling response to H$_2$O$_2$. These data implicate the **mitochondrion as a proximal component of redox-sensitive events in cell signaling** (K Chen, SR Thomas, A Albano, MP Murphy, and JF Keaney, Jr. Mitochondrial Function Is Required for Hydrogen Peroxide-induced Growth Factor Receptor Transactivation and Downstream Signaling. J. Biol. Chem., Vol. 279, Issue 33, 35079-35086, August 13, 2004).

Curiously, one of the sites of greatest production of **H$_2$O$_2$**, within the cell is the **mitochondrion and it does not contain catalase.** Yet, it usually survives and functions quite well and its DNA remains intact throughout a normal life time. **This could not be if peroxide was causing significant harm to the mitochondrion.**

H$_2$O$_2$ has emerged as a particularly important signaling molecule that is consistent with its chemical similarities to nitric oxide, a well characterized autocrine and paracrine signaling species (Thomas, S. R., Chen, K., and Keaney, J. F., Jr. (2003) Antioxid. Redox Signal. 5, 181-194). Like nitric oxide, **H$_2$O$_2$ has defined targets such as protein thiol moieties that produce a variety of sulfur oxidation products** that have the potential to produce distinct cellular responses (Kim, S. O., Merchant, K., Nudelman, R., Beyer, W. F., Jr., Keng, T., DeAngelo, J., Hausladen, A., and Stamler, J. S. (2002) Cell 109, 383-396).

H$_2$O$_2$ is a weak oxidant with a relatively long (seconds) half-life in biological systems. **H$_2$O$_2$ is soluble in both lipid and aqueous environments**, and thus, capable of traversing several cell diameters before it reacts with its target or is catabolized. Some authors say that **H$_2$O$_2$ serves as its own reductant (and oxidant) during dismutation.**

Halliwell states that H_2O_2 is widely regarded as a cytotoxic agent, whose levels must be minimized by the action of antioxidant defense enzymes. Actually, **H_2O_2 is poorly reactive in the absence of transition metal ions and exposure to certain human tissues to H_2O_2 may be greater than is commonly supposed.** Cell culture is frequently used for studies on "physiological" processes such as **signal transduction and regulation of gene expression** and chemical reactions involving the **culture media need to be considered because they may lead to the generation of substantial amounts of H_2O_2** in vitro. Some or all other reported effects of ascorbic and polyphenolics compounds (e.g., quercetin, catechins, epigallocatechin, epigallocatechin gallate) on cells in culture may be due to H_2O_2 generation by interaction of these compounds with cell culture media (Halliwell, B., Clement, M.V., Ramalingam, J. and Long, L.H. Hydrogen peroxide. Ubiquitous in cell culture and in vivo? IUBMB Life. 2000. Oct-Nov;50(4-5):251-257).

Others have found that mammalian cells are not killed by H_2O_2-generated .OH radicals (Ward JF, Blakey WF, Joner EL. Mammalian cells are not killed by DNA single-strand breaks caused by hydroxyl radicals from hydrogen peroxide endothelial cells against oxidant damage. Biochem Biophys Res Commun 1985;127-270-276).

Hydrogen Peroxide Production:
Also, Copper Containing Oxidases Produce H_2O_2

 Cytochrome oxidase
 Laccase
 Ferroxidase I
 2) **cytochrome P-450, cytochrome B5 and Xanthine oxidase** which produce superoxides;
 3) **oxidases** for fatty acids, urate, L-pipecolic acid, D-amino acids, alcohols, polyamines, a-hydroxy acids and cholestanoic acid which produce H_2O_2;

The major sites of **EMOD** production in the muscle, inside the cells, are:

>Mitochondria
>Sarcolemma
>Lysosomes
>and activation of neutrophils.

6.1   Cell H$_2$O$_2$ Reaction is Concentration Dependent

The following abstract by K.J. Davies contains very important information relative to a cell's response to varying concentrations of H$_2$O$_2$ and information of a time course over which these responses occur. Although I disagree with the use of the concept of "oxidative stress," I applaud his assemblage of data for this paper.

Proliferating mammalian cells exhibit a broad spectrum of responses to oxidative stress, depending on the stress level encountered.

Very low levels of hydrogen peroxide, e.g., 3 to 15 microM, or 0.1 to 0.5 micromol/10^7 cells, **cause a significant mitogenic response,** 25% to 45 % growth stimulation.

Greater concentrations of H$_2$O$_2$, 120 to 150 microM, or 2 to 5 micromol/10^7 cells, **cause a temporary growth arrest** that appears to protect cells from excess energy use and DNA damage. **After 4-6 h** of temporary growth arrest, many **cells will exhibit up to a 40-fold transient adaptive response in which genes for oxidant protection and damage repair are preferentially expressed. After 18 h of H$_2$O$_2$ adaptation** (including the 4-6 h of temporary growth arrest) **cells exhibit maximal protection against oxidative stress.**

The H_2O_2 originally added **is metabolized within 30-40 min**, and if no more is added the **cells will gradually de-adapt, so that by 36 h after the initial H_2O_2 stimulus they have returned to their original level of H_2O_2 sensitivity.** (Davies KJ. The broad spectrum of responses to oxidants in proliferating cells: a new paradigm for oxidative stress. IUBMB Life. 1999 Jul;48(1):41-7).

H_2O_2 and O_2^{-} **are in steady state in pico and nano-molar range and H_2O_2 concentration can be as high as 25 μM.**

5 μM H_2O_2 is non-toxic (O_2 Paradox, page 574).

H_2O_2 produciton (The Oxygen Paradox)
3.24×10^9 H_2O_2/cell - hr
Cellular fraction

> Mitochondria - 13.6%
> Microsomes - 47.7%
> Peroxisomes - 34.1%
> Supernatant - 4.6%

H_2O_2 production
8.1% of total O_2 consumed
> (liver cell)

5.3% of total O_2 consumed
> (-peroxisomes)

6.2   Low Levels of H_2O_2

Low levels of H_2O_2 are important to the cell because they regulate physiological processes such as:

- receptor-mediated cell signaling pathways
- normal cell proliferation and
- transcription activation (Simon, H.U. et al Role of reactive oxygen species (ROS) in apoptosis function. Apoptosis, 5: 415-418, 2000,

Huang, R.P. et al, UV activates growth factor receptors via reactive oxygen species. J Cell Biol., 133: 211-220, 1996).
Undoubtedly, **I predict that H$_2$O$_2$ will be proven to be one of the most important cellular secondary messengers and this will lead to new therapeutic applications and interventions. H$_2$O$_2$ will conform to this pattern of initial discovery, to be later followed by clinical application.**

Peroxide is becoming a recognized second messenger just like cAMP, Ca^{2+}, Ins 1,4,5-P3, and NO (Rhee, S.G. Redox signaling: hydrogen peroxide as intracellular messenger. Exp. and Mol. Med., Vol. 31, No. 2, 53-59, June 1999).

Hydrogen peroxide is used to cleanse and irrigate wounds. **As it decomposes immediately into water and oxygen on contact with organic tissue, it is usually regarded as a safe agent. (**Oxygen embolism due to hydrogen peroxide irrigation during cervical spinal surgery. Morikawa H, Mima H, Fujita H, Mishima S. Can J Anaesth. 1995 Mar;42(3):231-3). **When applied to tissue, solutions of H$_2$O$_2$ have poor penetrability** (HSDB. 1995. Hazardous Substances Data Bank. Medlars Online Information Retrieval System, National Library of Medicine).

2 ml of 3% H$_2$O$_2$ can release 20 ml of oxygen micro-bubbles. Hydrogen peroxide has a half-life of 0.75 to 2.0 seconds in human blood. Catalase breaks down peroxide into water and ground state oxygen, both of which are harmless and are needed by the body. Thus, H$_2$O$_2$ given by a peripheral vein is decomposed before it can leave the upper extremity.

In the body, hydrogen peroxide (H$_2$O$_2$) can be:

i) divalently reduced by catalase (CAT) or glutathione peroxidase (GSH-Px),
ii) divalently reduced by diverse peroxidases producing **singlet oxygen (^{1}O$_2$),**

iii) monovalently reduced to produce hydroxyl radical (°OH) through the Fenton reaction catalysed by transition metals (M) such as iron or copper,

iv) monovalently reduced by reaction with $O_2{}^-$ to produce $^1O_2$.

.OH can also convert themselves back into water by pulling off hydrogen atoms (hydrogen atom abstraction) from a biological molecule, as happens in lipid peroxidation. They can also combine with themselves and form **H_2O_2. To me, it seems likely that harmful hydroxyl radicals which are produced at a finite or specific cellular locus would have a tendency to react with other hydroxyl radicals (since they are being generated from the same locus) to produce beneficial hydrogen peroxide. .OH + .OH →H-O-O-H**

Nick Lane states that it is likely that both iron and H_2O_2 are present at steady-state concentrations of about 10^{-6} gm/kg body weight. He then uses Avogadro's number (6.023×10^{23} molecules in one mole of any substance) and calculates that **we produce about 50 .OH radicals in each cell every second or that in a day, each cell generates 4 million .OH radicals. Thus, in the average body of 100 trillion cells (figures vary), we would produce 4 X 10^{17} .OH radicals per day.** Again, I ask "How toxic are EMODs?" (Oxygen: The molecule that made the world. Nick Lane, Oxford University Press, 2002).

If two hydroxyl radicals ever meet, they can join their unpaired electrons and make an oxygen-oxygen covalent bond, giving H_2O_2 (hydrogen peroxide), a product with no unpaired electrons. I believe that this reaction saves the cell from rapid destruction by .OH and allows for the beneficial effects of hydrogen peroxide and electronic excitation states. In my opinion, this is another ingenious pathway for hydrogen peroxide formation, which, although it has been

known for many years, has basically gone unrecognized by most investigators.

$$.OH + .OH \rightarrow H\text{-}O\text{-}O\text{-}H$$

Another ingenious way for the **body to produce H_2O_2** is by the **deactivation of $^1O_2$** by NADPH as follows:

$$NADPH + {}^1O_2 + H^+ \rightarrow NADP^+ + H_2O_2$$

(Bodaness, R.S. and Chan, P.C. *FEBS Lett.* 1979; 105: 195-196).

It is frequently pointed out that H_2O_2 will react with iron to produce the .OH radical but curiously, it does not react with the iron contained in the heme proteins such as catalase, hemoglobin or NADPH oxidase.

It was proposed erroneously many years ago that the hydroxyl radical could be produced from the interaction of O_2^- and H_2O_2 by a chemical process known as the Haber-Weiss reaction. However, **detailed studies of the rate of this reaction have shown that the Haber-Weiss reaction could not take place under physiological conditions,** even though it is still referred to in the literature.

6.3 H_2O_2 and O_2^- Facts and Singlet Oxygen

Superoxide in the neutrophil can also serve as a source of **singlet oxygen** as follows:

$$H^+ + HO_2 + O_2^- \rightarrow H_2O_2 + {}^1O_2$$

This example of spontaneous dismutation to produce $^1O_2$ has been proven by Khan (Khan, A.U. J Am Chem Soc 1981; 103, 6516-6517). In biological tissues, **superoxide can be nonenzymatically converted into H_2O_2 and $^1O_2$** (Steinbeck, M.J., Khan, A.U. and

Karnovsky, M.J. Extracellular production of singlet oxygen by stimulated macrophages quantified using 9, 10-diphenylanthracene and perylene in a polystyrene film. J Biol Chem 268: 15649-15654). **70-90% of O_2 uptake during the respiratory burst goes to O_2^{-} formation but this goes to produce singlet oxygen.** Shift of oxygen to this system reduces electron transport and lactic acid accumulates and is transported to the lysosome. **Acid pH aids in the production of singlet oxygen.**

O_2 itself does not absorb UV light. Skin photosensitizers absorb UV and pass the energy to O_2 to form $^1O_2$.

Sunlight (UV light) is absorbed by surface waters and transient oxidants are formed such as $\cdot OH$, O_2^{-} and $^1O_2$. These species can degrade (oxidize) organic substances, i.e., phenols, polyaromatic hydrocarbons (PAHs) and pesticides.

The primary photosensitizers in cells are:

> Flavines
> Porphyrins
> Chlorophylls
> Quinones
> Bilirubin
> Retinal
> Furocoumarins

I feel that it needs to be pointed out that ultrasonic waves has been shown to generate EMODs, such as O_2^{-} and $^1O_2$, upon ultrasonic irradiation of sensitizers (e.g., porphyrins, chlorins, methylene-blue, fluorescein, acridine derivatives, rhodamines and tetracyclines).

All organic material is photodegradable at certain UV wavelengths and UV 100-280 nm destroys nearly all organics with ROS and $^1O_2$ and yields volatized CO_2 and H_2O.

    1) Dismutation of $O_2^{\cdot-}$

$$HO_2^{\cdot} + O_2^{\cdot-} + H^+ \rightarrow {}^1O_2 + H_2O_2$$

The generation of H_2O_2 and O_2 ($^1\Delta_g$) by the direct interaction of two molecules of $O_2^{\cdot-}$ is summarized:

$$O_2^{\cdot-} + O_2^{\cdot-} + 2H^+ \text{ à } H_2O_2 + O_2(^1\Delta_g)$$

7.0 PEROXIDE AND CANCER

Neoplasia is the ultimate, grandiose opportunist.
Like its chemical viral kin, it feeds off of its host,
till its parasitic extremes
silence the obliging hand that had fed it.
It lies in prolonged waiting, hidden in the deep,
shadowy recesses
of the cell's complex biochemical engine room.
Then, in a moment of prooxidant weakness,
it lethally crawls forth from its hiding place
to selfishly do its dirty work.
Spider venom-like, it gradually digests
its host-victim,
whilst deliriously cloning itself.
Its job is now done.
Its destiny is now realized.
R. M. Howes, M.D., Ph.D.
6/12/05

Our best understanding of the proneoplastic activity of **reactive oxygen and nitrogen** intermediates comes from their ability to **induce damage to DNA** (Aust, A.E., Eveleigh, J.F.: Mechanisms of DNA oxidation. Proc Soc Exp Biol Med 222:246-252, 1999) (Marnett, .L.J: Oxyradicals and DNA damage. Carcinogenesis 21:361-370, 2000). **Exposure of cells to activated phagocytes leads to oxidative and nitrosative modification of bases, and single-strand breaks** (Frenkel, K., Chrzan, K., Troll, W., et al: Radiation-like modification of bases in DNA exposed to tumor promoter-activated polymorphonuclear leukocytes. Cancer Res 46:5533-5540, 1986) (Schraufstätter, I., Hyslop, P.A., Jackson, J.H., et al: Oxidant-induced DNA damage of target cells. J Clin Invest 82:1040-1050, 1988) (Szabo, C., Ohshima, H.: DNA damage induced by peroxynitrite: Subsequent biological effects. Nitric Oxide 1:373-385, 1997). Despite the presence of a wide array of mechanisms to **repair oxidatively damaged DNA, the repair process is slow and not always complete** (Shacter, E., Beecham, E.J., Covey, J.M., et al: Activated neutrophils induce prolonged DNA damage in neighboring cells. Carcinogenesis 9:2297-2304, 1988). Further processing of **damaged DNA leads to proneoplastic mutations, including point mutations, deletions, sister chromatid exchanges, and chromosomal translocations** (Weitberg, A.B., Corvese, D.: Translocation of chromosomes 16 and 18 in oxygen radical-transformed human lung fibroblasts. Biochem Biophys Res Commun 169:70-74, 1990). **Other authors point out that neither superoxide anion nor hydrogen peroxide will produce DNA oxidative changes but singlet oxygen is capable of producing the 8-OH guanosine derivative.**

Reactive oxygen and nitrogen intermediates have varying degrees of reactivity and diffusability that influence their mutagenic potential (Aust, A.E., Eveleigh, J.F.: Mechanisms of DNA oxidation. Proc Soc Exp Biol Med 222:246-252, 1999). Superoxide is the primary product of the phagocytic oxidative burst and is generated by a membrane-associated nicotinamide adenine dinucleotide phosphate (NADPH) oxidase. **Superoxide is not particularly reactive with biomolecules and cannot diffuse across cell membranes.** It rapidly dismutates—either spontaneously or catalytically through the action of superoxide dismutase—to **hydrogen peroxide, which also is not particularly reactive on its own.** However, **hydrogen peroxide can diffuse significant distances** and cross cell membranes like water.

It is important to point out that antioxidants have failed to prevent, control or reverse cancer. Thus, the theory is wrong and it is time that researchers stop incriminating

EMODs as a mutagenic agent merely because artifactual in vitro data suggests that oxidative attacks on DNA may increase the risk of mutagenesis. We must never forget that in vitro studies may have little resemblance to the events occurring in the living/breathing cell.

I fact, I believe that it is possible that the current US epidemics of cancer, diabetes, obesity and fatigue may be related to increased ingestion of vitamins and dietary supplements. These agents are now commonly found as supplements or fortifiers of many foods and are aggressively marketed to an ever-growing segment of the population. These agents could be interfering with our prooxidant protective system.

Apoptosis, sometimes called "a guardian angel" or "cell policeman," is a cell suicidal altruistic mechanism targeted to **selectively eliminate cancerous and other cells that threaten our health and life.** It appears to be the sacrifice of the "bad" cells to save the integrity and life of the whole organism. Apoptosis is carried out by a multistage chain of reactions in which **EMODs act as triggers and essential mediators** (Kerr, J.F.R., Winterfold, C.M. and Harmon, B.V. Apoptosis, its significance in cancer and cancer therapy. Cancer 1994; 73: 2013-2026), (Blackstone, N.W. and Green, D.R. The evolution of a mechanism of cell suicide. Bio Essays 1999; 21: 84-88). Recently, it became evident that **mitochondria play a crucial role in apoptosis** (Kroemer, G., Zamzami, N. and Susin, S.A. Mitochondrial control of apoptosis. Immunol Today 1997; 18: 44-51). Schematically, apoptosis signals, which arise in cancer cells, promote accumulation of the p53 protein that triggers the release of ROS, cytochrome C and a few other regulators from mitochondria. The latter activate a cascade of proteolytic enzymes, called caspases, that digest a number of pivotal cell proteins and promote a caspase-activated deoxyribonuclease. Cleavage of the critical proteins and DNA results in apoptotic cell death. Importantly, **most anticancer drugs and radiation kill cancer**

cells by inducing apoptosis (Hickman, J.A. Apoptosis induced by anticancer drugs. Cancer Metast Rev 1992; 11: 121-139). Mutations in the p53 gene make cancer cells resistant to apoptosis and, accordingly, to anticancer drugs.

7.1   Hydrogen Peroxide and Hydroxyl Radical Antineoplastic Cytotoxicity

The **cytotoxicity** of the clinically important antineoplastic quinones doxorubicin, mitomycin C, and diaziridinylbenzoquinone for the Ehrlich ascites carcinoma was **significantly reduced or abolished by the antioxidant enzymes catalase and superoxide dismutase, the hydroxyl radical scavengers dimethyl sulfoxide, diethylurea, and thiourea, and the iron chelators deferoxamine, 2,2-bipyridine, and diethylenetriaminepentaacetic acid.** However, tumor cell killing by 5-iminodaunorubicin, a doxorubicin analog with a modified quinone function that prohibits oxidation-reduction cycling, was not ameliorated by any of the free radical scavengers tested. Furthermore, treatment of intact tumor cells with doxorubicin, mitomycin C, and diaziridinylbenzoquinone but not 5-iminodaunorubicin generated the hydroxyl radical, or a related chemical oxidant, in vitro in a process that required hydrogen peroxide, iron, and intact tumor cells. These results **suggest that drug-induced hydrogen peroxide and hydroxyl radical production may play a role in the antineoplastic action of redox active anticancer quinones** (J H. Doroshow. Role of Hydrogen Peroxide and Hydroxyl Radical Formation in the Killing of Ehrlich Tumor Cells by Anticancer Quinones. PNAS June 15, 1986, vol. 83, no. 12, 4514-4518).

The metabolism of quinone-containing antitumor agents involves enzymatic reduction of the quinone by one or two electrons. This reduction results in the formation of the semiquinone or the hydroquinone of the anticancer drug. The consequence of these enzymatic reductions is that **the semiquinone yields its extra**

electron to oxygen with the formation of superoxide radical anion and the original quinone. This reduction by a reductase followed by oxidation by molecular oxygen (dioxygen) is known as **redox-cycling and continues until the system becomes anaerobic.**

Quinone anticancer agents upon reduction can also set up an equilibrium between the hydroquinone, the parental quinone and the semiquinone which **results in a long-lived semiquinone.** Depending on the compound, aziridine quinones, for example, this equilibrium is long lasting thus allowing for the detection of the semiquinone under aerobic conditions. **This phenomenon is known as comproportionation-disporportionation equilibrium.** (Gutierrez PL. The metabolism of quinone-containing alkylating agents: free radical production and measurement. Front Biosci. 2000 Jul 1;5:D629-38).

The International Agency for Research on Cancer (IARC) has determined that hydrogen **peroxide is not classifiable as to its carcinogencity to humans. Even though accusations against H_2O_2 have been wide spread, there is no verified data, in man, that H_2O_2 in any way causes or promotes cancer in vivo. The WHO-IARC said, "There is inadequate evidence in humans for the carcinogenicity of hydrogen peroxide."**

Overall, although there is some disagreement as to whether phagocyte-derived oxidants contribute to tumorigenesis (Collins AR: Oxidative DNA damage, antioxidants, and cancer. Bioessays 21:238-246, 1999) there is a significant body of experimental data supporting the conclusion that they do. **Although the preponderance of the data supports the theory that reactive oxygen species contributes to mutagenesis, I do not believe that it is so. Presently, there is increasing evidence against the Free Radi-Crap theory of oxidative stress and aging, the most significant of which, is the simple fact that antioxidants do not prevent, control or reverse** cancer and atherosclerotic disease. If these diseases are due to oxidation, then antioxidants should stop them, but they do not. In fact, there is increasing evidence that patients taking various form of β-carotene and α-tocopherol and vitamin C, have had increasing strokes, cancers and fatal cardiovascular events.

Oxidants such as H_2O_2, have been found to mimic the intracellular signals initiated by TCR (T cell receptors) aggregation and have also been used to study this signaling pathway. In short, H_2O_2 can trigger T cell proliferation and activation. (Wange, R. L., and Samelson, L. E. (1996) Immunity 5, 197-205). T cells are one of the most important components of the human immune system, which protects us from pathogens. Patients with T Cell immunodeficiencies are prone to infections and to certain types of cancers, especially leukemias and lymphomas. The immune system is vital to protect us against infectious agents (bacteria, viruses, fungi, protozoa and cancer) and there is strong evidence that our immune system uses H_2O_2 to fight infectious diseases and cancer.

Lactobacilli-mediated control of vaginal cancer through specific reactive oxygen species interaction. Bauer G. Med Hypotheses 2001 Aug;57(2):252-7.

Abteilung Virologie, Institut fur Medizinische Mikrobiologie und Hygiene, Universitat Freiburg, Germany. tgfb@ukl.uni-freiburg.de

Klebanoff et al. proposed that hydrogen peroxide-producing lactobacilli and peroxidase in the vagina of healthy women might be responsible for the prevention of vaginosis and also might exert an antitumor effect (1). Based on recent evidence on superoxide anion generation by transformed cells (2,3) and on the potential of myeloperoxidase for selective apoptosis induction in transformed cells (4), a model for specific reactive oxygen species interaction during lactobacilli-mediated tumor control in the vagina is presented here. We propose that **peroxidase, which converts hydrogen peroxide into hypochlorous acid, is responsible for creating a microbicidal vaginal milieu by maintaining a balanced, non-toxic, steady state level of the microbicides H$_2$O$_2$ and HOCl.** In case individual superoxide anion-producing transformed cells eventually appear in the mucosa, they will be driven into apoptosis by **interaction of HOCl with superoxide anions which leads to the generation of hydroxyl radicals.** Hence selective apoptosis induction in transformed cells represents the key element of lactobacilli-mediated antitumor defense. Since papilloma virus infected cells are resistant to this pathway of apoptosis induction, they are plausible candidates for circumvention of lactobacilli-mediated control of oncogenesis.

I believe that this is a very important concept for both the control of pathogens and neoplastic cells. It illustrates the importance of adequate EMOD levels to maintain homeostasis.

Oxygen radicals are not only generated in the mitochondria. Neutrophils and macrophages produce EMODs via a plasma membrane bound nicotinamide adenine dinucleotide phosphate, reduced form (NADPH)-oxidase. The radicals are generated for cell killing and bactericidal activities. The NADPH-oxidase is not exclusive to these cells, however. A panel of human tumor cell lines was shown to produce large quantities of hydrogen peroxide *in vitro* (Szatrowski TP, Nathan CF. Production of large amounts of hydrogen peroxide by human tumor cells. Cancer Res 1991;51:794–798). The hydrogen peroxide production was prevented by diphenyleneiodonium, which is an inhibitor of the flavoprotein component of the NADPH-oxidase. **Tumor cells may overproduce EMODs because the NADPH-oxidase is regulated by the GTPase Rac1, which is itself downstream of the proto-oncogene *Ras*.**

I believe that cancer cells may produce such large quantities of H_2O_2 and EMODs to kill normal cells and aid in its invasiveness into the surrounding tissue. This may be analogous to the production of EMODs by hepatitis virus to kill normal cells and the production of EMODs by bacteria or their production of catalase to make them more effective pathogens.

Leukocytes may lyse tumor cells in vitro in at least **five** situations. With phagocytes, cytolysis can be triggered by pharmacologic or particulate agents that elicit the respiratory burst. One, such **cytotoxicity is oxidative** (Clark, R. A., and S. J. Klebanoff. 1975. Neutrophil-mediated tumor cell cytotoxicity: role of the peroxidase system.]. *Exp. Med.* 141:1442) (Nathan, C. F., L. H. Brukner, S. C. Silverstein, and Z. A. Cohn. 1979. Extracellular cytolysis by activated macrophages and granulocytes. I. Pharmacologic triggering of effector cells and the release of hydrogen peroxide. *J. Exp. Med.* 149:.84)

(Nathan, C. F., S. C. Silverstein, L. H. Brukner, and Z. A. Cohn. 1979. Extracellular cytolysis by activated macrophages and granulocytes. II. Hydrogen peroxide as a mediator of cytotoxicity. *J. Exp. Med.* 149. 100) (Weiss, S. J., A. F. LoBuglio, and M. B. Kessler. 1980. Oxidative mechanism of monocyte mediated cytotoxicity. *Proc. Natl. Acad. Sci. U. S. A.* 77:584).

Two, lectins can also initiate cytolysis. With neutrophils as effector cells, the mechanism appears **oxidative** (Clark, R. A., and S. J. Klebanoff. 1979. Role of the myeioperoxidase-H_2O_2-halide system in concanavalin A-induced tumor cell killing by human neutrophils. *J. Immunol.* 122:2605), but the biochemical basis of lectin-dependent cytolysis by lymphocytes is unknown. **Third,** non-immune leukocytes, such as activated macrophages and natural killer cells, may kill or inhibit tumor cells spontaneously. **Fourth,** several substances have been proposed to mediate spontaneous cytotoxicity by activated macrophages in vitro. **Fifth,** leukocytes may lyse tumor cells to which they are specifically immune, and cytotoxicity by non-immune leukocytes may be elicited by specific antibody against the tumor cells.

In earlier investigations into the basis of pharmacologically induced cytolysis by activated macrophages, we took two general approaches. First, we ascertained that target cells were susceptible to lysis by H_2O_2 in the amounts that the effector cells released in response to phorbol myristate acetate (PMA) under the conditions of the assay. Second, we learned that **deprivation of either oxygen or glucose prevented PMA-induced H_2O_2 release from the effector cells and abolished cytolysis** (Nathan, C. F., S. C. Silverstein, L. H. Brukner, and Z. A. Cohn. 1979. Extracellular cytolysis by activated macrophages and granulocytes. II. Hydrogen peroxide as a mediator of cytotoxicity. *J. Exp. Med.* 149. 100). **I believe that this is a most important observation, which illustrates the oxygen-dependent nature of WBC cytolysis.**

7.2   Scavengers of H_2O_2

Scavengers of H_2O_2 prevented cytolysis as well (Nathan, C. F., S. C. Silverstein, L. H. Brukner, and Z. A. Cohn. 1979. Extracellular cytolysis by activated macrophages and granulocytes. II. Hydrogen peroxide as a mediator of cytotoxicity. *J. Exp. Med.* 149. 100).

Previous work by other investigators makes it likely that **activated macrophages produce reactive metabolites of oxygen during interaction with antibody-coated tumor cells** (Hafeman, D. G., and Z.J. Lucas. 1979. Polymorphonuclear leukocyte-mediated, antibody-dependent, cellular cytotoxicity against tumor cells: dependence on oxygen and the respiratory burst. *J. Immunol.* 123:55). Therefore, in the experiments reported here, we used the second approach described above to study alloantiserum-dependent lysis of lymphoma cells by activated macrophages. The results suggest that **this form of cytolysis is predominantly oxidative** (Nathan C, Cohn Z. Role of oxygen-dependent mechanisms in antibody-induced lysis of tumor cells by activated macrophages. J Exp Med. 1980 Jul 1;**152**(1):198–208).

Hydrogen peroxide, a secretory product of mononuclear phagocytes (Nathan, C. F., and R. K. Root. 1977. Hydrogen peroxide release from mouse peritoneal macrophages. Dependence on sequential activation and triggering.]. *Exp. Med.* 146:1648), **accounts for a considerable portion of their nonphagocytic lysis of tumor cells** in at least three circumstances: **when certain secretagogues are added, when antitumor antibody is present, or when the tumor cells are coated with eosinophil peroxidase** (Nathan CF, Cohn ZA. Antitumor effects of hydrogen peroxide in vivo. J Exp Med. 1981 Nov 1;**154**(5):1539–1553).

Granulocytes also secrete H$_2$O$_2$, which may participate in their cytotoxic effects in a variety of situations. Finally, preformed or enzymatically generated H$_2$0$_2$, with or without a peroxidase, lyses tumor cells (Nathan, C. F., L, H. Brukner, S. C. Silverstein, and Z.A. Cohn. 1979. Extracellular cytolysis by activated macrophages and granulocytes. I. Pharmacologic triggering of effector cells and the release of hydrogen peroxide. *J. Exp. Med.* 149:84) (Philpott, G.W.,W. T. Shearer, R. J. Bower, and C.W. Parker. 1973. Selective cytotoxicity of hapten-substituted cells with an antibody-enzyme conjugate. *J. Immunol.* 111:921) (Edelson, P. J., and Z.A. Cohn. 1973. Peroxidase-mediated mammalian cell cytotoxicity. *J. Exp. Med.* 138:318) (Clark, R.A., S. J. Klebanoff,A. B. Einstein, and A. Fefer. 1975. Peroxidase-H20-halide system: cytotoxic effect on mammalian tumor cells. *Blood.* 45:161) (Nathan, C. F. 1979. The role of oxidative metabolism in the cytotoxicity of activated macrophages after pharmacologic triggering. *In* Immunobiology and Immunotherapy of Cancer.W. D. Terry and Y. Yamamura, editors. Elsevier North-Holland, Inc., New York. 59) (Philpott, G.W.,A. Kulczycki, Jr., E. H. Grass, and C.W. Parker. 1980. Selective binding and cytotoxicity of rat basophilic leukemia cells (RBL-1) with immunoglobulin E-biotin and avidin-glucose oxidase conjugates. *J. Immunol.* 125:1201) (Nathan, C. F., B. A. Arrick, H.W. Murray, N. M. DeSantis, and Z.A. Cohn. 1981. Tumor cell antioxidant defenses: inhibition of the glutathione redox cycle enhances macrophage mediated cytolysis. J. *Exp. Med.* 153:766) In the present study Nathan sought to devise a nontoxic way to deliver hydrogen peroxide to sites of malignancy in vivo and to test its antitumor efficacy. Glucose oxidase was chosen for this purpose because its substrates, glucose and oxygen, are abundant in the body fluids, because **its sole products are H_2O_2 and gluconic acid** (Keilin, D., and E. F. Hartree. 1948. Properties of glucose oxidase (notatin). *Biochem. J.* 42:221), and because a flux of H~O2 generated enzymatically *in situ* might be less toxic than injection of preformed H_2O_2. To prolong the retention of the H~O2-generating system at the site of administration, glucose oxidase was coupled covalently to polystyrene microspheres.

Glucose oxidase, covalently coupled to polystyrene microspheres (GOL), produced **H_2O_2** at an average rate of 3.6 nmol/min per 109 beads under standard assay conditions. Injection of 1.3 × 101° to 1.1 × 10 ix GOL i.p. prolonged the survival of mice by 27% after injection of 106 P388 lymphoma cells in the same site, consistent with destruction of 97.6% of the tumor cells. Placing mice for several hours in 100% O~, the probable rate-limiting substrate for GOL, afforded a 42% prolongation of survival from P388 lymphoma, consistent with destruction of 99.6% of the tumor cells. **A single injection of preformed H_2O_2 readily killed P388 cells in the peritoneal cavity**, but only at doses nearly lethal to the mice. In contrast, GOL had very little toxicity, as judged by the normal appearance of the mice for over 400 d, gross and microscopic findings at autopsy, and various blood tests. GOL injected i.p. remained in the peritoneal cavity, where it was gradually organized into granulomata by macrophages, without generalized inflammation. Thus, **an H_2O_2-generating system confined to the tumor bed exerted clear-cut antitumor effects with little toxicity to the host**.

However, the real question is, **"Is there a most basic, singular and essential biochemical step, reaction or mechanism**

that is the product of this immune response, and which can explain other forms of cancer cell kill, such as photodynamic therapy, radiation and chemotherapy?" I firmly believe that there is such a biochemical explanation that will unify the vast array of data relating to cancer causation and tumoricidal activity. Furthermore, I believe that I have found the specific agent responsible for both photodynamic therapy and spontaneous regression of cancer. **I believe that the Howes Singlet Oxygen Delivery System produces and delivers that agent to cancer cells. That agent and that step concerns the transformation of ground state triplet oxygen to its more reactive counterparts, such as singlet metastable delta oxygen, hydrogen peroxide, hypochlorous and hypobromous acid, superoxide, nitric oxide, peroxynitrite and the hydroxyl radical.**

There are a number of properties shared by cancer cells, which favor the selective toxicity of Artemisinin against cancer cell lines, and against cancer in vivo. In addition to higher rates of iron flux via transferrin receptors than normal cells, **cancers are particularly sensitive to oxygen radicals** (May, W.S. J Membr Biol 1985; 88: 205-215).

7.3   Hyperoxia

Under hyperoxia conditions, mitochondrial EMODs generation increases as a linear function of the oxygen tension (Turrens, J.F. (2003) J. Physiol. 552, 335-344) and this has been implicated in cell dysfunction and death associated with hyperoxia (Guidot, D.M., McCord, J.M., Wright, R.M., and Repine, J.E. (1993) J. bio. Chem. 268, 26699-26703).

Oxygen is critical to aerobic metabolism, but excessive **oxygen** (hyperoxia) can cause cell injury and death. **An oxygen-tolerant strain of HeLa cells, which proliferates even under 80% O_2, termed "HeLa-80,"** was derived from wild-type HeLa cells ("HeLa-20") by selection for resistance to stepwise increases of

oxygen partial pressure. Surprisingly, **antioxidant defenses and susceptibility to oxidant-mediated killing do not differ between these two strains of HeLa cells.** However, under both 20 and 80% O$_2$, intracellular reactive **oxygen** species (**EMODs**) production is significantly (~2-fold) less in HeLa-80 cells. In both cell lines the source of **EMODs** is evidently mitochondrial. Although HeLa-80 cells consume **oxygen** at the same rate as HeLa-20 cells, they consume less glucose and produce less lactic acid. Most importantly, the **oxygen**-tolerant HeLa-80 cells have significantly higher cytochrome c oxidase activity (~2-fold), which may act to deplete upstream electron-rich intermediates responsible for **EMODs** generation. Indeed, preferential inhibition of cytochrome c oxidase by treatment with n-methyl protoporphyrin (which selectively diminishes synthesis of heme a in cytochrome c oxidase) enhances **EMODs** production and abrogates the **oxygen tolerance** of the HeLa-80 cells. Thus, it appears that the remarkable **oxygen tolerance of these cells derives from tighter coupling of the electron transport chain** (Campian, J.L., Qian, M., Gao, X., and Eaton, J.W. Oxygen tolerance and coupling of mitochondrial electron transport. 279(45): 46580-46587, 2004).

This implies that this cell's tolerance to hyperoxia is not due to enhanced antioxidant defenses and many **of these antioxidant enzymes are induced by EMODs.**

7.4 Vitamin C

Dr. Hugh Riordan has suggested that very high doses of intravenous (IV) vitamin C can kill cancer cells via conversion of vitamin C to hydrogen peroxide and due to deficiency of catalase. For this procedure to work, very high levels of IV vitamin C are required to reach "kill concentrations." Intravenous (IV) vitamin C may be one of the best documented alternative cancer treatments (Journal of Orthomolecular Medicine, Special Edition, 1999).

The chemical behavior of O_2^- differs greatly depending on what it is dissolved in. **In water, O_2^- is not very reactive. It can sometimes act as a weak oxidizing agent, by accepting one more electron.** For example, it can oxidize **ascorbic acid (vitamin C).**

Ascorbic acid + O_2^- + H+$\rightarrow$ ascorbic acid radical + H_2O_2

hydrogen peroxide

Clearly, there are appropriate conventional treatments that seem able to remove the immediate threat to life. Surgery, chemotherapy and radiation can be used with some degree of success in killing cancerous tissue. However, that degree of success must be viewed in the context of and weighed against the possible side effects and after effects that are to be expected. **The ideal agent to treat cancer would be cytotoxic to tumour cells, but non-toxic to normal cells.** Vitamin C has long been known to fulfill these requirements but is obscured, ridiculed and criticized by conventional medicine in favor of more powerful and toxic chemotherapeutic agents (Riordan N, Riordan H and Casiari J. Clinical and experimental experiences with intravenous vitamin C. Journal of Orthomolecular Medicine, Special Issue: Proceedings from Vitamin C as Cancer Therapy Workshop, Montreal. 15(4): 201-13. 1999).

Riordan has done work showing that vitamin C is toxic to several cancer lines at doses that are non-toxic to normal cells. **He found that at a dose of 7.04mg/dl, vitamin C is completely toxic to cancer cells while being completely non-toxic to normal cells.** Only at eight times the dose needed to kill cancer cells does vitamin C become toxic to normal cells. Thus vitamin C has a very wide therapeutic window (Riordan N et al. Intravenous ascorbate as a tumour cytotoxic chemotherapeutic agent. Medical Hypothesis. 9(2): 207-13. 1994).

When vitamin C of any type acts as an antioxidant and neutralizes free radicals, it produces dehydroascorbate, DHA, an oxidant.

Normal cells need and take in DHA. The **DHA is then converted to ascorbate and hydrogen peroxide, H_2O_2,** by an oxidation/reduction process. Normal cells safely neutralize excess dehydroascorbate by a reaction with catalase.

DHA may be the key to vitamin therapy. Dr. Benade et al at the National Cancer Institute found that in cultures **vitamin C selectively destroyed cancer cells by generating excess intracellular H_2O_2** (Benade L, Howard T and Burke D. Synergistic killings of Ehrlich ascites carcinoma cells by ascorbate and 3 amino-1, 2, 4-triazole. *Oncology.* 1969;23:33-43).

Cancer cells are less able than normal cells to neutralize H_2O_2 because they are deficient in catalase. Dr. Agus et al reported that cancer cells have extra glucose channels that rapidly bring in glucose and excess DHA (Agus DB, Vera JC and Golde DW. Stromal cell oxidation: a mechanism by which tumors obtain vitamin C. *Cancer Research.* 1999;59:4555-4558). Cancer cells are defective in that they cannot fully distinguish between glucose and DHA. This may explain why vitamin C is safe in large doses for normal cells but toxic to cancer cells. The good results of Cameron and Hoffer with humans confirm the National Cancer Institute lab tests.

Mark Levine's group published on line for PNAS on September 12, 2005 results showing that, "**Pharmacologic ascorbic acid concentrations selectively kill cancer cells: Action as a pro-drug to deliver hydrogen peroxide to tissues.**"

Our goals here were to test whether ascorbate killed cancer cells selectively, and if so, to determine mechanisms, using clinically relevant conditions. Cell death in 10 cancer and 4 normal cell types was measured by using 1-h exposures. Normal cells were unaffected by 20 mM ascorbate, whereas 5 cancer lines had EC50 values of <4 mM, a concentration easily achievable i.v. Human lymphoma cells were studied in detail because of their sensitivity to ascorbate

(EC50 of 0.5 mM) and suitability for addressing mechanisms. **Extracellular but not intracellular ascorbate mediated cell death, which occurred by apoptosis and pyknosis/necrosis.**

Cell death was independent of metal chelators and absolutely dependent on H_2O_2 formation. Cell death from H_2O_2 added to cells was identical to that found when H_2O_2 was generated by ascorbate treatment. H_2O_2 generation was dependent on ascorbate concentration, incubation time, and the presence of 0.5-10% serum, and displayed a linear relationship with ascorbate radical formation.

Taken together, these data indicate that **ascorbate at concentrations achieved only by i.v. administration may be a pro-drug for formation of H_2O_2,** and that blood can be a delivery system of the pro-drug to tissues. These findings give plausibility to i.v. ascorbic acid in cancer treatment, and have unexpected implications for treatment of infections where H_2O_2 may be beneficial. **I believe that this again supports my EMOD theories regarding tumoricidal activity of EMODs, especially H_2O_2.**

Ascorbate treatment led to the formation of hydrogen peroxide (H_2O_2), a chemical known to be toxic to cells. Why it killed cancer cells but not normal cells was unknown, said the researchers. It was possible the hydrogen peroxide caused damage that was repaired in normal cells but not in sensitive cancer cells. **I believe that the cancer cells have higher levels of EMODs, due to low levels of antioxidants and antioxidant enzymes, and it therefore takes a smaller amount for it to reach apoptotic levels induced by EMODs than for normal cells. This is the point of selectivity for toxicity to cancer cells but no harm to normal cells.**

Ascorbic acid and ascorbic acid salts are preferentially toxic to tumour cells, which is thought to be related to intracellular generation of hydrogen peroxide (Tsao C, Dungham B and Ping

Y. In vivo antineoplastic activity of ascorbic acid for human mammary tumour. In vivo. 2: 147-50. 1988; Bram S et al. Vitamin C preferential toxicity for malignant melanoma cells. Nature. 284: 629-31. 1980).

The main mechanism thought to be responsible for this is the lack or relative deficiency of catalase in tumour cells (Maramag C et al. Effect of vitamin C on prostate cancer cells in vitro: effect on cell number, viability, and DNA synthesis. Prostate. 32: 188-95. 1997). **There is a reported 10- to 100-fold greater content of catalase in normal cells than in tumour cells** (Benade L, Howard T and Burk D. Synergistic killing of Ehrlich ascites carcinoma cells by ascorbate and 3-amino-1,2,4-triazole. Oncology. 23: 33-43. 1969).

The claim that vitamin C is useful in the treatment of cancer is largely attributable to Linus Pauling, PhD. In 1976 and 1978, he and a Scottish surgeon, Ewan Cameron, MB, ChB, **reported that patients treated with high doses of vitamin C had survived three to four times longer than similar patients who did not receive vitamin C supplements. However, since this has been an area of heated contention, I will avoid its discussion.**

Humans lack gulonolactone oxidase, which is necessary to synthesize vitamin C and H_2O_2 **is produced as a by-product in the process. I find it incredibly ironic that in the synthesis of one of the most touted of all of the antioxidants, ascorbate, that the dreaded H_2O_2 is generated. Again, I ask, "How could nature be so dumb?" Obviously, nature is not dumb and H_2O_2 is very important in maintaining homeostasis within the cell and as a secondary messenger.**

7.5   Increased CAT and GSH-Px Increase Cancer Rate

Investigators determined whether age- and gender-related changes in lipid peroxidation (LPO) were attributable to differences in hepatic antioxidant defense mechanisms of aging 1-, 4-, 10-or 18-month-old

male and female CBA mice. Specifically, total superoxide dismutase
(tSOD), glutathione peroxidase (GSH-Px) and catalase (CAT)
activities were examined. As an indicator of liver oxidative damage, we
determined LPO, expressed in terms of thiobarbituric acid reactive
substances (TBARS). **LPO increased in both sexes with age.**
tSOD seems to be a relatively inert antioxidative enzyme in both
sexes of mice. The main changes in antioxidant capacity of mice liver
during aging were associated with sex-related **CAT and GSH-Px
increments observed in males** but not in females. Surprisingly,
more than 60% of 18-month-old males (but none of females)
which started to appear at 10-months developed hepatic tumors.
The **results show that (1) the increased liver antioxidant
capacity of CAT and Gpx in male mice might be a sign of
oxidative stress; (2) the increase in CAT and Gpx activities
in male mice is strongly correlated with incidence of
hepatic tumors; (3) the significantly increased SOD activity
in tumor-bearing mice might have induced damage with
accumulated hydrogen peroxide.** (Sverko V, Sobocanec S, Balog
T, Marotti T. Age and gender differences in antioxidant enzyme
activity: potential relationship to liver carcinogenesis in male mice.
Biogerontology. 2004;5(4):235-42). **This important study shows
that increased cancer is "strongly" associated with increased
antioxidant enzymes (CAT and GSH-Px) and since both of
these breakdown H_2O_2, I interpret this to mean that this
caused a decreased level of EMODs and thus, "allowed" the
manifestation of cancer. The presence of the antioxidant
enzymes wiped out the body's prooxidant protection and
created a deficiency state of EMODs.**

7.6   MnSOD Increased in a Direct Relationship with Tumor Grade

The most important cellular protective mechanisms against
oxidative stress are antioxidant enzymes. Their action is based
on decomposal of reactive oxygen species (EMODs) and their
transformation to H_2O_2. Within the mitochondria manganese

superoxide dismutase (MnSOD) affords the major defense against EMODs. **Researchers investigated tissue sections from 101 breast carcinomas for the immunohistochemical expression of MnSOD protein and these results were assessed in relation to various clinicopathological parameters, in order to clarify the prognostic value of this enzyme.** The possible relationship to hormone receptor content, anti-apoptotic protein bcl-2, p53 and cell proliferation was also estimated. In this study **MnSOD increased in a direct relationship with tumor grade** and is therefore **inversely correlated with differentiation** (p=0.0004). Furthermore, there was a strong positive correlation between MnSOD expression and p53 protein immunoreactivity (p=0.0029). These results indicate that **neoplastic cells in breast carcinomas retain their capability to produce MnSOD** and thus protected from the possible cellular damage provoked by reactive oxygen species. **MnSOD content varies according to the degree of differentiation of breast carcinoma** (Tsanou E, Ioachim E, Briasoulis E, Damala K, Charchanti A, Karavasilis V, Pavlidis N, Agnantis NJ. Immunohistochemical expression of superoxide dismutase (MnSOD) anti-oxidant enzyme in invasive breast carcinoma. Histol Histopathol. 2004 Jul;19(3):807-13). **Again, I disagree with the conclusions of the authors. I believe that the increase in MnSOD means that EMODs (H$_2$O$_2$) has been increased and this creates a hostile environment for tumor cells and leads to less differentiated (less cancerous) tumors.**

7.7   Antioxidant Enzymes and Thyroid Cancer

To the contrary, researchers have reported a **decreased expression of glutathione peroxidase (GPx)** mRNA, an antioxidant enzyme, **in thyroid anaplastic carcinomas** (Hasegawa Y, Takano T, Miyauchi A, Matsuzuka F, Yoshida H, Kuma K, et al. Decreased expression of glutathione peroxidase mRNA in thyroid anaplastic carcinoma. Cancer Lett 2002;182:69–741). Other than GPx, **many enzymes, e.g., catalase (CAT), thyroid peroxidase**

(TPO) and superoxide dismutase (SOD), take part in the catalysis of EMODs. These antioxidant enzymes protect cell constituents from damage by oxygen free radicals and play crucial roles in neoplastic disease (Durak I, Bayram F, Kavutcu M, Canbolat O, Ozturk HS. Impaired enzymatic antioxidant defense mechanism in cancerous human thyroid tissues. J Endocrinol Invest 1996;19:312–5). This adds to the confusion but I believe that it is clear that enzymes which increase H_2O_2 production result in decreased mutagenicity.

7.8 Chronic Inflammation and Cancer

Some of the following materials were excerpted or modified from the following article:

Emily Shacter, PhD & Sigmund A. Weitzman, MD ONCOLOGY 16:217-232, 2002.

The various factors known to cause cancer also induce chronic inflammatory responses. These include bacterial, viral, and parasitic infections (e.g., H pylori, Epstein-Barr virus, human immunodeficiency virus, flukes, schistosomes), chemical irritants (i.e., tumor promoters, such as phorbol ester 12-O-tetradecanoyl-13-phorbol acetate, also known as phorbol myristate acetate), non-digestible particles (e.g., asbestos, silica), and other factors yet to be discovered. Also one could have added that chemical carcinogens, such as polycyclic aromatic hydrocarbons, which require oxidative metabolism for their activities, induce chronic inflammation with the attendant oxidative stress, macromolecular damage, and cytokine formation.

A substantial body of evidence **erroneously** supports the conclusion that chronic inflammation can predispose an individual to cancer, as demonstrated by the association between chronic inflammatory bowel diseases and the increased risk of colon carcinoma. **However, I believe that this assertion is wrong**

and that the inflammatory response is an unsuccessful attempt by the body to rid itself of the foreign invader or irritant. Chronic inflammation is caused by a variety of factors, including bacterial, viral, and parasitic infections, chemical irritants, and non-digestible particles. **The presence and the triggering of an inflammatory response is the body's natural way to deal with pathogens or pollutants. In fact, it is the only way in which the body can respond.** The longer the inflammation persists, the higher the risk of associated carcinogenesis. **I believe that this is due to the fact that the body can not generate sufficient EMODs to kill the invading pathogens and these deficient EMODs levels (which can not even kill invading bacteria could neither kill cancer) would most certainly be conducive to "allowing" the manifestation of cancer. If Ames is right, proneoplasia is always present due to oxidative genotoxic events.** The following section describes some of the underlying causes of the association between chronic inflammation and cancer. Inflammatory mediators contribute to neoplasia by inducing "proneoplastic" mutations, adaptive responses, resistance to apoptosis, and environmental changes such as stimulation of angiogenesis. **I believe that inflammatory cells migrate to the infected site to kill the pathogens and that they are not causative of neoplasia. In fact, they are there to kill neoplastic cells.** All these changes confer a survival advantage to a susceptible cell. This article, discusses the contribution of reactive oxygen and nitrogen intermediates, prostaglandins, and inflammatory cytokines to carcinogenesis. **A thorough understanding of the molecular basis of inflammation-associated neoplasia and progression, as I interpret it, may lead to novel approaches to the prevention and treatment of cancer.**

Allegedly, chronic inflammation may be a causative factor in a variety of cancers. In general, the longer the inflammation persists, the higher the risk of cancer. **I believe that this is due to the fact that the longer time period is an additional time of**

"allowance" for the manifestation or development of cancer. Hence, acute inflammation, such as occurs in response to a transient infection, is not regarded as a risk factor for the development of neoplasia, although many of the same molecular mediators are generated in both acute and chronic inflammation. **In the instance of acute inflammation, the body produces adequate EMODs levels to stop the invading pathogens and to keep preneoplasia in abeyance.** In general, inflammatory leukocytes such as neutrophils, monocytes, macrophages, and eosinophils provide the soluble factors that are thought to mediate the development of inflammation-associated cancer, although other cells, including the cancer cells themselves, also participate. However, **as we now know, the seeds for neoplasia are always present in all aerobic cells and I believe that the inflammatory cells are bringing with them, the necessary EMODs levels to kill cancerous cells. The body is responding in the only way that it has available to it.**

Inflammatory mediators include metabolites of arachidonic acid, cytokines, chemokines, and free radicals. Chronic exposure to these mediators **may lead** to increased cell proliferation, mutagenesis, oncogene activation, and angiogenesis. Researchers claim that the ultimate result is the proliferation of cells that have lost normal growth control. Animal models provide experimental evidence that chronic inflammation can promote cancer and further insights into possible mechanisms.

A wide array of chronic inflammatory conditions predisposes susceptible cells to neoplastic transformation. **Most of the resulting tumors are of epithelial cell origin (carcinomas).** The most widely studied and best established of these links are colon carcinoma associated with inflammatory bowel disease (chronic ulcerative colitis and Crohn's disease), esophageal adenocarcinoma associated with reflux esophagitis (Barrett's esophagus), hepatitis predisposing to liver cancer, schistosomiasis causing an increased risk of bladder and colon carcinomas, and chronic *Helicobacter* infection leading to cancer of the stomach. Some increase in the incidence of lymphoma is also seen, particularly **mucosa-associated lymphoid tissue (MALT)** lymphoma.

The types of chronic inflammation that lead to cancer are varied. In some cases, the **"progenitors of the inflammation"** are known. **These include chronic bacterial and parasitic infections, chemical irritants, and non-digestible particles.** In other cases, the underlying cause of the chronic inflammation is **unknown.** This is true for **inflammatory bowel disease, sialadenitis, and lichen sclerosis.** Some of the known chronic inflammatory agents will be described below. Of these, parasitic infections are perhaps the best described. It seems that **any parasitic infection that persists or recurs over many years can predispose to cancer.** Thus, **bacterial, viral, and parasitic infections can all lead to cancer if left unchecked. Of course, the fact that an infection is chronic indicates that the body can not generate adequate EMODs levels to clear it up and thus, there is a relative deficiency level of EMODs at that site. This deficiency level of EMODs is what leads to the "allowance" of cancer manifestation at that site.**

7.9   Helicobacter Pylori

The strongest association between chronic bacterial infection and the development of cancer involves the organism *Helicobacter pylori*, which is associated with at least a **twofold increased risk of adenocarcinoma of the stomach** (Correa, P.: Helicobacter pylori and gastric carcinogenesis. Am J Surg Pathol 19:S37-43, 1995) (Parsonnet, J.: Bacterial infection as a cause of cancer. Environ Health Perspect 103(suppl 8):263-268, 1995). In addition, *H pylori* infection is thought to increase the incidence of MALT lymphoma. Strong experimental evidence that *Helicobacter* infection is carcinogenic comes from studies showing that gerbils infected with *H pylori* develop active chronic gastritis followed by a high incidence of gastric adenocarcinoma. *Helicobacter* infection in humans is always accompanied by mucosal inflammation (gastritis) with an influx of lymphocytes, plasma cells, and neutrophils. The robust immune response to *H pylori* generally fails to clear the infection, thus resulting in a chronic inflammatory response thought to be a key element of the carcinogenic activity of the bacterium. **This is exactly what I have been indicating. The body fails to clear the infection, due to inadequate generation of EMODs and consequently, the conditions are conducive to the "allowance" of cancer formation.**

Unless treated, *H pylori* infection and the associated gastritis persist for decades, **which I interpret to mean that the body has to keep trying to rid itself of the invading pathogen but that it can not quite manage to generate enough EMODs to do so.** Eradication of *H pylori* infection with antibiotics may also eliminate the excess risk for cancer, but this has not yet been established.

7.10 Viral Infections

Many different viruses cause an increased incidence of cancer. Those **most commonly associated with chronic inflammation are the hepatitis B and C viruses, which lead to chronic active hepatitis and hepatocellular carcinoma** (Hayashi, P.H., Zeldis, J.B.: Molecular biology of viral hepatitis and hepatocellular carcinoma. Compr Ther 19:188-196, 1993). **Epstein-Barr virus (EBV) is associated with B-cell non-Hodgkin's lymphoma,** and may contain a chronic inflammatory component (Copie-Bergman, C., Niedobitek, G., Mangham, D.C., et al: Epstein-Barr virus in B-cell lymphomas associated with chronic suppurative inflammation. J Pathol 183:287-292, 1997). Other viral infections can also increase the incidence of cancer, but the role of inflammatory mediators is less clear. **Our prooxidant protective reaction is the same oxidative response to any pathogen or pollutant e.g., bacteria, virus, fungus, parasite or cancer. We generate EMODs to deal with these situations.** For example, the **human papillomavirus, herpes simplex virus**

2, and cytomegalovirus have been implicated in cervical and other carcinomas (Bornstein, J., Rahat, M.A., Abramovici, H.: Etiology of cervical cancer: Current concepts. Obstet Gynecol Surg 50:146-154, 1995). Among RNA retroviruses, the human immunodeficiency virus **(HIV) predisposes to the development of non-Hodgkin's lymphoma, squamous cell carcinomas, and Kaposi's sarcoma** (Goedert, J.J.: The epidemiology of acquired immunodeficiency syndrome malignancies. Semin Oncol 27:390-401, 2000) while the human T-cell lymphoma virus causes adult T-cell leukemia.

Unlike the other parasitic infections described here, **viruses implicated in inducing neoplasia directly infect the cells that ultimately undergo neoplastic transformation.** Hence, it is difficult to determine whether these agents act by causing a chronic inflammatory condition, by directly transforming the cells that they infect, or both. **I believe that this demonstrates that the virus is the causative agent and it has been shown that even the genotype specifically results in specific types of cancer causation. The products of the inflammatory response, as it relates to reactive oxygen species, are the same for responses to various genotypes of viruses or strains of bacteria. The specificity comes from the invading pathogen and not from the oxidative assault upon the invader.** Most of these viruses induce chronic increased proliferation of the infected cells, thus predisposing to neoplastic transformation. For example, EBV causes sustained proliferation of peripheral B lymphocytes, but when coupled with a secondary mutation can result in malignant transformation, such as occurs with the chromosomal translocations that activate the c-myc oncogene in Burkitt's lymphoma. The hepatitis viruses are thought to give rise to hepatocellular carcinoma by causing liver damage and regeneration together with the generation of secondary inflammatory mediators (Hayashi PH, Zeldis JB: Molecular biology of viral hepatitis and hepatocellular carcinoma. Compr Ther 19:188-196, 1993).

7.11 Noninfectious Causes of Chronic Inflammation

Various noninfectious agents also cause chronic inflammation associated with an increased risk of cancer. For example, esophageal reflux causes chronic exposure of the esophageal epidermis to **irritation by gastric acids.** This leads to reflux esophagitis, or Barrett's esophagus, and subsequent development of esophageal carcinoma (Pera, M., Trastek, V.F., Pairolero, P.C., et al: Barrett's disease: Pathophysiology of metaplasia and adenocarcinoma. Ann Thorac Surg 56:1191-1197, 1993). **Please remember that the body is responding to injury in the only way that it can and that is with an attempt at oxidative healing of the injury. This is the same response as the one to vascular injury with stents or angioplasty balloons or whatever because it is the only response available to the body.**

Excess fecal bile acids in patients with primary sclerosing cholangitis and ulcerative colitis are associated with an increased risk of colorectal carcinoma. **Again, the body responds to an injury with an attempt at oxidative healing. The inflammatory response cells which produce EMODs are at the site due to the injury and not as a causative factor in carcinogenesis. I believe that the body may be thinking that it can possibly detoxify the injurious chemicals at the site, with mechanisms such as the cytochrome P450 detoxifying system. I believe that the concentrations of the injurious chemicals and acids are the mutagens and not the EMODs.** A recent publication demonstrated that ursodiol (Actigall), a drug that reduces the colonic levels of deoxycholate and other bile acids (used to treat cholangitis), significantly reduces the incidence of neoplasia (Tung, B.Y., Emond, M.J., Haggitt, R.C., et al: Ursodiol use is associated with lower prevalence of colonic neoplasia in patients with ulcerative colitis and primary sclerosing cholangitis. Ann Intern Med 134:89-95, 2001). **Chronic irritation of the liver by alcohol causes cirrhosis and hepatocellular carcinoma** and again, **I believe that the body is responding to the injury with an inflammatory EMODs response**. (Seitz, H.K., Poschl, G., Simanowski, U.A.: Alcohol and cancer. Recent Dev Alcohol 14:67-95, 1998).

Nondigestible agents such as asbestos, coal, and silica dust lead to chronic inflammation in the lung because of the inability of the immune system to remove the substances. **Again, the body is not quite capable of successfully detoxifying or removing the chemical irritant, mutagen or pollutant and it responds to the presence of this agent with the only mechanism available to it, e.g., the inflammatory response and generation of EMODs.** Such **sterile inflammations** increase the incidence of epithelial cancers including mesothelioma and lung carcinoma (Steenland, K., Stayner, L.: Silica, asbestos, man-made mineral fibers, and cancer. Cancer Causes Control 8:491-503, 1997). Experimental evidence that chronic sterile inflammation can cause cancer comes from studies in BALB/c mice that received intraperitoneal administration of nondigestible, non-genotoxic mineral oils or plastic disks. The mice developed a high incidence of B lymphocytic (plasma cell) tumors but no epithelial cancers.

8.0 ACUTE H₂O₂ TOXICITY

Hydrogen peroxide has proven to be an extremely safe topical, oral or intravenous medicinal.

I have found a total of 13 deaths due to the accidental or intentional use of H₂O₂ in the entire history of recorded medical literature available on the internet. Caveat: Some references do not provide access to the original article or to an abstract. None of the references available to me on the internet go beyond 1979. thus, there may be cases of which I am unaware. Many of the articles concerning ingestion or infusion of peroxide are non-conclusive. Clinical histories are incomplete and documentation is scanty. One thing for certain is that many cases of over-zealous or accidental ingestion of concentrated hydrogen peroxide (20-40%) have had a surprisingly uneventful recovery. Incredibly, as can be seen for the ingestion or infusion of 3% H₂O₂ have produced very few patients with serious complications or severe outcomes.

Isolated case reports have documented that **hydrogen peroxide exposure** can be associated with serious toxicity by various routes of exposure. The purpose of this study was to better delineate the epidemiology, medical outcome, and potential health hazards of hydrogen peroxide exposures to the general public. We performed **a retrospective review of all exposures reported to a regional poison center over a 36 month period and found that of 95,052 exposures reported, 325 (.34%) were due to hydrogen peroxide.** The pediatric population (< 18 years) accounted for 71% of hydrogen peroxide exposures and ingestion was the most common route of exposure (83%). Nausea and vomiting were the most common symptoms secondary to ingestion. **Ocular and dermal exposures to dilute solutions resulted in transient symptoms without permanent sequelae. While most exposures by all routes resulted in a benign outcome (no effect or minor effect), there was a trend toward more severe outcomes in those who ingested a concentration**

Prof Randolph Michael Howes MD,PhD

greater than 10% (p = 0.011). **RMH:** This equals 2,640 exposures/ month or 88/day. (Abstract: Hydrogen peroxide exposure--325 exposures reported to a regional poison control center. Dickson KF, Caravati EM. J Toxicol Clin Toxicol. 1994;32(6):705-14).Division of Emergency Medicine, University of Utah School of Medicine, Utah Poison Control Center, Salt Lake City.

This as a retrospective chart review of exposures to **hydrogen peroxide 3%** reported to the Long Island Regional Poison Control Center from **January 1992 to April 1995 (39 months) was conducted**. Data extracted included age, route of exposure, amount of agent, symptoms, therapy, and medical outcome.

RESULTS: **There were 670 exposures to hydrogen peroxide 3% of 81,126 total exposures reported during the 40 months. Most exposures were by oral route (77%), occurred in children < 17 years old (67%), and were asymptomatic (85.6%). All but one exposure resulted in a benign outcome.** One child, who presented with bloody emesis, developed multiple gastric ulcers and duodenal erosions after ingestion of hydrogen peroxide 2-4 oz. CONCLUSIONS: **Exposure to hydrogen peroxide 3% is usually benign;** however, severe gastric injury may occur following small ingestions in children. Patients who report persistent vomiting or bloody emesis require medical evaluation and consideration of endoscopy to evaluate gastrointestinal injury.
RMH: This equals 2,081 H_2O_2 exposures/month or 69/day. (Abstract: Hydrogen peroxide 3% exposures. Henry MC, Wheeler J, Mofenson HC, Caraccio TR, Marsh M, Comer GM, Singer AJ. J Toxicol Clin Toxicol. 1996;34(3):323-7).

Hydrogen peroxide is a readily available clear, odorless liquid that is commonly used as an irrigant for superficial wounds. It is not widely thought of as a poison; however, **it may rarely be the cause of accidental death.** (Hydrogen peroxide: a source of lethal oxygen embolism. Case report and review of the literature. Cina SJ, Downs JC, Conradi SE. Am J Forensic Med Pathol. 1994 Mar;15(1):44-50).

In 5 persons who accidentally drank 50 mL of a 33% H$_2$O$_2$ solution, symptoms included stomach and chest pain, retention of breath, foaming at the mouth and loss of consciousness. Later, motor and sensory disorders, fever, micro-hemorrhages and moderate leukocytosis were noted. **All recovered completely within 2-3 weeks** (IARC. 1985. International Agency for Research on Cancer. Hydrogen Peroxide. In: IARC Monographs on the Evaluation of Carcinogenic Risk if Chemicals to Humans: Allyl compounds, Aldehydes, Epoxides and Peroxides, Vol. 36. IARC, Lyon, pp. 285-314).

In my opinion, this represents the low toxicity of H$_2$O$_2$ and demonstrates the body's ability to handle excess amounts of H$_2$O$_2$. **Alternative medicine clinics around the world have given thousands upon thousands of I.V. doses of H$_2$O$_2$ without untoward effects.**

Information from the Hazardous Substances Data Bank (HSDB), a database of the National Library of Medicine's TOXNET system (http://toxnet.nlm.nih.gov) **indicates in general, ingestion, ocular or dermal exposure to small amounts of dilute hydrogen peroxide will cause no serious problems.**

However, in treatment of corneal ulcerations, particularly in herpetic dendritic keratitis, 20% solution has been applied, after local anesthetic, every two hours as a localized cautery to the ulcer, and **has been reported to have had good effect in numerous patients**. In one instance a 10% solution was dropped on one eye of a patient after application of cocaine, and **this eye was normal** by the next day. (Grant, W.M. Toxicology of the Eye. 3rd ed. Springfield, IL, Charles C. Thomas Publisher, 1986: 493). Ocular exposure to household strength (3%) solutions usually requires little

Prof Randolph Michael Howes MD,PhD

more than thorough irrigation, **since serious complications are rare.**

Recent reports have suggested that **hydrogen peroxide released by mononuclear phagocytes and neutrophils may extend the antimicrobial, antitumor,** and oxidant-injury activities of these cells to adjacent tissues (Nathan CF, Brukner LH, Silverstein SC, Cohn ZA. Extracellular cytolysis by activated macrophages and granulocytes. I. Pharmacologic triggering of effector cells and the release of hydrogen peroxide. J Exp Med. 1979 Jan 1;**149**(1):84–99) (Nathan CF, Silverstein SC, Brukner LH, Cohn ZA. Extracellular cytolysis by activated macrophages and granulocytes. II. Hydrogen peroxide as a mediator of cytotoxicity. J Exp Med. 1979 Jan 1;**149**(1):100–113).

Providing additional support for a potential therapeutic role for parenterally administered hydrogen peroxide, (Dockrell, HJ. M., and J. H. L. Playfair. 1983. Killing of blood-stage murine malaria parasites by hydrogen peroxide. Infect. Immun. 16:75-80) reported that **murine Plasmodium yoelii parasitemia was reduced after the intravenous administration of hydrogen peroxide.**

However, the fivefold lower level of catalase activity present in hemolysate prepared from mice compared with hemolysate from humans (Lorinez, A.I., J.J. Jacoby and H. M. Livingstone, 1948. Studies on the parenteral administration of hydrogen peroxide. Anesthesiology 9:162-174) and the use of intracellular parasites as markers of hydrogen peroxide activity limit the implications of this study. We therefore employed circulating hydrogen peroxide-susceptible Escherichia coli to assess the therapeutic potential of intravenously administered hydrogen peroxide in **the rabbit, an animal whose levels of catalase activity in blood closely parallel those of humans.**

Physiological tolerance of rabbits for intravenous hydrogen peroxide infusion. Rabbits tolerated the intravenous infusion

150

of 0.225% saline with 5% glucose containing 0.0125, 0.025, and 0.05 M hydrogen-peroxide at 20 ml/h (0.25, 0.50, and 1.0, umol/h, respectively) for 30 min with no significant change in arterial blood gases, heart rate, or mean arterial blood pressure (Fig. 1). Increasing the concentration of hydrogen peroxide in the infusion to 0.10 M (2.0, umol/h) for 30 min significantly decreased the heart rate ($P < 0.05$) without significantly affecting the other monitored parameters (Fig. 1). After a 0.5-h infusion of 0.20 M hydrogen peroxide at 20 ml/h (4.0, umol/h), the mean PO_2 decreased sharply ($P < 0.05$), the mean arterial blood pressure decreased ($P < 0.05$), and the heart rate increased toward the baseline rate. However, 0.5 h after discontinuing the 4.0 p.mol/h hydrogen peroxide infusion, the PO_2 and mean arterial blood pressure returned to baseline levels, indicating that the observed effects of hydrogen peroxide infusion were rapidly reversible.

Some of the following materials were taken from: Howes, R. M. 2004. U.T.O.P.I.A. - Unified Theory of Oxygen Participation in Aerobiosis. (767 page text) Free Radical Publishing Co. Kentwood, LA.

9.0 GENERAL INFORMATION ON HYDROGEN PEROXIDE

Hydrogen peroxide is only one of the many components that help regulate the amount of oxygen getting to your cells. Its presence is vital for many other functions as well. **It is required for the production of thyroid hormone and sexual hormones** (Mol Cell Endocrinol 86;46(2): 149-154) (Steroids 82;40(5):5690579). **It stimulates the production of interferon** (J Immunol 85;134(4):24492455). **It dilates blood vessels in the heart and brain** (Am J Physiol 86;250 (5 pt 2): H815-821 and (2 pt 2):H157-162). **It improves glucose utilization in diabetics** (Proceedings of the IBOM Conference 1989, 1990, 1991).

Superoxide (O_2^-) can undergo monovalent reduction to produce peroxide (O_2^{-2}), an activated form of oxygen that carries a negative charge of -2. Usually peroxide is termed "hydrogen peroxide" (H_2O_2) since in biological systems the negative charge of -2 is neutralized by two protons (two hydrogen atoms, each with a positive charge).

superoxide + monovalent reduction = hydrogen peroxide

Hydrogen peroxide is important in biological systems because it **can pass readily through cell membranes and cannot be excluded from cells**. Hydrogen peroxide is actually necessary for the function of many enzymes, and thus **is required (like oxygen itself) for health**. Hydrogen peroxide is not as reactive as a product it can form, the hydroxyl radical.

Endogenous hydrogen peroxide has been found in plant tissues at the following levels (mg/kg frozen weight):

potato tubers, 7.6
Green tomatoes, 3.5
Red tomatoes, 3.5
Castor beans in water, 4.7 (IARC, 1985)

Reportedly, the best way to get H_2O_2 from your fruits is to use a juicer and drink the juice within 10 minutes before the H_2O_2 auto-oxidizes such as with carrots. Cranberry juice is said to be loaded with H_2O_2 as is the tops of beets and watermelon. Uncooked vegetables and fruits contain natural H_2O_2 and cooking breaks it down. This is likely one of the major factors which responsible for the frequent articles recommending a high intake of fresh fruits and vegetables. **The colostrum of mother's milk is high in H_2O_2, which is thought to activate the newborn's immune system and protect the undeveloped immune protective system of the baby.** Perhaps this is a corollary to the formation of bactericidal amounts of H_2O_2 when glucose is oxidized in the presence of penicillium notatum (General Biochemistry, Fruton & Simmonds 577.1 F944 p. 339).

H_2O_2 as a human food additive is generally regarded as safe and may be used as a component of articles for use in packaging, handling, transporting or holding food in accordance with prescribed conditions [FDA 21 CFR 175.105 (4/1/93)].

H_2O_2 has been used on fresh fruits and vegetables for decades. It has been used in dentistry and oral hygiene for decade upon decade. **All of these umpteen examples of H_2O_2 application and ingestion have been essentially without adverse effects and only a handful of patients have suffered serious or adverse reactions or fatalities from use of hydrogen peroxide.**

The consumption of oxygen during cellular respiration is the fundamental pathway that sustains aerobic life, which always and continually produces electronically modified oxygen derivatives (EMODs), especially superoxide anion and hydrogen peroxide.

Hydrogen peroxide is involved in all of life's vital processes, and is crucial for the immune system to function properly. The cells in the body that fight infection (known as granulocytes, monocytes and leucocytes) produce hydrogen peroxide as a **first line of defense** against invading organisms like parasites, viruses, bacteria, yeast and neoplasia. It is also required for the metabolism of protein, carbohydrates, fats, vitamins and minerals. As a hormonal regulator, **hydrogen peroxide is necessary for the body's production of thyroxine (tetraiodothyronine);** it also helps regulate blood sugar and the production of energy in cells. Hydrogen peroxide has long been used medically as a disinfectant, antiseptic and oxidizer, with a minimum of harmful side effects.

In addition to the multitude of peroxide production documented in other sections of this book, hydrogen peroxide is also produced by:

> Sodium perborate
> Glycerol oxidase
> Lipoxygenase and
> Glucose oxidases

Hydrogen peroxide (H_2O_2) is actually quite abundant in nature. It is formed mainly by the action of sunlight on water and is thus found in traces in rain and snow. Hydrogen peroxide (H_2O_2) is present in the atmosphere. **On a sunny day, there are over 1 billion hydroxyl radicals in a liter of air. Gaseous H_2O_2 is recognized to be a key component and product of the earth's lower atmospheric photochemical reactions**, in both clean and polluted atmospheres. (IARC. 1985. International Agency for Research on Cancer. Hydrogen Peroxide. In: IARC Monographs on the Evaluation of Carcinogenic Risk if Chemicals to Humans: Allyl compounds, Aldehydes, Epoxides and Peroxides, Vol. 36. IARC, Lyon, pp. 285-314). **RMH Note: even with the hydroxyl radials significantly present in the air, the birds are not falling from the sky and people are not keeling over, while breathing the air on a sunny day.**

Today, over a billion pounds of H_2O_2 are produced annually in the United States (US Peroxide Inc.) (US Peroxide Inc. Introduction to hydrogen peroxide, environmental application overview. http://www.H2O2.com/intro/overview.html**).**

H_2O_2 is a ubiquitous, naturally occurring substance. Surface water concentrations of H_2O_2 have been found to vary between 51-231 mg/L, increasing both with exposure to sunlight and the presence of dissolved organic matter (IARC. 1985. International Agency for Research on Cancer. Hydrogen Peroxide. In: IARC Monographs on the Evaluation of Carcinogenic Risk if Chemicals to Humans: Allyl compounds, Aldehydes, Epoxides and Peroxides, Vol. 36. IARC, Lyon, pp. 285-314).

Probably no single substance has been applied to open wounds with greater frequency than H_2O_2. For over a century, wounds have been and continue to be washed, bathed, scrubbed, debrided and cleaned with 3% H_2O_2. In short, wounds have been flooded with peroxide. **H_2O_2 is a pale blue liquid, which mixes readily with water, diffusing easily in the body and crossing membranes.** Since it does not have unpaired electrons, **hydrogen peroxide is not a free radical.** It has been used for many years as a bleach or oxidizing agent to disinfect wounds. **When applied to tissue, solutions of H_2O_2 have poor penetrability** (HSDB. 1995. Hazardous Substances Data Bank. Medlars Online Information Retrieval System, National Library of Medicine).

Oxidizing bleaches kill microbes by reacting with cell membranes and cell proteins. The most widely used are hydrogen peroxide and **sodium hypochlorite for household and hospital uses,** and **calcium hypochlorite for drinking water and swimming pool disinfecting.** H_2O_2 as a topical gel or a liquid is used to cleanse minor wounds or minor gum inflammation (HSDB, 1995).

Ozone, hydrogen peroxide, sodium hypochlorite and UV light kill pathogens on the outside of the body and likewise, they kill them on the inside of the body.

Ergo, we have an excellent clinical study model and, according to the free radical theory, all of these open wounds, with iron containing hemoglobin (blood), dripping from them, should be producing the hydroxyl radical, DNA mutations and cancer, at these wound sites; but that has not happened! **Millions upon millions of wounds have been directly and repeatedly exposed to H_2O_2 and instead of becoming cancerous, the wounds have healed. It is frequently pointed out that H_2O_2 will react with iron to produce the .OH radical but curiously, it does not react with the iron contained in the heme proteins, such as catalase.**

Basically, hydrogen peroxide (peroxide or H_2O_2) is a non-radical of rather low reactivity and has a proven record of safety for over a century, especially when compared to modern pharmaceuticals which are responsible for significant numbers of adverse reactions (reportedly, millions annually) and over 100,000 deaths (Dr. Barbara Starfield). We must keep in mind that **any substance, medicine, substrate, co-factor, nutrient, supplement, mineral chemical or reagent can be harmful**, if administered to a cell, tissue, organ or an organism and if it is in the wrong concentration, location, etc. (too much or too little or in the wrong place at the wrong time).

EMODs are also intentionally produced in the body and used for synthesis and detoxification processes as well as for immune defense. **H_2O_2 is produced** in the **thyroid gland** as a substrate for thyroperoxidase, which catalyzes the attachment of iodine to thryoglobulin, an important protein for the synthesis of thyroid hormone. **H_2O_2 is generated in peroxisomes to aid in the degradation of fatty acids** and other molecules, and **H_2O_2 is used for detoxification reactions involving the liver cytochrome P-450 system.**

Prof Randolph Michael Howes MD, PhD

Some cells, such as phagocytic leukocytes, have evolved the use of **H_2O_2 as a bactericidal defense chemical, a phenomenon known as the oxidative burst, which** are important in protecting us from infection. I refer to the oxidative burst as the "peroxide spike."

The alleged damaging power of peroxide comes from the transition to highly reactive hydroxyl radicals that may indiscriminately react with a wide variety of organic substrates causing peroxidation of lipids, cross-linking and inactivation of proteins, and mutations in DNA (Knievel, 2004) (Knievel DP. Oxidative Stress. In: Response of plants to environmental stress. PennState, AGRO518, http://www.agronomy.psu.edu/courses/AGRO518/Oxygen.html).

The reactions leading to **H_2O_2** are minimized by sequestering the metal ions that would otherwise act as catalysts into proteins. Ferritin, transferrin, hemosiderin and heme are examples of proteins that enclose iron and thus play a role in protecting the cell against oxidative damage (Nappi & Vass, 2000) (Nappi AJ, Vass E. Iron, metalloenzymes and cytotoxic reactions. Cell Mol Biol 46(3):637-647, 2000). **(RMH Note: The iron is also there to form a binding mechanism for oxygen and to carry out the role of the heme proteins.)**

A major problem of antioxidant therapies is the lack of specificity. Extensive radical scavenging, or delivery of oxygen boosts via the blood, perturbs the body's **natural redox balance**, and unwanted, often unpredictable, side effects are common.

Information from the Hazardous Substances Data Bank (HSDB), a database of the National Library of Medicine's TOXNET system (http://toxnet.nlm.nih.gov) **indicates in general, ingestion, ocular or dermal exposure to small amounts of dilute hydrogen peroxide will cause no serious problems.**

A Ca^{2+}-activated NADPH Oxidase in Testis, Spleen, and Lymph Nodes. (Botond Bánfi, Gergely Molnár, Andres Maturana,

Klaus Steger, Balázs Hegedûs, Nicolas Demaurex, and Karl-Heinz Krause. J. Biol. Chem., Vol. 276, Issue 40, 37594-37601, October 5, 2001).

Superoxide and its derivatives are increasingly implicated in the regulation of physiological functions from oxygen sensing and blood pressure regulation to lymphocyte activation and sperm-oocyte fusion. Here we describe a novel superoxide-generating NADPH oxidase referred to as NADPH oxidase 5 (NOX5). NOX5 is distantly related to the gp91^{phox} subunit of the phagocyte NADPH oxidase with conserved regions crucial for the electron transport (NADPH, FAD and heme binding sites). However, NOX5 has a unique N-terminal extension that contains three EF hand motifs. The mRNA of NOX5 is expressed in pachytene spermatocytes of testis and in B- and T-lymphocyte-rich areas of spleen and lymph nodes. When heterologously expressed, NOX5 was quiescent in unstimulated cells. However, in response to elevations of the cytosolic Ca^{2+} concentration it generated large amounts of superoxide. Upon Ca^{2+} activation, NOX5 also displayed a second function: it became a proton channel, presumably to compensate charge and pH alterations due to electron export. In summary, **we have identified a novel NADPH oxidase that generates superoxide and functions as an H$^+$ channel in a Ca^{2+}-dependent manner. NOX5 is likely to be involved in Ca^{2+}-activated, redox-dependent processes of spermatozoa and lymphocytes such as sperm-oocyte fusion, cell proliferation, and cytokine secretion. I believe that this is another example of the extreme importance of EMODs.**

Some of the following material was excerpted, abstracted or modified from: The superoxide-producing NAD(P)H oxidase Nox4 in the nucleus of human vascular endothelial cells (Junya Kuroda, Kazunori Nakagawa, Tomoko Yamasaki, Kei-ichiro Nakamura, Ryu Takeya, Futoshi Kuribayashi, Shinobu Imajoh-Ohmi, Kazuhiko Igarashi, Yosaburo Shibata, Katsuo Sueishi and Hideki Sumimoto. Genes to Cells (2005) **10**, 1139-1151).

The superoxide-producing NAD(P)H oxidase **Nox4 was initially identified as an enzyme that is highly expressed in the kidney and is possibly involved in oxygen sensing and cellular senescence.** Although **the oxidase is also abundant in vascular endothelial cells**, its role remains to be elucidated. Here we show that **Nox4 preferentially localizes to the nucleus of human umbilical vein endothelial cells** (HUVECs), by immunocytochemistry and immunoelectron microscopy using three kinds of affinity-purified antibodies raised against distinct immunogens from human Nox4. Silencing of Nox4 by RNA interference (RNAi) abrogates nuclear signals given with the antibodies, confirming the nuclear localization of Nox4. The nuclear fraction of HUVECs exhibits an NAD(P)H-dependent superoxide-producing activity in a manner dependent on Nox4, which activity can be enhanced upon cell stimulation with phorbol 12-myristate 13-acetate. This stimulant also facilitates gene expression as estimated in the present transfection assay of HUVECs using a reporter regulated by the Maf-recognition element MARE, a DNA sequence that constitutes a part of oxidative stress response. **Both basal and stimulated transcriptional activities are impaired by RNAi-mediated Nox4 silencing. Thus Nox4 appears to produce superoxide in the nucleus of HUVECs, thereby regulating gene expression via a mechanism for oxidative stress response. I believe that this again illustrates the essential presence of EMODs, even in the cellular nucleus.**

Under normal physiological conditions, EMODs are tightly regulated and can serve as cellular messengers (Topper, J.N., Cai, J., Falb, D. and Gimbrone, M.A., Jr. Identification of vascular endothelial genes differentially responsive to fluid mechanical stimuli: Cyclooxygenase-2, manganese superoxide dismutase and endothelial cell nitric oxide synthase are selectively upregulated by steady laminar shear stress. Proc Natl Acad Sci USA 1996; 93: 10417-10422), (Wung, B.S., Cheng, J.J., Chao, Y.J., Hsieh, H.J. and Wang, D.L. Modulation of Ras/Raf/extracellular signal-regulated kinase pathway by reactive oxygen species is involved in cyclic strain-induced early growth response-1 gene expression in endothelial cells. Circ Res 1999; 84: 804-812).

9.1 The Central Nervous System

EMODs have recently been implicated in a variety of redox-based signaling mechanisms that can mediate changes in neural plasticity including:

> **activation of oxidative stress-responsive transcription factors**
> **modulation of LTP induction**
> **and mediation of nonsynaptic communication between neurons and glia.**

In addition, **EMODs have been implicated as modulators of synaptic transmission,** following demonstration that H_2O_2 can reversibly depress evoked population spikes in slices of guinea pig hippocampus.

Oxidative metabolism in brain tissue occurs in the mitochondria as in all cells. During the process of oxidative phosphorylation, a significant amount of O_2 consumed is diverted to from superoxide $(O_2^{\cdot-})$, **which is the stoichiometric precursor of H_2O_2. The amount of H_2O_2 produced by brain mitochondria is up to 5% of the amount of O_2 consumed** (Arnaiz, S.L., Coronel, M.F. and Boveris, A. Nitric oxide, superoxide and hydrogen peroxide production in brain mitochondria after haloperidol treatment. Nitric Oxide 1999; 3: 235-243). Given that the rate of O_2 consumption in gray matter is 2-5 mmol/g tissue wet weight per minute; or 2-5mM (assuming 1 g = 1 mL), this would mean that **concentrations of up to 250 mM H_2O_2 could be generated every minute within brain neutrophils.** Because **the rate of O_2 consumption is roughly 10-fold higher in neurons than in glia,** however, this H_2O_2 would be produced predominantly in the neuronal compartment, which could lead to higher, intra-neuronal concentrations. Moreover, the presence of mitochondria within 250 nm of the synapse in **DA (dopamine)** terminals suggests that even higher levels could be reached in the restricted, intracellular compartment of a synaptic terminal. It is relevant to note, however, that such local increases are likely to be transient because H_2O_2 is membrane permeable and thus can readily leave the compartment in which it is produced.

In addition to mitochondrial sources, H_2O_2 will also be produced in DA terminals by **monoamine oxidase (MAO),** which is a metabolizing enzyme for DA. Importantly, **MAO is localized on the outer membrane of mitochondria**, which would further enhance H_2O_2 concentrations near DA synapses.

Actual concentration of H_2O_2 at a given location will depend not only on the activity of sources of H_2O_2 and the size of the compartment it enters, but also on the activity of the local antioxidant network. **In brain tissue, H_2O_2 levels are regulated largely by the intracellular enzyme, glutathione (GSH) peroxidase, and by endogenous catalase in peroxisomes**. Importantly, the present results with exogenous catalase indicate that **cellular antioxidant regulation does not completely remove endogenously generated H_2O_2.** Rather these processes **appear to permit levels of H_2O_2 that are sufficient to exert modulatory actions.** The lack of effect of up to 10 mM exogenous H_2O_2 in elevated $[Ca^{2+}]$, however, indicates that H_2O_2-mediated effects are saturable; this is also consistent with the calculation that competing levels of endogenous H_2O_2 might be milli- molar. Indeed, the concentration of exogenous H_2O_2 used in the present studies (1.5 mM) is **within the range (1-3 mM) found to have biological effects in many other studies in the literature.**

Catalase is present in trace quantities in brain and is localized in peroxisomes, which in the brain are referred to as "microperoxisomes." **In contrast to glutathione peroxidase** and catalase, which exhibit relatively low enzymatic activity in brain, superoxide dismutase is relatively abundant (Sies, H. Oxidative Stress. Academic Press 1985; 388).

I believe that the above fact "that the antioxidant enzymes in the brain do not completely deplete H_2O_2 levels" is again evidence of the need for these RONS for normal brain function. According to the Free Radi-Crap theory, leaving steady state levels of H_2O_2 and extremely dangerous RONS would have disastrous consequences, especially a chain reaction involving lipid peroxidation, but ....under normal physiological conditions, that does not happen.

It was recently shown that H_2O_2 caused a decrease in ATP production, which interfered with stimulus secretion in pancreatic cells.

There is evidence in the literature to suggest that H_2O_2 application can cause membrane hyperpolarization mediated by an increased K^+ in some cell types, including CA1 pyramidal neurons, which could lead to a decrease in transmitter release.

Independent of the possible mechanisms by which H_2O_2 may act, the finding that H_2O_2 can inhibit transmitter release reveals a novel process by which synaptic transmission might be modulated physiologically (Chen, B.T., Avshalumov, M.V. and Rice, M.E. H_2O_2 is a novel, endogenous modulator of synaptic dopamine release. J Neurophysiol 2001; 85: 2468-2476).

I am amazed at the number of instances in which EMODs are acting as sensitive and crucial signaling and regulating agents in cellular metabolism.

9.2　Pancreatic Beta Cells and H_2O_2

The control of insulin secretion in the pancreatic beta cell depends on the precise tuning of glucose metabolism leading to signal transduction. Insulin stimulates H_2O_2 production in fat cells and **H_2O_2 acts as a secondary messenger for insulin.** .OH mediates the induction of diabetes in mice by alloxan.

Type I diabetes, or insulin dependent diabetes mellitus, is an autoimmune disease characterized by altered function and beta cell death subsequent to exposure to inflammation products. During insulitis, macrophages infiltrate the islets of Langerhans and generate reactive oxygen species such as hydrogen peroxide (H_2O_2), which exert alleged deleterious actions on the beta cells and on mitochondrial oxidative metabolism. **Activated phagocytes can produce as much as 47 nmol of $H_2O_2/10^6$ cells within 30 minutes corresponding to a concentration of 47 mM H_2O_2 in a diluted volume of I ml** (Anderson, R. J Immunol Methods 1992; 155: 49-55). Nitric oxide (NO), another free radical precursor produced by macrophages, suppresses mitochondrial activity leading to a defective insulin release in response to nutrient secretagogues (Welsh, N., Eizirik, D.L., Bendtzen, K. and Sandler, S. Endocrinology 1991; 129: 3167-3173). Moreover, it has been shown that **NO damages islet cell DNA and mitochondrial DNA in beta cells.** In general, mitochondrial DNA is more sensitive to oxidative stress than nuclear DNA (Yakes, F.M. and Van Houten, B. Proc Natl Acad Sci USA 1997; 94: 514-519), (Beckman, K.B. and Ames, B.N. Physiol Rev 1998; 78: 547-581).

In cells, the mitochondrion is the main source of oxidants. Indeed, imperfect electron transport generates superoxide anions, which are spontaneously dismutated to H_2O_2. Thus, the mitochondria are pivotal in the control of insulin secretion, whereas at the same time generating reactive oxygen species in the cell mostly in the form of H_2O_2.

Of particular importance is the high sensitivity of pancreatic beta cells to oxidative stress. Moreover, the diabetic state is associated with increased oxidative stress and free radical damage (Yu, B.P. Physiol Rev 1994; 74: 139-162). In fact, **the expression of the H_2O_2-inactivating enzymes catalase and glutathione peroxidase in rat pancreatic islets is twenty times lower than in the liver** (Tiedge, M., Lortz, S., Drinkgern, J. and Lenizen, S. Diabetes 1997; 46: 1733-1742).

In mouse pancreatic beta cells, H_2O_2 hyperpolarizes the cell membrane coupled with an increase of cell membrane conductance (Krippeit-Drews, P., Lang, F., Haussinger, D. and Drews, G. Pflugers Arch Eur J Physiol 1994; 426: 552-554).

Moreover, it has recently been shown that H_2O_2:

> **increases intracellular Ca^{2+}**
> **decreases the ATP/ADP ratio**
> **and inhibits glucose-stimulated insulin secretion**
from isolated mouse islets (Krippeit-Drews, P., Kramer, C., Welker, S., Lang, F., Ammon, H.P. and Drews, G. J Physiol (Lond) 1999; 514: 471-481).

The cells were exposed to **200 μM H_2O_2 which is a level seen during activation of phagocytes in vitro. The diabetogenic compound alloxan is known to generate H_2O_2 and free radicals** (Maechler, P., Jornot, L. and Wollheim, C.B. Hydrogen peroxide alters mitochondrial activation and insulin secretion in pancreatic beta cells. J Biol Chem 1999; 274: 27905-27913).

9.3   Pharmacokinetics

This amazing molecule, hydrogen peroxide, is developing an image as a very important signaling molecule. In fact, H_2O_2 **seems to be one of the most important EMODs** that acts as a signaling molecule. H_2O_2 **is as important for cell functioning**

as other ubiquitous signaling molecules such as cAMP, nitric oxide and calcium.

It is now certain that just as EMODs and H_2O_2 have been considered "death molecules", they are now called "molecules of life" (Droege, 2001) (Droege, W. Free radicals in the physiological control of cell function. Physiol Rev 82:47-95, 2001) (Rhee et al., 2003) (Rhee SG, Chang TS, Bae YS, Lee SR, Kang SW. Cellular regulation by hydrogen peroxide. J Am Soc. Nephrol 14:S211-S215, 2003).

The stability of H_2O_2 further depends on the cell's redox state. H_2O_2 is more stable in an oxidizing environment, such as the extracellular space, than in a reducing environment like the cell interior. Therefore, H_2O_2 has also been proposed to act as an inter-cellular messenger (Reth, 2002) (Reth M. Hydrogen peroxide as second messenger in lymphocyte activation. Nature Immunol 3(12):1129-1134, 2002).

The hepatocytes steady state H_2O_2 concentration can be up to 25 μM.

The net H_2O_2 concentration depends on the site and source of H_2O_2 production, the numerous H_2O_2 activities within the cell, the spontaneous and enzymatic dismutation of H_2O_2, as well as the concentration of protective agents. Dependent on the presence and interaction of the redox sensitive molecules in the cell, and dependent on the activation state of the cell, H_2O_2 signaling can lead to cell activation or cell inhibition.

H_2O_2 is well suited to act as cellular messenger since it does not randomly react with all molecules, as most other ROS do, but instead primarily targets cysteine residues. It oxidizes the -SH group of cysteine to $-OH$ which is then reduced by cellular reducing agents such as glutathione and thioredoxin. However, these reactions are only possible when the cysteine is deprotonated (-S-), which is not often the case at physiological pH. Only a positively charged amino acid in the vicinity of the cysteine can keep it in an oxidizable form, which means that only selected proteins are targets for H_2O_2 (Reth, 2002) (Reth M. Hydrogen peroxide as second messenger in lymphocyte activation. Nature Immunol 3(12):1129-1134, 2002).

The H_2O_2-dependent modifications of the target proteins can cause their activation or inactivation. For instance, **H_2O_2 down regulates transcription factors such as p53, Jun, and Fos, but leads to activation of NF-kappa B and c-Jun N-terminal kinase (JNK) pathways** (Chen et al., 2001) (Chen YR, Shrivastava A, Tan TH. Down-regulation of the c-Jun N-terminal kinase (JNK) phosphatase M3/6 and activation of JNK by hydrogen peroxide and pyrrolidine dithiocarbamate. Oncogene 20(3):367-374, 2001) (Livolsi et al., 2001) (Livolsi A, Busuttil V, Imbert V, Abraham RT, Peyron JF. Tyrosine phosphorylation-dependent activation of NF-kappa B. Requirement of p56 LCK and ZAP-70 protein tyrosine kinases. Eur J Biochem 268(5):1508-1515, 2001) (Reth, 2002) (Reth, 2002) (Reth M. Hydrogen peroxide as second messenger in lymphocyte activation. Nature Immunol 3(12):1129-1134, 2002).

An important group of molecules that are downregulated by H_2O_2 is the **protein tyrosine phosphatase (PTP)** group, **evolutionarily conserved molecules that play a central role for transmitting signals from cell surface receptors to the nucleus.** It was shown that stimulation of cells from a human epidermal cell line by endothelial growth factor (EGF) caused **H_2O_2** oxidation of PTP-1B in a reversible way, with maximal activation 10 minutes after receptor stimulation (Lee et al., 1998) (Lee SR, Kwon KS, Kim R, Rhee SG. Reversible inactivation of protein-tyrosine phosphatase 1B in A431 cells stimulated with epidermal growth factor. J Biol Chem 273:15366-15372, 1998).

The phosphorylation state, and thus activation state, of any cellular protein is the net effect of tyrosine kinase activity, which phosphorylates the protein, and corresponding PTP activity, which reverses the reaction. Thus, activation of tyrosine kinase by EGF binding to the EGF receptor, and inhibition of PTP activity by H_2O_2 can lead to similar effects, promotion of growth factor signaling.

Elegant experiments provided additional *in vivo* evidence of the reversible regulation of other growth factor receptors such as PDGF and insulin by H_2O_2 (Li & Dixon, 2000) (Li L, Dixon JE. Form, function and regulation of protein tyrosine phosphatases and their involvement in human diseases. Sem in Immunol 12:75-84, 2000) (Meng et al., 2002) (Meng TC, Fukada T, Tonks NK. Reversible oxidation and inactivation of protein tyrosine phosphatases *in vivo*. Mol Cell 9:387-399, 2002). It seems accepted that PTP oxidation by H_2O_2 is an important physiological signaling event.

Regulation of vascular tone, sensing of oxygen tension, and enhancement of membrane receptor signal transduction are only a few examples of non-detrimental processes that involve ROS (Droege, 2001) (Droege, W. Free radicals in the physiological control of cell function. Physiol Rev 82:47-95, 2001) (Lander, 1997) (Lander HM. An essential role for free radicals and derived species in signal transduction. FASEB J 11:188-124, 1997).

The International Agency for Research on Cancer (IARC) has determined that hydrogen peroxide is not classifiable as to its carcinogencity to humans. Even though accusations against H_2O_2 have been wide spread, there is no verified data, in man, that H_2O_2 in any way causes or promotes cancer in vivo. The WHO-IARC said, "There is inadequate evidence in humans for the carcinogenicity of hydrogen peroxide."

H_2O_2 is produced metabolically in intact cells and tissues. It is formed by the reduction of O_2 either directly in a two-electron transfer reaction, often catalyzed by lipoproteins, or by an initial one-electron step to O_2 followed by dismutation to H_2O_2 (IARC, 1985). **H_2O_2 has been detected in serum and in intact liver** (IARC, 1985).

Typical intra-arterial administration produces only 2.9 ml of oxygen per 100 ml of blood per minute, an insignificant addition considering that normal adult metabolism requires between 200 and 250 ml of oxygen each. However, **they fail to point out that 2 ml of 3% H_2O_2 can release 20 ml of oxygen micro-bubbles. As stated earlier, hydrogen peroxide has a half-life of 0.75 to 2.0 seconds in human blood.**

In the early sixties, Baylor University Medical Center investigators studied five dogs, rats with Walker 256 rat sarcoma and four human patients and found that:

- none of the patients showed adverse clinical effects secondary to intra-arterial hydrogen peroxide
- no adverse local or systemic toxic effects were encountered in animals or humans
- there was no significant imbalance in acid-base or cation-anion equilibrium
- early evidence in these studies would suggest an increased therapeutic ratio in malignant tumors to ionizing irradiation.

(Mallams, J.T., Finney, J.W. and Balla, G.A. The use of hydrogen peroxide as a source of oxygen in a regional intra-arterial infusion system. Southern Med J 1962; 55: 230-232).

Studies by Nathan and Cohn have shown that **hydrogen peroxide contributes to the lysis of tumor cells by macrophages and granulocytes in a variety of experimental conditions.** (Nathan, C.F. and Cohn, Z.A. Antitumor effects of hydrogen peroxide in vivo. J Exp Med 1981; 154: 1539-1553). They also found that **an H$_2$O$_2$-generating system confined to the tumor bed exerted clear-cut antitumor effects with little toxicity to the host.**

9.4   Interferon Inducing Activity of H$_2$O$_2$

The activated macrophages have a major role in the immune response as regulatory cells which can enhance or suppress immune reactions. (Rosenthal, A.S. Regulation of the immune response - role of the macrophage. N Engl J Med 1980; 303: 1153). With natural killer (NK) cells, the activated macrophages induced by various stimulants, including adjuvants such as bacillus Calmette-Guerin (BCG), Corynebacterium parvum, or polyanions, show dual effects of suppression and augmentation on the activity of NK cells. Also, **these activated macrophages produce oxidative metabolites such as hydrogen peroxide, which is responsible for sterilizing action against microorganisms and cytotoxic activity against tumor cells** (Murray, H.W., Juangbhanich, C.W., Nathan, C.F. and Cohn, Z.A. Macrophage oxygen-dependent anti-microbial activity: The role of oxygen intermediates. J Exp Med 1979; 150: 950), (Nathan, C.F., Silverstein, S.C., Brukner, L.H. and Cohn, Z.A. Extracellular cytolysis by activated macrophages and granulocytes: Hydrogen peroxide as a mediator of cytotoxicity. J Exp Med 1979; 149: 100). **These reports suggest that hydrogen peroxide regulates immune responses.**

9.5   Tumoricidal Activity of H$_2$O$_2$

Investigators have shown that hydrogen peroxide-generated by TNF-activated PMNs was also cytotoxic and tumoricidal. (Shau, H. Cytostatic and tumoricidal activities of tumor necrosis factor-treated neutrophils. Immunol Lett 1988 17(1): 47-51).

Studies support the internalization and degradation of receptor bound C-reactive protein by U-937 cells (human monocytic cell line): **induction of H$_2$O$_2$ production and tumoricidal activity.** (Tebo, J.M. and Mortensen, R.F. Internalization and degradation of

receptor bound C-reactive protein by U-937 cells: Induction of
H_2O_2 production and tumoricidal activity. Biochem Biophys Acta
1991; 1095(3): 210-216).

**Hydrogen peroxide is routinely used during microsurgical
procedures to augment hemostasis after intracranial tissue
resection. Elsewhere in the body, hydrogen peroxide is
used to kill the resection margin of tumor cells; in vitro
studies support these clinical uses.** Hydrogen peroxide may
prove most beneficial for discrete lesions, such as pituitary tumors
and metastases. (Mesiwala, A.H., Farrell, L., Santiago, P., Ghatan, S. and
Silbergeld, D.L. The effects of hydrogen peroxide on brain and brain
tumors. Surg Neurol 2003; 59(5): 398-407).

**Mast cells, when supplemented with H_2O_2 and iodide,
are cytotoxic to mammalian tumor** cells as determined
by 51Cr release, and transmission and scanning electron
microscopy. H_2O_2 at the concentration employed (10(-4)M)
initiates mast cell degranulation, and mast cell granules (MCG),
which contain a small amount of endogenous peroxidase
activity, are toxic to tumor cells when combined with H_2O_2 and
iodide. This toxicity is greatly increased by binding eosinophil
peroxidase (EPO) to MCG surface. These reactions may play a
role in the host defense against neoplasms. (Henderson, W.R.,
Chi, E.Y., Jong, E.C. and Klebanoff, S.J. Mast cell-mediated tumor-
cell cytotoxicity. Role of the peroxidase system. J Exp Med
1981; 153(3): 520-533).

**Several anti-cancer drugs are known to bring about
their tumoricidal actions by a free radical dependent
mechanism.** A majority of the studies reported that adriamycin,
mitocmycin C, etc., augment free radical generation (**superoxide
anion and hydrogen peroxide**) and lipid peroxidation process
in vitro. **These results confirm that many anti-cancer drugs
augment free radical generation and lipid peroxidation
even in an in vivo situation.** (Sangeetha, P., Das, U.N., Koratkar,

R. and Suryaprabha, P. Increase in free radical generation and lipid peroxidation following chemotherapy in patients with cancer. Free Radic Biol Med 1990; 8(1): 15-19).

It is hypothesized **that ascorbic acid exhibits cytotoxic tumoricidal activity via a prooxidant effect. There is a 10 to 100 fold greater content of catalase in normal cells than in tumor cells.** Due to this, **cancer cells reach high levels of intracellular hydrogen peroxide leading to their destruction, while normal cells are protected.** (Matsuda, T., Kuroyanagi, M., Sugiyama, S., Umehara, K., Ueno, A. and Nishi, K. Role of hydrogen peroxide for cell death induction by sodium 5,6-Benzylidene-L-ascorbate. Chem Pharm Bull 1994; 6: 1216-1225), (Mizuno, M., Minato, K., Ito, H., Kawade, M., Terai, H. and Tsuchida, H. Anti-tumor polysaccharide from the mycelium of liquid-cultured Agaricus Blazel Mill. Biochem Mol Biol Int 1999; 47: 707-714).

Various investigators have studied the value of H_2O_2 and shrinking the size of tumors (Aronoff, B.L., et al. Cancer 1965; 18: 1250), and have studied treatment advantages and **increased tumor cytotoxicity by the use of regional H_2O_2 infusion**. (Mallams, J.T., Balla, G.A. and Finney, J.W. Regional oxygenation and irradiation in the treatment of malignant tumors. Prog in Clin Cancer 1965; 1: 137).

Lactobacilli-mediated control of vaginal cancer through specific reactive oxygen species interaction. Bauer G. Med Hypotheses 2001 Aug;57(2):252-7.

Abteilung Virologie, Institut fur Medizinische Mikrobiologie und Hygiene, Universitat Freiburg, Germany. tgfb@ukl.uni-freiburg.de

Klebanoff et al. proposed that hydrogen peroxide-producing lactobacilli and peroxidase in the vagina of healthy women might be responsible for the prevention of vaginosis and also might exert an antitumor effect (1). Based on recent evidence on superoxide anion generation by transformed cells (2,3) and on the potential of myeloperoxidase for selective apoptosis induction in transformed cells (4), a model for specific reactive oxygen species interaction during lactobacilli-mediated tumor control in the vagina is presented here. We propose that **peroxidase, which converts hydrogen peroxide into hypochlorous acid, is responsible for creating a microbicidal vaginal milieu by maintaining a balanced, non-toxic, steady state level of the microbicides H(2)O(2) and HOCl.** In case individual superoxide anion-producing transformed cells eventually appear in the mucosa, they will be driven into apoptosis by **interaction of HOCl with superoxide anions which leads to the generation of hydroxyl radicals.** Hence selective apoptosis induction in transformed cells represents the key element of lactobacilli-mediated antitumor defense. Since papilloma virus infected cells are resistant to this pathway of apoptosis induction, they are plausible candidates for circumvention of lactobacilli-mediated control of oncogenesis.

I believe that this is a very important concept for both the control of pathogens and neoplastic cells. It illustrates the importance of adequate EMOD levels to maintain homeostasis.

Polymorphonuclear leukocytes (PMN) of mice can destroy tumor cells effectively in vitro in the presence of antitumor polysaccharide, linear beta-1, 3-D-glucan from Alcaligenes faecalis var, myxogenes IFO 13140 (TAK), and some other immonomodulators. **Hydrogen peroxide is important for these cytotoxicities** whereas, unlike the results with TAK, **the H_2O_2: halide:myeloperoxidase system may partly participate in the cytotoxicity with some immunomodulators.** (Morikawa, K., Kamegaya, S., Yamazaki, M. and Mizuno, D. Hydrogen peroxide as a tumoricidal mediator of murine polymorphonuclear leukocytes induced by a linear beta-1,3-D-glucan and some other immonomodulators. Cancer Res 1985; 45(8): 3482-3486).

Prof Randolph Michael Howes MD,PhD

It was found that the (Nitric Oxide) NO-mediated loss of cell viability was dependent on both NO and hydrogen peroxide (H_2O_2). Somewhat surprisingly, superoxide ($O_2.-$) and its reaction product with NO, peroxynitrite (-OONO), did not appear to be directly involved in the observed NO-mediated cytotoxicity against this cancer cell line. A recent report utilizing NO donor compounds indicated that **NO was particularly tumoricidal in the presence of hydrogen peroxide (H_2O_2) and not $O_2.^-$.** There is evidence confirming the original observations of Ioannidis and de Groot (Ioannidis, I. And de Grott, H. Cytotoxicity of nitric oxide in Fu5 rat hepatoma cells: evidence for cooperative action with hydrogen peroxide. Biochem J 1993; 296(Pt2): 341-345), indicating **that the combination of NO and H_2O_2 was particularly cytotoxic to a human ovarian cancer cell line.** (Farias-Eisner, R., Chaudhuri, G., Aeberhard, E. and Fukuto, J.M. The chemistry and tumoricidal activity of nitric oxide/hydrogen peroxide and the implications to cell resistance/susceptibility. J Biol Chem 1996; 271(11): 6144-6151).

Studies demonstrate that **a combination of sub-lytic concentrations of chemically generated NO and H_2O_2 leads to death of murine lymphoma cells, in part, via induction of apoptosis.** (Filep, J.G., Lapierre, C., Lachance, S. and Chan, J.S.D. Nitric oxide cooperates with hydrogen peroxide in inducing DNA fragmentation and cell lysis in murine lymphoma cells. Biochem J 1997; 321: 887-901). In vitro studies have suggested that a reaction of **NO gas and H_2O_2 produces singlet oxygen or hydroxyl radicals.** (Kanner, J., Harel, S. and Granit, R. Arch Biochem Biophys 1991; 289: 130-136), (Noronha-Dutra, A.A., Epperlein, M.M. and Woolf, N. FEBS Lett 1993; 321: 59-62). Nevertheless, this has not yet been demonstrated in cell cultures.

In many non-phagocytotic cells, including epithelial, endothelial, and smooth muscle cells, new proteins that are

homologous to gp91-phox have been described. They seem to play the role that **NADPH oxidase plays in phagocytotic cells, i.e. intentional production of ROS** (Hoidal, 2001) (Hoidal JR. Reactive oxygen species and cell signaling. Am J Respir Cell Mol Biol 25:661-663, 2001) (Lambeth, 2004) (Lambeth JD. Nox enzymes and the biology of reactive oxygen. Nature Rev Immunol 4:181-189, 2004).

The **NOX family is involved in regulation of cell growth and proliferation (NOX 1, NOX 5), participates in host defense (NOX 1) and mediates oxygen sensing (NOX 3/4).**

A second family of non-phagocytic **NADPH oxidase similar enzymes has a dual redox function and is thus called DUOX enzymes. It was shown that DUOX 1 and 2 play a role in thyroid hormone synthesis.**

9.6 H_2O_2 Regulation of T Cells

The immune system is vital to protect us against infectious agents (bacteria, viruses, fungi, protozoa and cancer). **Patients with T Cell immunodeficiencies are prone to infections and to certain types of cancers, especially leukemias and lymphomas.**

T cells are exposed to H_2O_2 at sites of inflammation where activated macrophages and neutrophils produce large amounts of superoxide **and its derivatives via the phagocytic isoform of NADPH oxidase. It is estimated that** during this oxidative burst the local H_2O_2 concentration may reach 10-100 μM in the vicinity of T cells **(Nathan & Root, 1977) (Nathan CF, Root RK. Hydrogen peroxide release from mouse peritoneal macrophages: dependence on sequential activation and triggering. J Exp med 146:1648-1662, 1977). A large body of evidence, accumulated since the late seventies, indicates that T cells are able to sense these redox changes and to respond by activation of certain T signal cascades and**

transcription factors (Droege, 2001) (Droege, W. Free radicals in the physiological control of cell function. Physiol Rev 82:47-95, 2001).

T lymphocytes play an important role in the defense against environmental pathogens. **A growing body of evidence demonstrates that T lymphocytes are strongly regulated in their activities by ROS such as H_2O_2.** T lymphocytes respond to H_2O_2 that is released by phagocytic leukocytes (such as macrophages) after inflammatory activation by antigenic peptides. T lymphocytes also produce H_2O_2 leading to regulation of distinct **T cell receptor (TCR)** pathways such as MAPK pathways. H_2O_2 is produced by a recently discovered phagocyte-type NADPH oxidase, however, additional sources are likely. For instance, **there is evidence that the TCR itself produces H_2O_2,** either amplifying signaling cascades after relatively weak receptor stimulation, or bypassing TCR activation by antigenic peptides. H_2O_2 produced during metabolism contributes to the **cellular redox state of T lymphocytes,** similar like in other cells.

It has been known for some time that H_2O_2 at low concentrations has T cell mitogenic effects and promotes IL-2 production (Roth & Droege, 1987) (Roth S, Droege W. Regulation of T-cell activation and T-cell growth factor (TCGF) production by hydrogen peroxide. Cell Imunol 108:417-424, 1987) (Hehner et al., 2000) (Hehner SP, Breitkreutz R, Shubinshky G, Unsoeld H, Schulze-Osthoff K, Lienhard Schmitz M, Droege, W. Enhancement of T cell receptor signaling by a mild oxidative shift in the intracellular thiol pool. J Immunol 165:4319-4328, 2000).

T cell responses in general are highly regulated by tyrosine phosphorylation. It is thus not astonishing that H_2O_2 affects T cell **activity by balancing the activities of tyrosine kinases and phosphatases.** For instance, H_2O_2 results in the activation of the SRC-family protein tyrosine kinase p56(lck) and of the SYK-family protein tyrosine kinase ZAP-70, similar to the signaling events that take place after stimulation of the T cell receptor (Livolsi et al., 2001) (Livolsi A, Busuttil V, Imbert V, Abraham RT, Peyron JF. Tyrosine phosphorylation-dependent activation of NF-kappa B. Requirement of p56 LCK and ZAP-70 protein tyrosine kinases. Eur J Biochem 268(5):1508-1515, 2001).

The activation of T cell receptor signal pathways seems to occur via inhibition of PTPs by H_2O_2 and to result in activation of all three members of the MAPK family: ERK, p38, and JNK (Lee & Esselman. 2002) (Lee K, Esselman WJ. Inhibition of PTPs by H_2O_2 regulates the activation of distinct MAPK pathways. Free Rad Biol Med 33(8):1121-1132, 2002).

It is proposed that the **oxidative activation of T cells** not only occurs during pathological conditions of chronic oxidative stress, but also **regularly as a very early response of the immune system to an invading pathogen** (Hehner et al., 2000) (Hehner SP, Breitkreutz R, Shubinshky G, Unsoeld H, Schulze-Osthoff K, Lienhard Schmitz M, Droege, W. Enhancement of T cell receptor signaling by a mild oxidative shift in the intracellular thiol pool. J Immunol 165:4319-4328, 2000).

It may be that T cells sense small quantities of ROS (H_2O_2) long before inflammatory stages are reached.

There is evidence that T cells themselves produce H_2O_2 upon stimulation of their antigen receptor (Devadas et al., 2002) (Devadas S, Zaritskaya L, Rhee SG, Oberley L, Williams MS. Discrete generation of superoxide and hydrogen peroxide by T cell receptor stimulation: selective regulation of mitogen-activated protein kinase activation and Fas ligand expression. J Exp Med 195(1):59-70, 2002) (Williams & Kwon, 2004) (Williams MS, Kwon J. T cell receptor stimulation, reactive oxygen species and cell signaling. Free Rad Biol Med 37(8):1144-1151, 2004).

It is proposed that not only H_2O_2 is produced, but also superoxide anion ($O_2\cdot-$). Both then act as second messenger, each activating different T cell receptor signaling pathways. In these studies using the transformed Jurkat T cell line, $O_2\cdot-$ activated an apoptotic signaling pathway, while H_2O_2 activated a proliferative pathway. The T cell receptor dependent H_2O_2 production by Jurkat cells was reproduced in activated proliferating human T blast cells (Kwon et al., 2003) (Kwon J, Devadas S, Williams MS. T cell receptor-stimulated generation of hydrogen peroxide inhibits MEK-ERK activation and lck serine phosphorylation. Free Rad Biol Med 35(4):406-417, 2003). However, in the non-transformed human cells the production of H_2O_2 resulted in cellular inhibition.

It is thus likely that the overall response of cells to changes in the cells' redox status will very much depend on the metabolic cell state in which the changes occurred.

Discoveries that T cell receptors catalytically generate substantial amounts of H_2O_2 are seminal observations (Reth, 2002) (Reth M. Hydrogen peroxide as second messenger in lymphocyte activation. Nature Immunol 3(12):1129-1134, 2002).

The activation of such an enzyme after T cell receptor stimulation and recruitment of apoptotic signals such as Fas ligand and Fas. Kinetic studies indicate that in addition to this sustained H_2O_2 production, there seems to be a rapid transient H_2O_2 production, independent of Fas or NADPH oxidase. Since H_2O_2 production can be measured before $O_2\cdot-$ is detected, and since $O_2\cdot-$ generation can be measured even when H_2O_2 is dismutated by catalase or thioredoxin peroxidase, H_2O_2 does not seem to be derived from $O_2\cdot-$ as is believed to be the case in most other known systems (Devadas et al., 2002) (Devadas S, Zaritskaya L, Rhee SG, Oberley L, Williams MS. Discrete generation of superoxide and hydrogen peroxide by T cell receptor stimulation:

selective regulation of mitogen-activated protein kinase activation and Fas ligand expression. J Exp Med 195(1):59-70, 2002).

A potential source for the unique production of H_2O_2 is the T cell receptor itself. This idea comes from studies with isolated antibodies, which have the ability to catalyze **a light-dependent reaction between molecular oxygen and water that leads to the production of H_2O_2** (Wentworth et al., 2000) (Wentworth AD, Jones LH, Wentworth P Jr, Janda KD, Lerner RA. Antibodies have the intrinsic capacity to destroy antigens. PNAS 97(20):10930-10935, 2000) (2001) (Wentworth P Jr, Jones LH, Wentworth AD, Zhu X, Larsen NA, Wilson IA, Xu X, Goddard WA III, Janda KD, Eschenmoser A, Lerner RA. Antibody catalysis of the oxidation of water. Science 293 (5536):1806-1811, 2001).

These events occur in all antibodies, regardless of source or antigenic specificity, and are being investigated at the molecular level. **The reaction is initiated by singlet oxygen that reacts with H_2O to ultimately produce H_2O_2 via intermediates such as H_2O3 and ozone** (Wentworth et al., 2003) (Wentworth P Jr, Wentworth AD, Zhu X, Wislon IA, Janda KD, Eschenmoser A, Lerner RA. Evidence for the production of trioxygen species during antibody-catalyzed chemical modification of antigens. PNAS 100(4):1490-1493, 2003).

The catalytic site of this reaction is at the interface between the variable and constant Ig domains, **where H_2O_2 molecules are trapped in a hydrophobic pocket** (Zhu et al., 2004) (Zhu X, Wentworth P Jr, Wentworth AD, Eschenmoser A, Lerner RA, Wilson IA. Probing the antibody-catalyzed water-oxidation pathway at atomic resolution. PNAS 101(8):2247-2252, 2004). When Wentworth and colleagues tested the ability of a wide variety of non-antibody proteins to catalyze H_2O_2 production, **the only other protein that produced H_2O_2 at a physiologically significant rate was the purified $\alpha\beta$ T cell receptor.**

Human T cell blasts indeed produce H_2O_2 under metabolically favorable conditions in a membrane-associated, **light dependent** event (unpublished data) (Nindl G, Peterson NR, Hughes EF, Waite LR, OHnson MT Effect of hydrogen peroxide on proliferation, apoptosis and interleukin-2 production of Jurkat T cells. Biomed Sci Instrum 40:123-128, 2004) (Hydrogen Peroxide - From Oxidative Stressor to Redox Regulator. Gabi Nindl. Cell Science Reviews. Vol 1. No. 2. Received 5th October © Cellscience 2004.).

H_2O_2 may play a ubiquitous role as an intracellular and/or intercellular second messenger much like nitric oxide or calcium. ROS and H_2O_2 seem to be used by cells mainly as regulators of signal transduction by cell surface receptors. H_2O_2 is able to promote either proliferation or death of inflammatory T cells, depending upon the circumstances. **There is also substantial evidence that T cells can produce H_2O_2 in response to various activating stimuli.**

Oxidants such as H_2O_2, pervanadate, and ultraviolet light have been found to mimic the intracellular signals initiated by TCR aggregation and have also been used to study this signaling pathway. **In short, H_2O_2 can trigger T cell proliferation and activation.** (Wange, R. L., and Samelson, L. E. (1996) Immunity 5, 197-205).

Treatment of T cells with either H_2O_2 or thiol-modulating agents such as diamide results in the tyrosine phosphorylation of multiple proteins (Nakamura K, Hori T, Sato N, Sugie K, Kawakami T, and Yodoi J. Redox regulation of a src family protein tyrosine kinase p56lck in T cells. *Oncogene* 8: 3133–3139, 1993), **including Src, Lck, and Fyn.**

As mentioned before, one source of H_2O_2 production is the phagocyte-type NADPH oxidase, but other sources such as the T cell receptor itself are likely.

9.7   Protein Tyrosine Phosphatases

Treatment with H_2O_2 leads to inactivation of many phosphatases via cysteine oxidation to a sulfenic acid, both with the isolated protein (Lee SR, Kwon KS, Kim SR, and Rhee SG. Reversible inactivation of protein-tyrosine phosphatase 1B in A431 cells stimulated with epidermal growth factor. J Biol Chem 273: 15366–15372, 1998) **and in cells in response to epidermal growth factor** (532). **These studies suggest that at least part of H_2O_2 signaling is mediated through the inactivation of protein tyrosine phosphatases**.

In addition to inactivation, H_2O_2 may also alter the cellular content of protein tyrosine phosphatases. In particular, **treatment of HeLa cells with H_2O_2 is characterized by rapid degradation of the Cdc25C** (Savitsky PA and Finkel T. Redox regulation of Cdc25C. J Biol Chem 277: 20535–20540, 2002), **a phosphatase involved in the cell cycle progression and checkpoint control.** This effect of H_2O_2 is due to cysteine disulfide formation in Cdc25C, as it can be recapitulated by mutation of either cysteine residues at positions 377 and 330 in the protein. Thus **H_2O_2 may impair protein tyrosine phosphatase activity through either enzymatic inactivation or protein degradation.**

Little is known about the specific mechanisms involved in H_2O_2-mediated protein tyrosine phosphatase inactivation. Although reagent H_2O_2 inactivates multiple forms of protein tyrosine phosphatases, engagement of platelet-derived growth factor with its receptor specifically inactivates SHP-2 (Meng TC, Fukada T, and Tonks NK. Reversible oxidation and inactivation of protein tyrosine phosphatases in vivo. Mol Cell 9: 387–399, 2002), **and the basis for this selectivity is not clear.** As is the case for other signaling micro-domains, the source(s) of ROS stimulated by ligand engagement might

181

be expected to bear some spatial or vectorial arrangement to their intended targets. **Although many features of H_2O_2 as a signaling molecule parallel that of NO, we have little knowledge at present of how H_2O_2 may function as a paracrine mediator.**

9.8   Transcription Factors and H_2O_2

Within the vessel wall, the transcription factor nuclear factor B (NF- B) plays a critical role in the regulation of inflammatory and immune response genes relevant to atherosclerosis. It has been proposed that H_2O_2 activates NF- B in certain cell lines via this mechanism (Schreck R, Rieber P, and Baeuerle PA. Reactive oxygen intermediates as apparently widely used messengers in the activation of the NF-kappa B transcription factor and HIV-1. *EMBO J* 10: 2247–2258, 1991).

Also, **H_2O_2 promotes phosphorylation of human ribonuclear protein-U** (Stone JR and Collins T. Rapid phosphorylation of heterogeneous nuclear ribonucleoprotein C1/C2 in response to physiologic levels of hydrogen peroxide in human endothelial cells. *J Biol Chem* 277: 15621–15628, 2002) **that regulates specific SCF (Skp-1/Cul/F box) family ubiquitin ligase involved in I- B degradation** (Davis M, Hatzubai A, Andersen JS, Ben-Shushan E, Fisher GZ, Yaron A, Bauskin A, Mercurio F, Mann M, and Ben-Neriah Y. Pseudosubstrate regulation of the SCF(-TrCP) ubiquitin ligase by hnRNP-U. *Genes Dev* 16: 439–451, 2002). These observations lend plausibility to the notion that ubiquitination of I- B may be a redox-sensitive step for NF- B activation.

c-Jun amino-terminal kinase is activated by H_2O_2 leading to both c-Jun phosphorylation with concomitant increased AP-1 transactivation (Chen K, Vita JA, Berk BC, and Keaney JF Jr. c-Jun N-terminal kinase activation by hydrogen peroxide in endothelial cells involves SRC-dependent epidermal growth factor receptor transactivation. *J Biol Chem* 276: 16045–16050, 2001) **and activation**

of ATF2, which enhances transcription of c-Jun. The two major pathways of H_2O_2-induced AP-1 activation involve MAPK stimulation through either apoptosis signal-regulating kinase 1 (ASK1) or inhibition of MAPK phosphatases.

It is now clear that EMODs may also mediate a number of physiological responses that are pervasive in nature. Roles for EMODs are best established for H_2O_2 that has been implicated in the vascular injury response and, perhaps, various forms of hypertrophy for both smooth muscle cells and cardiac myocytes.

9.9 Cellular Proliferation and H_2O_2

Actually, human cells respond to H_2O_2 in a complex manner, with a multitude of genes affected. For example, cells with 10-fold increase in cellular H_2O_2 concentration due to overexpression of Nox1 show increased expression of some 200 genes, whereas overexpression of Nox1 plus catalase reverts 70% of the altered genes to normal (Arnold RS, Shi J, Murad E, Whalen AM, Sun CQ, Polavarapu R, Parthasarathy S, Petros JA, and Lambeth JD. Hydrogen peroxide mediates the cell growth and transformation caused by the mitogenic oxidase Nox1. *Proc Natl Acad Sci USA* 98: 5550–5555, 2001). Many of the genetic changes seen are in proteins related to cell cycle, signal transduction, and transcription rather than antioxidant defense, indicating that the response triggered by H_2O_2 is specific and different from the stress response seen in bacteria.

In vascular smooth muscle cells in vitro, cell growth-enhancing, low concentrations of H_2O_2 activate multiple intracellular proteins and enzymes, including the epidermal growth factor receptor, c-Src, p38 MAPK, Ras, and Akt/ protein kinase B (Griendling KK, Sorescu D, Lassègue B, and Ushio-Fukai M. Modulation of protein kinase activity and gene expression by reactive oxygen species and their role in vascular physiology and pathophysiology. *Arterioscler Thromb Vasc Biol* 20: 2175–2183, 2000).

Conversely, **intermediate concentrations of added H_2O_2 (100 µM) inhibit serum-induced progression through the cell cycle via a decrease in cyclin A expression and cyclin-dependent kinase 2 activity, as well as upregulation of p21 and p53, whereas higher concentrations of H_2O_2 (500 µM) cause apoptosis of vascular smooth muscle cells** (Deshpande NN, Sorescu D, Seshiah P, Ushio-Fukai M, Akers M, Yin Q, and Griendling KK. Mechanism of hydrogen peroxide-induced cell cycle arrest in vascular smooth muscle. *Antioxid Redox Signal* 4: 845–854, 2002).

Growth factors including platelet-derived growth factor (Sundaresan M, Yu ZX, Ferrans VJ, Irani K, and Finkel T. Requirement for generation of H_2O_2 for platelet-derived growth factor signal transduction. *Science* 270: 296–299, 1995**) and epidermal growth factor trigger H_2O_2 production.** Similarly, **vascular endothelial growth factor-mediated proliferation and migration of endothelial cells appear to depend on EMOD production.**

A role of ROS in the control of growth of vascular cells is supported best for H_2O_2 mediating a proliferative phenotype in vascular smooth muscle cells. In fact, **H_2O_2 may be required for smooth muscle cell survival, as overexpression of catalase inhibits proliferation and can induce apopotosis** (Brown MR, Miller FJ Jr, Li WG, Ellingson AN, Mozena JD, Chatterjee P, Engelhardt JF, Zwacka RM, Oberley LW, Fang X, Spector AA, and Weintraub NL. Overexpression of human catalase inhibits proliferation and promotes apoptosis in vascular smooth muscle cells. *Circ Res* 85: 524–533, 1999). **I believe that this is an incredibly important role for H_2O_2.**

Low concentrations (i.e., <10 µM) of added H_2O_2, but not O_2^-; are also mitogenic to or enhance the survival of other

cells (Burdon RH. Superoxide and hydrogen peroxide in relation to mammalian cell proliferation. *Free Radic Biol Med* 18: 775–794, 1995**) including endothelial cells** (Stone JR and Collins T. The role of hydrogen peroxide in endothelial proliferative responses. *Endothelium* 9: 231–238, 2002).

In contrast, high concentrations, **H_2O_2 at >50 µM, corresponding to intracellular concentrations of >1 µM (**Boveris A, Alvarez S, Bustamante J, and Valdez L. Measurement of superoxide radical and hydrogen peroxide production in isolated cells and subcellular organelles. *Methods Enzymol* 349: 280–287, 2002**), can cause cultured cells to undergo growth arrest, apoptosis, or necrosis** (Li PF, Dietz R, and von Harsdorf R. Reactive oxygen species induce apoptosis of vascular smooth muscle cell. *FEBS Lett* 404: 249–252, 1997).

Also, the presence of H_2O_2 at low micromolar concentrations inhibits the aggregation (Stuart MJ and Holmsen H. Hydrogen peroxide, an inhibitor of platelet function: effect on adenine nucleotide metabolism, and the release reaction. *Am J Hematol* 2: 53–63, 1977).

Higher concentrations of H_2O_2, in the millimolar range, appear to stimulate platelet aggregation (Rodvien R, Lindon JN, and Levine P. Physiology and ultrastructure of the blood platelet following exposure to hydrogen peroxide. *Br J Haematol* 33: 19–24, 1976). This observation may be physiologically relevant to certain platelet agonists. For example, **collagen appears to stimulate considerable platelet H_2O_2 production.**

In fact, **H_2O_2 has also been implicated in platelet "priming" that facilitates tyrosine phosphorylation of the fibrinogen receptor that is ultimately required for aggregation** (Irani K, Pham Y, Coleman LD, Roos C, Cooke GE, Miodovnik A, Karim N, Wilhide CC, Bray PF, and Goldschmidt-Clermont PJ. Priming of platelet aIIb 3 by oxidants is associated with tyrosine phosphorylation of   3. *Arterioscler Thromb Vasc Biol* 18: 1698–1706, 1998).This latter contention is supported by data that **ultraviolet irradiation enhances platelet aggregation** through the upregulation of fibrinogen binding sites as a direct result of activation of protein kinase C mediated by EMODs.Thus **the role of EMODs in modulating platelet function is dependent on the particular type and concentration of ROS involved.I believe that this is classic redox regulation.**

10.0 BAYLOR UNIVERSITY SCHOOL OF MEDICINE STUDIES OF H_2O_2

10.1 Intra-Arterial H_2O_2 Regional Oxygenation

The intra-arterial infusion of hydrogen peroxide has been employed by Baylor University investigators as a method of regional oxygenation in the management of a variety of diseases (Urschel, H.C., Jr., Finney, J.W., Balla, G.A. and Mallams, J.T. Regional oxygenation of the ischemic myocardium with hydrogen peroxide. Surgical Forum, Amer Coll of Surg Cling Congress XV 1964; 273), (Urschel, H.C., Jr., Finney, J.W., Morales, A.R., Balla, G.A., Race, G.J. and Mallams, J.T. Cardiac resuscitation with hydrogen peroxide. Ann of Thorac Surg 1966; 2: 665), (Urschel, H.C., Jr., Finney, J.W., Balla, G.A., Race, G.J. and Mallams, J.T. Effects of hydrogen peroxide on the cardiovascular system. Proc Third Intl Conf on Hyperbaric Med 1966; 307), (Finney, J.W., Balla, G.A., Jay, B.E., Race, G.J., Urschel, H.C., Jr., Greenlee, R.G. and Mallams, J.T. Removal of cholesterol and other lipids from human athermanous arteries by dilute hydrogen peroxide. Angiology 1966; 17: 233), (Finney, J.W., Urschel, H.C., Jr., Balla, G.A., Race, G.J. and Mallams, J.T,. Protection of the ischemic heart with DMSO alone or in combination with hydrogen peroxide oxide. Ann of the NY Acad Sci 1967; 151: 231-241), (Balla, G.A., Finney, J.W., Aronoff, B.L., Byrd, D.L., Race, G.J., Mallams, J.T. and Davis, G. Use of intra-arterial hydrogen peroxide to promote wound healing. I. Regional intra-arterial therapy - technical surgical aspects. II. Wound healing - clinical aspects. Amer J Surg 1964; 108: 621), (Finney, J.W., Collier, R.E., Balla, G.A., Tomme, J.W., Wakely, J., Race, G.J., Urschel, H.C., D'Errico, A.D. and Mallams, J.T. The preferential localization of radioisotopes in malignant tissue by regional oxygenation. Nature 1964; 202: 1172). In some **patients so treated with hydrogen peroxide, a decrease in the severity of their atherosclerosis was observed.** This phenomenon was studied and confirmed by both in vitro and in vivo experimentation. (Finney, J.W., Jay, B.E., Race, G.J., Urschel, H.C., Mallams, J.T. and Balla, G.A. Removal of cholesterol and other lipids from experimental animal and human atheromatous arteries by dilute hydrogen peroxide. Angiology 1966;17:223-228).

Several patients who have been infused intra-arterially with hydrogen peroxide as an adjunct to irradiation therapy in the management of their malignant disease have undergone postmortem examination. In all cases studied to date, the patients received hydrogen peroxide infusion through a retrograde catheter in the abdominal aorta as an adjunct to irradiation therapy over periods of time ranging from 4 - 16 weeks. During this time, **the individuals were given daily infusions of 250 ml of hydrogen peroxide in "Ionosol-T" with a peroxide concentration ranging from 0.24% to 0.48%.**

Upon gross examination, **the segment of the aorta being infused with hydrogen peroxide was found to be different from the area not being infused. This difference was marked by a decrease in the number and severity of atheromatous plaques and an increase in flexibility and elasticity of the vessel.** Ordinarily one expects to find an increase in number and severity of the atheromatous lesions from the thoracic to the abdominal aorta. In these patients, **where the H_2O_2 infusion catheter was in the abdominal aorta below the renal arteries, there was lack of raised lesions from the point of the catheter to the bifurcation, and the iliacs were relatively free of gross disease except from some intimal and subintimal fibrosis.** In my opinion, this observation is of most importance since it is both dramatic and in humans.

Histologic evaluation of Oil Red O stained sections showed a decrease in total subliminal lipid deposits in the aorta below as compared to that above the H_2O_2 infusion catheter tip. When weighed samples of the vessels were extracted and total lipids determined, it was found that approximately a 50% reduction in total lipids (10 - 40% decrease in cholesterol and 20 - 50% decrease in cholesterol

esters) had occurred in the area being infused with hydrogen peroxide. This data further emphasizes the importance of this research data. Obviously, H_2O_2 has unique clinical importance in the treatment of arteriosclerosis that has thus far been over-looked or ignored.

In vitro studies confirmed the elution of lipid from human atheromatous aortas when incubated with either hydrogen peroxide or saline under high oxygen tension.

Serum lipid studies were conducted in various patients being infused intra-arterially with hydrogen peroxide. Venous blood samples were collected from the cubital vein immediately before and after the infusions with a total time lapse between the two sample of 20 - 30 minutes. **It was noted that the total increase in circulating lipids following the intra-arterial infusion of H_2O_2 seemed to be directly proportional to both the severity of disease and concentration of hydrogen peroxide infused.**

Routine blood work was done on alternate days; this included complete blood count (CBC) and platelet and reticulocyte counts. They demonstrated elevation in all the formed elements as noted previously when the carotid arteries have been infused by hydrogen peroxide.

Although the early clinical improvement was slight and the changes subtle, it can be stated that the patient was in no way clinically worse and it not demonstrate progression of the patient's symptoms which were marked prior to H_2O_2 infusion. **Apparent diminution of the vertebral artery stenosis and less delay in filling time of the vertebral compared to the carotid artery were observed.** This occurred with the severest limitations for infusion which probably will be encountered. These included minimal blood flow past a severe stenosis in a small vessel system which has a higher susceptibility to spasm and with the catheter a moderate distance from the lesion.

Human Studies: (Finney, J.W., George, M.S., Balla, A, Race, G.J. and Mallams, J.T. Peripheral blood changes in humans and experimental animals following the infusion of hydrogen peroxide into the carotid artery. Angiology 1965; 16: 62). In the human series studied (137 patients), the catheter varied in size and location, depending upon the tumor site. To March 1, 1964, 33 patients have been treated for malignant tumors of the head and neck, 13 of whom had the catheter placed in either the **common or internal carotid artery**. In the other 20, the catheter was placed into **the external carotid** via either the superficial temporal or superior thyroid artery. For the most part, the remaining 104 patients have been **treated for malignancies involving the liver, bladder, ovary, pancreas, endometrium, colon or cervix, with the catheters passed retrograde through the femoral artery to the appropriate level in the aorta**.

10.2 H_2O_2 Cardiac Resuscitation

The following information was excerpted from a paper by Urschel et al., (Urschel, H.C., Jr., Morales, A.R., Finney, J.W., Balla, G.A., Race, G.J. and Mallams, J.T. **Cardiac Resuscitation with Hydrogen Peroxide**. 1966; 2(5): 665-682).

Many clinical cardiac arrhythmias or situations of cardiac arrest are associated either primarily or secondarily with local or systemic hypoxia and anoxia. In addition to standard methods of cardiac resuscitation, hyperbaric oxygenation (OHP) has been employed both experimentally and clinically to improve myocardial oxygenation in these situation. Due to the technical and physiological problems inherent with OHP, studies were undertaken in Baylor University Medical Center laboratory to determine the feasibility of administering intravascular oxygen in a regional or systemic system. This approach employs dilute concentrations of hydrogen peroxide given by a variety of routes to provide oxygen.

Hydrogen peroxide under the influence of catalase and peroxidases is degraded to oxygen and water.

The H_2O_2-consuming enzymes catalase and glutathione peroxidase (GPx) strongly limit the action of H_2O_2.

Human blood and tissues contain excess quantities of both enzyme systems. **Hydrogen peroxide provides from 3 to 8 atmosphere equivalents of oxygen which is administered in solution**, thus avoiding the necessity of lung transport. Therapy can be provided regionally, avoiding the pulmonary and CNS toxicity problems of hyperbaric chambers. It can be given continuously over long periods of time by a single physician without expensive equipment and large teams, and also avoids the compression-decompression hazards of OHP.

Many clinical and experimental applications of hydrogen peroxide have been demonstrated. In over 300 patients regional intra-arterial hydrogen peroxide has potentiated the effect of radiation therapy in situations of malignancy involving the head, neck, pelvis and retro-peritoneum (Mallams, J.T., Balla, G.A. and Finney, J.W. Regional oxygenation and irradiation in the treatment of malignant tumors. Prog Clin Cancer 1965; 1: 137).

Increased localization of radioactive isotopes in malignant tumors has been achieved by regional and intra-arterial infusion of hydrogen peroxide (Finney, J.W., Collier, R.E., Balla, G.A., Tomme, J.W., Wakley, J., Race, G.J., Urschel, H.C., D'Errico, A.D. and Mallams, J.T. The preferential localization of radioisotopes in malignant tissue by regional oxygenation. Nature 1961; 202: 1172) (Finney, J.W., Balla, G.A., Collier, R.E., Wakely, J., Urschel, H.C. and Mallams, J.T. Differential localization of isotopes in tumors through the use of intra-arterial hydrogen peroxide: Part 1: Basic science. Amer J Roentgen 1965; 94: 783).

Peripheral bone marrow stimulation has been obtained by carotid artery infusion of hydrogen peroxide experimentally and clinically. (Finney, J.W., Balla, G.A., Mallams, J.T. and Race, G.J. Peripheral blood changes in humans and experimental animals following the infusion of hydrogen peroxide into the internal carotid artery. Angiology 1965; 16: 62).

10.3 Wound Healing

Wound healing has been markedly accelerated by the intra-arterial administration of hydrogen peroxide (Balla, G.A., Finney, J.W., Aronoff, B.L., Byrd, D.L., Race, G.J., Mallams, J.T. and Davis, G. Use of intra-arterial hydrogen peroxide to promote wound healing: Part 1: Regional intra-arterial therapy - technical surgical aspects. Part II: wound healing - clinical aspects. Amer J Surg 1964; 108: 621).

Significant reduction in the morbidity and mortality of experimental and clinical Clostridium welchii infections has been achieved by intra-arterial hydrogen peroxide (Bradley, B.E., Jr., Vedros, N.A., Defalco, A.J., Lawson, D.W., Vineyard, G.C. and Urschel, H.C. The effect of intra-arterial hydrogen peroxide in rabbits infected with clostridum perfringens. J Trauma 1965; 6: 799).

10.4 Arteriosclerotic Plaques

Arteriosclerotic plaques have been markedly reduced and have even disappeared following the intra-arterial infusion of hydrogen peroxide (Finney, J.W., Balla, G.A., Jay, B.E., Race, G.J., Urschel, H.C., Greenlee, R.G. and Mallams, J.T. Removal of cholesterol and other lipids from human atheromatous arteries by dilute hydrogen peroxide. Angiology 1966; 17: 223).

10.5 Shock Reversal

The reversal of many types of shock has been achieved by infusion of hydrogen peroxide into the thoracic aorta

(Urschel, H.C., Jr., Finney, J.W., Morales, A.R., Balla, G.A., Mallams, J.T. and Race, G.J. Myocardial protection during aortic cross clamping with hydrogen peroxide [Abstract], Circulation 1964; 30: 172), (Urschel, H.C., Jr., Finney, J.W., Balla, G.A., Race, G.J. and Mallams, J.T. Effects of hydrogen peroxide on the cardiovascular system. In Proceedings of the Third International Conference of Hyperbaric Medicine; 1965).

The time required to remove all hydrogen peroxide from the blood system when one-sixth of the total volume is 0.5% hydrogen peroxide is less than 0.1 second in human blood and 0.2 second in rabbit blood. This total peroxide volume would not be encountered under in vivo conditions; therefore, the life of the peroxide molecule in the vascular system would be considerably shorter than this.

It has also been shown that **the time of maximum oxygen concentration in a dilute blood system was at a point immediately following the complete disappearance of hydrogen peroxide from the solution.**

Elevated oxygen tensions have been observed during the intra-arterial infusion of hydrogen peroxide under a variety of experimental conditions in both animals and humans. In animals being infused into the thoracic aorta, samples collected from the femoral artery revealed **a total oxygen content equivalent to 4 to 6 atmospheres of pressure. In humans who were being infused into the thoracic aorta, blood samples were collected from the femoral artery and showed an oxygen content equivalent from 2 to 4 atmospheres of pure oxygen.**

It has been repeatedly observed that high concentrations of oxygen are present on both the arterial and venous side of a regional system being infused with dilute hydrogen peroxide solutions. The rate of the diffusion and final concentration in a given tissue will ultimately govern the degree to which the peroxide will exert its beneficial effect.

Studies indicate that exogenously generated superoxide anion by xanthine/xanthine oxidase reaction is spontaneously converted to **H_2O_2, which dilates human coronary arteries through vascular smooth muscle hyperpolarization**. Superoxide is converted to H_2O_2 likely by superoxide dismutase within vascular cells and dilates human coronary arterioles through a different pathway involving the activation of guanylate cyclase. These findings suggest that exogenously and endogenously produced H_2O_2 may elicit vasodilation by different mechanisms (Sato, A., Sakuma, I. and Gutterman, D.D. mechanism of dilation of reactive oxygen species in human coronary arterioles. Am J Physiol, 2003, 285: H_2345-H_2354).

10.6 Oxygenation of the Ischemic or Anoxic Myocardium of Small Animals

Employing 5- to 7-pound giant New Zealand rabbits, the myocardium was rendered anoxic by tracheal cross-clamp. **In all control animals, ischemic changes in the electrocardiograms, as noted by nodal block or arrhythmias, appeared in an average of cardiac arrest was 13 minutes, the range being from 10 to 16 minutes. All animals developed cardiac arrest and following failure to standard resuscitative methods, most of them could be resuscitated by simply adding hydrogen peroxide to the heart by whichever route of carrier solution administration was being employed.**

In 10 rabbits, a catheter was inserted retrograde through the right carotid artery into the base of the aorta. The left chest was opened, the pericardium opened and a variety of coronary arteries were ligated, including the circumflex, the anterior descending, the right coronary, or a combination of these. **Dilute hydrogen peroxide in concentrations ranging from 0.06% to 0.72% was infused** retrograde into the coronary arteries by a slow drip at the time of ligation. Ionosol-T was used as the carrier solution. Specific cardiographic abnormalities, associated myocardial ischemia such as S-T segment elevation, elevation or depression of the T-wave, nodal block and ventricular tachycardia or fibrillation could readily be reversed and often repeatedly so in a given animal by application of the peroxide. A drop in blood pressure associated with cardiac arrhythmias could also be reversed with similar therapy, but less consistently.

In another group of 10 animals, the left chest was opened, the pericardium was incised and a similar group of coronary arteries and branches were ligated. Ventricular fibrillation usually followed in several minutes. After cardiac massage, which was carried on for 15 minutes with no reversal of fibrillation, hydrogen peroxide in concentrations from 0.06% - 0.72% in Ionosol-T carrier solution at normal temperature was added directly to the epicardium. Reversal of arythmia to regular sinus rhythm in 7 to 10 animals was accomplished. Blood pressure was frequently reversed simultaneously.

In another group of 10 animals, the left chest was opened, the pericardium was incised and a similar group of coronary arteries and branches were ligated. Ventricular fibrillation usually followed in several minutes. After cardiac massage, which was carried on for 15 minutes with no reversal of fibrillation, hydrogen peroxide in concentrations from 0.06% - 0.72% in Ionosol-T carrier solution at normal temperature was added directly to the epicardium. Reversal of arythmia to regular sinus rhythm in 7 to 10 animals was accomplished. Blood pressure was frequently reversed simultaneously.

Two groups of 10 pigs each were studied, one group to evaluate the effect of hydrogen peroxide during coronary artery ligation and the other to serve as the control. In animals treated with

0.06% hydrogen peroxide in Hank's solution, ventricular fibrillation occurred in only one-half of the animals between 5 and 30 minutes, with an **average time of 20 minutes. Five animals never developed ventricular fibrillation. All of those which did were easily resuscitable with cardiac massage and electrical defibrillation. All except I maintained normal blood pressures with a mean of 100 mm Hg. Nine H$_2$O$_2$-treated animals lived 3 hours and were sacrificed.** One animal with an average blood pressure of 75 mm Hg died 2 hours after coronary artery ligation.

In all the animals used as controls, following a terminal episode when no blood pressure or cardiac activity could be obtained with the standard methods of resuscitation, dilute solutions of hydrogen peroxide were added to the myocardium. In 4 animals resuscitation could be obtained in spite of massive infarctions and systemic acidosis. No toxicity was demonstrated during the period of therapy.

10.7 Human Observations

Because of the apparent advantages in myocardial support during situations of anoxia, hydrogen peroxide was employed in a 60-year old white female. She developed vascular collapse of unknown etiology and was unresponsive to the conventional methods of resuscitation. A cardiac catheter was passed through the right brachial artery to the root of the aorta. Electrocardiogram and blood pressure were monitored. **Within I minute after the infusion of 0.12% hydrogen peroxide, the electrocardiogram reverted from a nodal rhythm to a regular sinus rhythm, and the mean arterial pressure increased 35 to 70 mm Hg within 3 minutes.** In 10 minutes after cessation of the infusion, the electrocardiogram again reverted to nodal rhythm and the blood pressure dropped. This sequence of events was carried out six times during the course of one evening. Each time the reversal of the electrocardiographic abnormalities and hypotension was achieved with hydrogen peroxide.

10.8 Ventilation of Rabbits with a H_2O_2 Aerosol

In these studies, rabbits were anesthetized with pentobarbital sodium, intubated and placed on 100% oxygen on a Byrd respirator. The chest was opened between the fourth and fifth intercostals space. The pericardium was slit and a flanged PE-90 catheter was secured into the left atrium by a purse-string suture. The chest was closed and the animal was allowed to breath 100% oxygen for 30 minutes prior to the aerosol. **Concentrations of hydrogen peroxide from 1% to 6% in normal saline were nebulized as an aerosol. Following nebulization therapy, the left atrial blood of these animals was found to be "supersaturated" with oxygen, containing quantities equivalent to that expected with oxygen at 3 atmospheres absolute pressure.** If this value were exceeded, small bubbles began to appear in the samples collected. **The 1% aerosol, which was least irritating, provided as good arterial oxygen concentration as did the higher concentrations.**

Although this report is involved predominantly with pilot data, certain observations warrant comment. Dilute solutions of hydrogen peroxide provide a supersaturation of oxygen in plasma and tissue fluids equivalent to from 2 to 12 atmospheres.

In the concentrations and rates of application employed in these experiments, no evidence of intravascular emboli or capillary obstruction have been noted, nor has oxidation of tissue been a problem. It is necessary to employ vasodilators with the intra-arterial use of hydrogen peroxide, since arterial spasm is produced by this method.

Both peritoneal and rectal perfusion of hydrogen peroxide provide high concentrations of oxygen in the portal vein and inferior vena cava. If the lungs are intact, this oxygen is promptly lost in one passage through the pulmonary circulation.

Long-term toxicity studies employing hydrogen peroxide intravascular or by direct application to organs on twenty four hours of constant therapy do not demonstrate significant changes in rabbits followed for two months.

Hydrogen peroxide is broken down very rapidly when introduced into the blood stream in both rabbits and humans; **in dilute solutions, intravascular hydrogen peroxide has no unacceptable deleterious effect on formed blood elements** (with the exception of dogs, where, due to an apparent deficient in RBC and plasma catalase, methemoglobin is produced); (Mallams, J.T., Balla, G.A. and Finney, J.W. Regional oxygenation and irradiation in the treatment of malignant tumors. Progress in Clinc Cancer 1965; 1: 137), and **the breakdown of hydrogen peroxide by biological fluids results in the supersaturation of these fluids with oxygen** (Jay, B.E., Finney, J.W., Balla, G.A. and Mallams, J.T. The supersaturation of biologic fluids with oxygen by decomposition of hydrogen peroxide. Texas Rep Biol & Med 1964; 22: 106). **The magnitude of the supersaturation is equivalent to several atmospheres of oxygen.**

Kann, Mengel, and others have shown that the formation of lipid peroxides is one sequela to exposure to oxygen at high pressure. The authors have noted a reduction in the subintimal lipid deposits and atheromatous plaques in the arteries of individuals being infused intra-arterially with hydrogen peroxide.

Several patients who have been infused intra-arterially with hydrogen peroxide as an adjunct to irradiation therapy in the management of their malignant disease have undergone postmortem examination. During the autopsy, the catheter was left in place, the aorta was split longitudinally, and the tip of the catheter marked.

Sections were prepared from the aorta immediately above and below tip for comparative histologic evaluation by oil red-O and H and E stains.

All patients were being **infused into the abdominal aorta with 0.48 percent hydrogen peroxide in Ionosol T**. Venous samples were taken before and during the last minute of infusion and the results of the two samples compared. During the entire infusion period (20 minutes), the patient was reclined and relaxed.

The evaluation of aortas taken at postmortem from patients who had been treated with intra-arterial hydrogen peroxide showed the following changes:

In all cases studied to date, the patients have received hydrogen peroxide infusion alone as an adjunct to other modes of therapy for a variety of conditions over extended periods of time ranging from 4 to 16 weeks. During this time, the individuals received daily infusions of 250 ml of hydrogen peroxide in Ionosol T with **a peroxide concentration ranging from 0.36 to 0.48 percent.**

Upon gross examination, the segment of the aorta being infused was found to be different from the area not being infused. **This difference was marked by a decrease in the number and severity of atheromatous plaques, and an increase in flexibility and elasticity of the vessel.** Histologic evaluation by oil red-O stained sections **showed a decrease in total subliminal lipid deposits.** When weighed samples of the vessels were extracted and total lipids determined, **it was found that approximately a 50 percent reduction in total lipids had occurred in the area being infused with hydrogen peroxide.** In my opinion, this work is some of the most exciting work in the last 50 years!

In vitro studies on human aortas incubated with hydrogen peroxide, the results indicate a bi- or multiphase reaction

which starts immediately with the elution of relatively large quantities of cholesterol, cholesterol esters, phospholipid, triglyceride and free fatty acids: the total concentration of these components in the supernatant fluid decreases over a period of the next few hours. This decrease if followed by a subsequent increase in total concentration at 12 to 24 hours. **The same general results have been obtained with human aorta in saline exposed to oxygen at five atmospheres absolute pressure. (**: Finney, J.W., Jay, B.E., Race, G.J., Urschel, H.C., Mallams, J.T. and Balla, G.A. **Removal of cholesterol and other lipids from experimental animal and human atheromatous arteries by dilute hydrogen peroxide.** Angiology 1966; 17: 223-228.). **I believe that this data indicates the signaling capability of H$_2$O$_2$ because, even though it is present for a very short time, it can activate processes which occur sometime later. This effect is being reported with increasing frequency for many of the EMODs.**

10.9 Wound Healing with Hydrogen Peroxide Infusion

During the early studies in the treatment of patients with intra-arterial hydrogen peroxide and irradiation therapy, two observations were made. In some of the patients, **not only did the tumor respond more rapidly to irradiation, but also it was found that the wounds would heal at a much faster rate and with less scar formation.** As a result of this, wounds that were refractory to conventional modes of therapy were treated with intra-arterial hydrogen peroxide either alone or in combination with intra-arterial antibiotics. The major reasons given for delays in wound healing are: 1) inadequate nutrition, 2) necrotic tissue, 3) foreign bodies, 4) bacterial infections, 5) interference with blood supply, 6) lymphatic blockage and 7) diabetes mellitus. Many of these factors that interfere with wound healing can be combined under the broad, general term of "tissue anoxia." It was believed that if tissue anoxia could be altered by regional super oxygenation, an increased healing rate could be achieved. The patients used in this study were those who have exhibited delayed wound healing that has been refractory to conventional modes of therapy. The techniques used were daily or twice daily infusions of intra-arterial antibiotics (Mallams, J.T., Finney, J.W. and Balla, G.A. The use of hydrogen peroxide as a source of oxygen in regional intra-arterial infusion system. South Med J 1962; 55: 230), (Balla, G.A., Hutton, S.B., Mallams, J.T., Aronoff, B.L., Byrd, D.L., Finney, J.W. and Race, G.J. Retrograde catheterization of the external carotid artery via the superficial temporal artery for the treatment of head and neck malignancies by continuous intra-arterial infusion. Am Surgeon 1963; 29: 265), (Balla, G.A., Finney, J.W. and Mallams, J.T. A method for selective tissue oxygenation utilizing regional intra-arterial infusion techniques. Am Surgeon 1963; 29: 496), (Finney, J.W., Mallams, J.T. and Balla, G.A. Increased available oxygen through regional intra-arterial infusion. Proc Am Assoc Cancer Res 1962; 3: 318), (Mallams, J.T., Balla, G.A., Finney, J.W. and Aronoff, B.L. Regional oxygenation and irradiation. Head and Neck. Arch Otol 1964; 79: 155), (Balla, G.A., Mallams, J.T., Hutton, S.B., Aronoff, B.L. and Byrd, D.L. The treatment of head and neck malignancies by continuous intra-arterial infusion of methotrexate. Am J Surg 1962; 104: 699).

10.10 H_2O_2 Cardiac Resuscitation

Ventricular fibrillation or cardiac arrest was produced in 40 rabbits by tracheal occlusion or circumflex coronary artery ligation. **Regional application of 0.12 to .24% hydrogen peroxide via coronary artery infusion or epicardial application returned the heart to regular sinus rhythm and elevated blood pressure to normal, in contrast to ten control animals who could not be resuscitated with standard methods.** The procedure was repeated in ten goats undergoing anterior descending coronary artery ligation. The electrocardiogram, arterial and venous pressure, pH and myocardial tissue oxygen tension were monitored. Myocardial tissue oxygen tension values increased from two to six times control values following hydrogen peroxide application. Low molecular weight dextran and papaverine improved effective coronary artery infusion of hydrogen peroxide. Dimethyl sulfoxide (DMSO) may improve diffusion in the thick myocardium.

Following the failure of conventional resuscitation methods, hydrogen peroxide was employed in one human case with temporary reversal of ventricular fibrillation to regular sinus rhythm and elevation of the blood pressure to normal (Urschel, H.C., Jr., Finney, J.W., Morales, A.R., Balla, G.A. and Mallams, J.T. Cardiac resuscitation with hydrogen peroxide. Abstract of the 38th Scientific Sessions. 1965; Suppl II, Vol. 31 & 32).

10.11 Regional H_2O_2 for Clostridia Myositis

The intra-arterial infusion of hydrogen peroxide has been used as a method for producing a hyperoxic environment in experimental animals for the treatment of experimentally induced clostridia myositis. Eighty-five rabbits were employed in this study; 43 were controls and 42 were experimental animals. In the experimental study, 21 animals were treated with hydrogen peroxide by each route of administration. In this group, **52.4% of the animals receiving the intra-arterial H_2O_2 infusion and 66.6% receiving intramuscular clysis with H_2O_2 survived. There were no survivors past 72 hours in the control group.** (Finney, J.W., Haberman, S., Race, G.J., Bala, G.A. and Mallams, J.T. Local and regional application of hydrogen peroxide in the control of clostridia myositis in rabbits. J Bacterio 1967; 93: 1430-1437).

It has been shown in vivo that the breakdown of hydrogen peroxide progresses at a sufficiently rapid rate to prevent any unacceptable side reactions, and that oxygen supplied in this fashion is in a form which is metabolically usable by the animal.

It became evident during the study that the rate at which the spread of the disease was halted and at which the disease subsequently healed was more rapid than expected in the hydrogen peroxide-treated animals. (Balla, G.A., Finney, J.W., Aronoff, B.L., Byrd, D.L., Race, G.J., Mallams, J.T. and Davis, G. Use of intra-arterial hydrogen peroxide to promote wound. Part II. Wound healing, clinical aspects. Am J Surg 1964; 108: 625-629), (Finney, J.W., Balla, G.A., Collier, R.E., Wakley, J., Urschel, H.C. and Mallams, J.T. Differential localization of isotopes in tumors through the use of intra-arterial hydrogen peroxide. Part 1. Basic Science. Am J Roentgenol Radium Therapy Nucl Med 1965; 94: 783-788), (Jay, B.W., Finney, J.W., Balla, G.A. and Mallams, J.T. The supersaturation of biologic fluids with oxygen by the decomposition of hydrogen peroxide. Tex Rept Biol Med 1964; 22: 106-109), (Mallams, J.T., Balla, G.A., Finney, J.W. and Aronoff, B.L. Regional oxygenation and irradiation. Head and neck. Arch Otolaryngology 1964; 79: 155-159).

The heme-containing protein complex, NADPH oxidase, can produce large amounts of O_2^{-} and its derivative upon activation. In an inflammatory environment, **H_2O_2 is produced by activated macrophages at an estimated rate of 2-6 X 10^{-14} mol/h^{-1}/cell^{-1} and can reach as high as 10-100 μM in the vicinity of these cells** (Nathan, C.F. and Root, R.K. Hydrogen peroxide release from mouse peritoneal macrophages: dependence on sequential activation and triggering. J Exp Med 146: 1648-1662).

When body tissues are damaged, neutrophils and other phagocytes enter the damaged area. These cells become activated, releasing O_2^{-} and HOCl that can help to remove foreign organisms at the injury site. For example, **HOCl can oxidize thiol (~SH) groups on proteins**. When tissues are crushed or torn, iron can be released from cells, both a free iron and in the form of heme-containing proteins (such as myoglobin), and as the storage protein ferritin. **Free iron can convert O_2^{-} and H_2O_2 into highly damaging .OH. O_2^{-} can cause a limited release of iron from ferritin, and H_2O_2 can release iron from heme proteins.**

PART II - HYDROGEN PEROXIDE AND SUPEROXIDE:

Essentials for Aerobic Life, Prooxidant Protection and Oxidative Self-Healing

11.0 NADPH OXIDASE (NOX) BRIEF REVIEW

The view of **EMODs as an unintended consequence of life on an aerobic planet is altered in a fundamental way by the recent discovery of a family of enzymes, the sole function of which is to generate reactive oxygen and hydrogen peroxide.**

Because of **the rapid dismutation of $O_2^{\cdot-}$ to H_2O_2 (spontaneous, 10^5 $[mol/L]^{-1} \cdot s^{-1}$, SOD-catalyzed, 10^9 $[mol/L]^{-1} \times s^{-1}$),** endogenous rates of cellular H_2O_2 production can be used as an indirect measure of $O_2^{\cdot-}$ formation, recognizing that such measurements will also reflect direct divalent reduction of molecular oxygen to H_2O_2. Intracellular steady state H_2O_2 can be estimated by aminotriazole-mediated catalase inactivation (Royall, J.A., Gwin, P.D., Parks, D.A. and Freeman, B.A. Responses of vascular endothelial oxidant metabolism to lipopolysaccharide and tumor necrosis factor-*a* (TNF-α). Arch Biochem Biophys 1992; 294: 686-694).

Some of the following material was abstracted, excerpted or modified from: **The Nox Family of NAD(P)H Oxidases: Host Defense and Beyond.** Miklós Geiszt and Thomas L. Leto. **J. Biol. Chem., Vol. 279, Issue 50, 51715-51718, December 10, 2004.**

Reactive oxygen species (ROS) **EMODs** (Leto, T. L. (1999) in *Inflammation Basic Principles and Clinical Correlates* (Gallin, J. I., and Snyderman, R., eds) pp. 769–787, Lippincott Williams & Wilkins, Philadelphia) **play diverse roles in biology, including host defense, hormone biosynthesis, fertilization, and redox signaling involved in mitogenesis, apoptosis, or oxygen sensing.** Until recently, much of our understanding of the mechanisms of EMOD generation and their functions in man was based on studies of phagocytic cells, where abundant microbicidal oxidants released during engulfment of microbes serve as a **first line of host defense**. In phagocytic cells the ROS precursor superoxide is produced by a NADPH oxidase complex (Leto, T. L. (1999) in *Inflammation Basic Principles and Clinical Correlates* (Gallin, J. I., and Snyderman, R., eds) pp. 769–787, Lippincott Williams & Wilkins, Philadelphia) (Quinn, M. T., and Gauss, K. A. (2004) *J. Leukocyte Biol.* **76,** 760–781) (Cross, A. R., and Segal, A. W. (2004) *Biochim. Biophys. Acta* **1657,** 1–22).

The phagocytic oxidase (phox) consists of a membrane-bound flavocytochrome b_{558}, several modular cytosolic regulators ($p47^{phox}$, $p67^{phox}$, $p40^{phox}$), and a small GTPase, Rac1 or Rac2. The cytochrome is a complex of two proteins: a flavin- and heme-binding glycoprotein ($gp91^{phox}$) and a smaller subunit ($p22^{phox}$). With the recent expansion of information available in human genome databases, several novel $gp91^{phox}$ homologues have been recognized, suggesting that **enzymes similar to the phagocytic oxidase function in a variety of tissues, notably the colon, kidney, thyroid gland, testis, salivary glands, airways, and lymphoid organs** (Suh, Y. A., Arnold, R. S., Lassegue, B., Shi, J., Xu, X., Sorescu, D., Chung, A. B., Griendling, K. K., and Lambeth, J. D. (1999) *Nature* **401,** 79–82) (Geiszt, M., Kopp, J. B., Varnai, P., and Leto, T. L. (2000) *Proc. Natl. Acad. Sci. U. S. A.* **97,** 8010–8014) (Dupuy, C., Ohayon, R., Valent, A., Noel-Hudson, M. S., Deme, D., and Virion, A. (1999) *J. Biol. Chem.* **274,** 37265–37269) (De Deken, X., Wang, D., Many, M. C., Costagliola, S., Libert, F., Vassart, G., Dumont, J. E., and Miot, F. (2000) *J. Biol. Chem.* **275,** 23227–23233) (Shiose, A., Kuroda, J., Tsuruya, K., Hirai, M., Hirakata, H., Naito, S., Hattori, M., Sakaki, Y., and Sumimoto, H. (2001) *J. Biol. Chem.* **276,** 1417–1423) (Banfi, B., Molnar, G., Maturana, A., Steger, K., Hegedus, B., Demaurex, N., and Krause, K. H. (2001) *J. Biol. Chem.* **276,** 37594–37601).

The physiological functions of these novel NADPH oxidases, now designated the Nox family, are currently under intensive investigation.

11.1 NAD(P)H Oxidase 1 (Nox1)

Nox1, the first recognized homologue of gp91[phox], **now termed Nox2,** is **detected in abundance in the colon and at lower levels in uterus, prostate, and vascular smooth muscle cells** (Suh, Y. A., Arnold, R. S., Lassegue, B., Shi, J., Xu, X., Sorescu, D., Chung, A. B., Griendling, K. K., and Lambeth, J. D. (1999) *Nature* **401,** 79–82).

In early work exploring the function of Nox1, heterologous **overexpression of Nox1 in NIH-3T3 cells was associated with increased cell proliferation and resulted in tumor formation when these cells were injected into nude mice** (Suh, Y. A., Arnold, R. S., Lassegue, B., Shi, J., Xu, X., Sorescu, D., Chung, A. B., Griendling, K. K., and Lambeth, J. D. (1999) *Nature* **401,** 79–82). Subsequent reports proposed **that hydrogen peroxide (H_2O_2) formation in these Nox1-expressing cells is responsible for the increased mitogenesis** (Arnold, R. S., Shi, J., Murad, E., Whalen, A. M., Sun, C. Q., Polavarapu, R., Parthasarathy, S., Petros, J. A., and Lambeth, J. D. (2001) *Proc. Natl. Acad. Sci. U. S. A.* **98,** 5550–5555).

These findings were enthusiastically received because enhanced cellular ROS generation has been linked to the enhanced growth triggered by growth factor stimulation or tumorigenesis (Sundaresan, M., Yu, Z.-X., Ferrans, V. J., Irani, K., and Finkel, T. (1995) *Science* **270,** 296–299) (Irani, K., Xia, Y., Zweier, J., Sollott, S., Der, C., Rearon, E., Sundaresan, M., Finkel, T., and Goldschmidt-Clermont, P. (1997) *Science* **275,** 1649–1652) (Szatrowski, T. P., and Nathan, C. F. (1991) *Cancer Res.* **51,** 794–798).

Cells **overexpressing Nox1 also showed increased vascular endothelial growth factor expression, suggesting that ROS produced by Nox1 also stimulates angiogenesis in these tumors** (Arbiser, J. L., Petros, J., Klafter, R., Govindajaran, B., McLaughlin, E. R., Brown, L. F., Cohen, C., Moses, M., Kilroy, S., Arnold, R. S., and Lambeth, J. D. (2002) *Proc. Natl. Acad. Sci. U. S. A.* **99,** 715–720). **Further studies revealed, however, that these Nox1-transfected**

209

Prof Randolph Michael Howes MD,PhD

NIH-3T3 cell lines also carry a mutant form of Ras that can account for the enhanced proliferation and transformation (Lambeth, J. D. (2004) *Nat. Rev. Immunol.* **4,** 181–189).

Observations in colon-derived epithelial cells, which naturally express Nox1, do not support the proposed role of Nox1 as a mitogenic oxidase. In HT29 colon cancer cells, **the suppression of Nox1 levels does not affect cell proliferation** (Geiszt, M., Lekstrom, K., Brenner, S., Hewitt, S. M., Dana, R., Malech, H. L., and Leto, T. L. (2003) *J. Immunol.* **171,** 299–306). Furthermore, significantly higher Nox1 expression occurs when HT29 or CaCo$_2$ cells are induced to differentiate by interferon-γ or by calcitriol (Geiszt, M., Lekstrom, K., Brenner, S., Hewitt, S. M., Dana, R., Malech, H. L., and Leto, T. L. (2003) *J. Immunol.* **171,** 299–306). Finally, a survey of various human cancerous tissues showed **Nox1 expression is limited to colon tumors and the highest Nox1 expression occurs in more differentiated tumors** (Geiszt, M., Lekstrom, K., Brenner, S., Hewitt, S. M., Dana, R., Malech, H. L., and Leto, T. L. (2003) *J. Immunol.* **171,** 299–306). **Together, these findings suggest that Nox1 serves some other specialized function in differentiated colon epithelium unrelated to mitogenesis.**

Several observations suggest that **Nox1 could serve as a host defense oxidase.** Nox1 induction, along with increased ROS release, was detected in guinea pig gastric pit cells primed with *Helico-bacter pylori* lipopolysaccharides (LPS) (Kawahara, T., Teshima, S., Oka, A., Sugiyama, T., Kishi, K., and Rokutan, K. (2001) *Infect. Immun.* **69,** 4382–4389). Kawahara et al. (Kawahara, T., Kuwano, Y., Teshima-Kondo, S., Takeya, R., Sumimoto, H., Kishi, K., Tsunawaki, S., Hirayama, T., and Rokutan, K. (2004) *J. Immunol.* **172,** 3051–3058) proposed that **LPS from pathogenic H. pylori strains potently stimulates ROS production** through a toll-like receptor 4 (TLR4) pathway. In contrast, colon epithelial cells, which lack TLR4 receptors and do not respond to LPS, exhibit high Nox1-mediated ROS production in response to flagellin from *Salmonella enteritides,* acting through TLR5-dependent pathways (Kawahara, T., Kuwano, Y., Teshima-Kondo, S., Takeya, R., Sumimoto, H., Kishi, K., Tsunawaki, S., Hirayama, T., and Rokutan, K. (2004) *J. Immunol.* **172**, 3051–3058).

A role for Nox1 in innate immunity was also suggested by experiments showing that **Nox1 could replace Nox2 (gp91phox) in the regulated production of superoxide**, thereby partially rescuing the deficiency in superoxide production observed in chronic **granulomatous disease neutrophils** (Geiszt, M., Lekstrom, K., Brenner, S., Hewitt, S. M., Dana, R., Malech, H. L., and Leto, T. L. (2003) *J. Immunol.* **171**, 299–306). Together, these findings demonstrate that Nox1 is functionally similar to gp91^{phox}/Nox2.

Although few reports have explored the role of Nox1 in the colon, where it is most abundant, several groups have examined **the possible involvement of Nox1 in ROS production in vascular tissue.** Nox1 expression in cultured smooth muscle cells was described by Suh et al., and several other groups confirmed these findings. Several agonists, including platelet-derived growth factor, angiotensin II, and prostaglandin F2α, appear to up-regulate Nox1 mRNA levels in cultured smooth muscle cells, whereas suppression of Nox1 expression by antisense techniques inhibited superoxide production (Suh, Y. A., Arnold, R. S., Lassegue, B., Shi, J., Xu, X., Sorescu, D., Chung, A. B., Griendling, K. K., and Lambeth, J. D. (1999) *Nature* **401**, 79–82). Thus, production of ROS by Nox1 in these cells could have roles in angiotensin II- and growth factor-induced cell hypertrophy or proliferation.

11.2 NAD(P)H Oxidase 3 (Nox3)

Nox3, a 568-amino acid protein, also has close similarities to gp91^{phox}/Nox2 (58% sequence identity) (Kikuchi, H., Hikage, M., Miyashita, H., and Fukumoto, M. (2000) *Gene (Amst.)* **254**, 237–243). Nox3 mRNA was not detected in adult or in fetal tissues by Northern blotting; however, reverse transcription-PCR experiments **detected Nox3 mRNA in several fetal**

tissues, including kidney, liver, lung, and spleen (Kikuchi, H., Hikage, M., Miyashita, H., and Fukumoto, M. (2000) *Gene (Amst.)* **254,** 237–243) (Cheng, G., Cao, Z., Xu, X., van Meir, E. G., and Lambeth, J. D. (2001) *Gene (Amst.)* **269,** 131–140). Recently, a unique role for this oxidase within the inner ear was revealed by positional cloning studies that mapped genetic lesions causing the *head tilt* (*het*) phenotype in mice (Paffenholz, R., Bergstrom, R. A., Pasutto, F., Wabnitz, P., Munroe, R. J., Jagla, W., Heinzmann, U., Marquardt, A., Bareiss, A., Laufs, J., Russ, A., Stumm, G., Schimenti, J. C., and Bergstrom, D. E. (2004) *Genes Dev.* **18,** 486–491). **Mice with *Nox3* mutations exhibit impaired otoconial morphogenesis and defects in perception of gravity and balance.** It was proposed that this oxidase mediates ROS-dependent conformation changes in otoconin 90 involved in the nucleation of calcite crystal formation during the development of otoconia.

11.3 NAD(P)H Oxidase 4 (Nox4)

Nox4, a 578-amino acid protein with 39% sequence identity to gp91^{phox}/Nox2 was originally described as a **renal oxidase (Renox)** because **its expression at high levels is limited to the kidney** (Geiszt, M., Kopp, J. B., Varnai, P., and Leto, T. L. (2000) *Proc. Natl. Acad. Sci. U. S. A.* **97,** 8010–8014) (Shiose, A., Kuroda, J., Tsuruya, K., Hirai, M., Hirakata, H., Naito, S., Hattori, M., Sakaki, Y., and Sumimoto, H. (2001) *J. Biol. Chem.* **276,** 1417–1423). However, **the specific intrarenal distribution of Nox4 mRNA differs significantly in mice and humans.** *In situ* hybridization in mouse kidney sections demonstrated the highest levels in proximal tubules, whereas immunohistochemical and *in situ* hybridization studies on human kidneys detected Nox4 expression in distal portions of the nephron. When overexpressed in NIH-3T3 fibroblasts, **Nox4 increased superoxide production and induced a cellular senescence phenotype.**

Expression of antisense Nox4 mRNA in HEK293 cells, which contain endogenous Nox4, resulted in a decreased NADH- and NADPH- dependent superoxide production *in vitro*.

The expression pattern of Nox4 is consistent with several renal-specific functions. One proposed role in oxygen sensing and regulation of erythropoietin (EPO) synthesis (Geiszt, M., Kopp, J. B., Varnai, P., and Leto, T. L. (2000) *Proc. Natl. Acad. Sci. U. S. A.* **97**, 8010–8014) (Shiose, A., Kuroda, J., Tsuruya, K., Hirai, M., Hirakata, H., Naito, S., Hattori, M., Sakaki, Y., and Sumimoto, H. (2001) *J. Biol. Chem.* **276**, 1417–1423) is based on several findings. **The phagocyte cell homologue of Nox4, gp91phox/Nox2, was described as an oxygen sensor in the lung** (Wang, D., Youngson, C., Wong, V., Yeger, H., Dinauer, M. C., Vega-Saenz Miera, E., Rudy, B., and Cutz, E. (1996) *Proc. Natl. Acad. Sci. U. S. A.* **93**, 13182–13187).

In the kidney, EPO synthesis also occurs in proximal tubules, and **ROS are implicated as negative feedback signals regulating EPO synthesis** (Elbert, B. L., and Bunn, H. F. (1999) *Blood* **94**, 1864–1877). Although the hypoxia-inducible factor-1α, which regulates EPO synthesis, is regulated by proline hydroxylases (Bruick, R. K. (2003) *Genes Dev.* **17**, 2614–2623), **other hypoxia-inducible factor-1α-independent transcription factors, such as GATA-2, are direct H_2O_2-sensitive targets that suppress EPO expression** (Imagawa, S., Yamamoto, M., and Miura, T. (1997) *Blood* **89**, 1430–1439).

Finally, recent knock-out studies indicate that **superoxide dismutase 3**, which is also expressed in renal proximal tubules, **has a role in erythroid responses to hypoxia** (Suliman, H. B., Ali, M., and Piantadosi, C. A. (2004) *Blood* **104**, 43–50). These observations along with the high constitutive activity of Nox4 are consistent with a **role for Nox4 in oxygen sensing.**

A distinct possibility related to high renal Nox4 expression is that it serves as a phox-like antimicrobial system by releasing ROS into the glomerular filtrate; this might explain **significant (*i.e.* 100 µM) urinary hydrogen peroxide levels** (Varma, S. D., and Devamanoharan, P. S. (1990) *Free Radic. Res.* **8**, 73–78). **Other possible functions of the renal oxidase include roles in oxidation or detoxification of urine wastes or in renal pH or electrolyte homeostasis, based on the proton-generating and electrogenic activities of all NADPH oxidases.** Finally, Gorin *et al.* (Gorin, Y., Ricono, J. M., Wagner, B., Kim, N. H., Bhandari, B., Ghosh Choudhury, G., and Abboud, H. E. (2004) *Biochem. J.* **381**, 231–239) suggested that a Nox4-based oxidase is stimulated in response to angiotensin II in mesangial cells.

Several groups have also explored possible extra-renal functions of Nox4. According to Yang *et al.* (Yang, S., Madyastha, P., Bingel, S., Ries, W., and Key, L. (2001) *J. Biol. Chem.* **276**, 5452–5458), **Nox4** and gp91^{phox} (Nox2) **are present in murine osteoclasts, where they may provide an oxidative basis for bone resorption.** Low Nox4 expression is detected in vascular smooth muscle cells, where it appears to be down-regulated by agonists that increase Nox1 expression. Although the relative contribution of Nox4 to vascular ROS production remains unclear, **Nox4 was also suggested as the major component of an endothelial NAD(P)H oxidase** (Ago, T., Kitazono, T., Ooboshi, H., Iyama, T., Han, Y. H., Takada, J., Wakisaka, M., Ibayashi, S., Utsumi, H., and Iida, M. (2004) *Circulation* **109**, 227–233). In several cell lines, **growth factor or insulin receptor stimulation increases ROS production, which has an enhancing effect on tyrosine phosphorylation in part through inhibition of protein-tyrosine phosphatases** (Rhee, S. G., Chang, T. S., Bae, Y. S., Lee, S. R., Kang, S. W. (2003) *J. Am. Soc. Nephrol.* **14**, S211–S215).

A recent study indicates that **Nox4 mediates insulin-stimulated ROS production in 3T3-L1 adipocytes** (Mahadev, K., Motoshima, H., Wu, X., Ruddy, J. M., Arnold, R. S., Cheng, G., Lambeth,

J. D., and Goldstein, B. J. (2004) *Mol. Cell. Biol.* **24**, 1844–1854). Further studies in gene-targeted animals may confirm roles for Nox4 in insulin signaling.

11.4 NAD(P)H Oxidase 5 (Nox5)

NADPH oxidase 5 (Nox5) is more distantly related to the other Nox proteins, with an overall homology to gp91^{phox} of 27%. The protein consists of 737 amino acids and contains an additional N-terminal extension comprising four calcium-binding, EF-hand motifs that appear to render the enzyme directly responsive to calcium. **Superoxide production by Nox5-expressing cells is induced by the calcium ionophore ionomycin** (Banfi, B., Molnar, G., Maturana, A., Steger, K., Hegedus, B., Demaurex, N., and Krause, K. H. (2001) *J. Biol. Chem.* **276**, 37594–37601).

Recent work demonstrated that the EF-hands engage in direct, calcium-dependent interactions with the C-terminal domain of Nox5. **In testis, Nox5 mRNA was detected in pachytene spermatocytes** (Banfi, B., Molnar, G., Maturana, A., Steger, K., Hegedus, B., Demaurex, N., and Krause, K. H. (2001) *J. Biol. Chem.* **276**, 37594–37601), **raising the possibility that it may function in mature spermatozoa, such as in oxidative changes associated with human sperm capacitation or the acrosome reaction** (Baker, M. A., and Aitken, R. J. (2004) *Mol. Cell. Endocrinol.* **216**, 47–54). **In the spleen,** Nox5 message localizes to the mantle zone surrounding germinal centers (areas rich in B cells) and to periarterial lymphoid sheets (where mostly T cells are present) (Banfi, B., Molnar, G., Maturana, A., Steger, K., Hegedus, B., Demaurex, N., and Krause, K. H. (2001) *J. Biol. Chem.* **276**, 37594–37601).

T and B lymphocytes produce ROS when stimulated by some receptor agonists (Devadas, S., Zaritskaya, L., Rhee, S. G., Oberley, L., and Williams, M. S. (2002) *J. Exp. Med.* **195**, 59–70) (Lee, J. R., and Koretzky, G. A. (1998) *Eur. J. Immunol.* **28**, 4188–4197).

A role for Nox5 in cell proliferation was suggested by Brar *et al.*
(Brar, S. S., Corbin, Z., Kennedy, T. P., Hemendinger, R., Thornton,
L., Bommarius, B., Arnold, R. S., Whorton, A. R., Sturrock, A. B.,
Huecksteadt, T. P., Quinn, M. T., Krenitsky, K., Ardie, K. G., Lambeth,
J. D., and Hoidal, J. R. (2003) *Am. J. Physiol.* **285,** C353–C369), who
**demonstrated that antisense oligonucleotide-mediated
down-regulation of Nox5 expression in DU 145 prostate
cancer cells inhibits cell proliferation**.

11.5 Dual Oxidases (Duox1 and Duox2)

Dual oxidases, originally designated thyroid oxidases (thOX
or tox), were **cloned from human and porcine thyroid glands
and proposed to serve in iodide organification during
thyroxine synthesis** (Dupuy, C., Ohayon, R., Valent, A., Noel-
Hudson, M. S., Deme, D., and Virion, A. (1999) *J. Biol. Chem.* **274,**
37265–37269) (De Deken, X., Wang, D., Many, M. C., Costagliola, S.,
Libert, F., Vassart, G., Dumont, J. E., and Miot, F. (2000) *J. Biol. Chem.*
275, 23227–23233). The Duox (<u>du</u>al <u>ox</u>idase) nomenclature was
suggested as these proteins contain an N-terminal extracellular
peroxidase-like domain and a gp91^{phox}-like oxidase portion (Dupuy,
C., Ohayon, R., Valent, A., Noel-Hudson, M. S., Deme, D., and Virion,
A. (1999) *J. Biol. Chem.* **274,** 37265–37269) (Edens, W. A., Sharling,
L., Cheng, G., Shapira, R., Kinkade, J. M., Lee, T., Edens, H. A., Tang, X.,
Sullards, C., Flaherty, D. B., Benian, G. M., and Lambeth, J. D. (2001) *J.
Cell Biol.* **154,** 879–891).

Human Duox1 and Duox2 proteins contain 1551 and 1548 amino
acids, respectively, and show 83% sequence similarity. Separating the
peroxidase-like domain and the NADPH oxidase portion are an
additional transmembrane segment and two EF-hand motifs. The
peroxidase-like domains of Duox proteins are unusual in that they
lack conserved histidine residues found in all other peroxidases,
considered essential for heme binding. The presence of EF-hands
suggests that calcium directly regulates these enzymes, consistent
with early observations showing **that calcium ionophores**

stimulate H$_2$O$_2$ production in thyroid cells (Dupuy, C., Deme, D., Kaniewski, J., Pommier, J., and Virion, A. (1988) *FEBS Lett. 233,* 74–78).

Heterologous Duox expression in several mammalian cell lines fails to reconstitute ROS release, suggesting other tissue-specific oxidase components are needed for Duox activity (De Deken, X., Wangm, D., Dumont, J. E., and Miot, F. (2002) *Exp. Cell Res.* **273,** 187–196).

In thyroid follicles, **the Duox proteins are detected on the thyrocyte apical surface, where they could supply H$_2$O$_2$ for thyroperoxidase-mediated iodination and cross-linking of thyroglobulin tyrosine residues.** Duox2 is clearly essential for thyroxine biosynthesis because **Duox2 mutations result in congenital hypothyroidism,** even in heterozygotes (Moreno, J. C., Bikker, H., Kempers, M. J., van Trotsenburg, A. S., Baas, F., de Vijlder, J. J., Vulsma, T., and Ris-Stalpers, C. (2002) *N. Engl. J. Med.* **347,** 95–102).

The role of Duox1 in thyroid tissue has not been clarified. Duox proteins are also encoded by the genomes of lower species, such as *Caenorhabditis elegans.* Defective cuticle formation was observed during *C. elegans* development following inhibition of Duox expression by RNA interference. **It was proposed that Duox provides the ROS for oxidative cross-linking of extracellular matrix tyrosine residues in a reaction thought to involve the extracellular peroxidase-like domain.** The isolated *C. elegans* peroxidase-like domain produced in *Escherichia coli* appears to catalyze cross-linking of tyrosine residues *in vitro.*

Novel roles for **Duox enzymes in host defense were recently proposed in several non-thyroid tissues** (Geiszt, M., Witta, J., Baffi, J., Lekstrom, K., and Leto, T. L. (2003) *FASEB J.* **17,** 1502–1504).

Based on the high levels of Duox in epithelial cells of salivary gland ducts and along mucosal surfaces of colon,

rectum, and major airways, these enzymes were proposed to serve as sources of H_2O_2 supporting the anti-microbial activity of lactoperoxidase. Lactoperoxidase, abundant in milk, saliva, tears, and mucosal secretions, uses H_2O_2 to oxidize thiocyanate to hypothiocyanite, an oxidant effective against both Gram-negative and Gram-positive bacterial species (Reiter, B. A., and Oram, J. D. (1967) *Nature* **216**, 328–330). Thus, the dual oxidases may represent "missing links" that complete an oxidant-dependant microbicidal system that has been long recognized in many body fluids.

Duox 1 & 2 serve as a source of H_2O_2 that is utilized by thyroid peroxidase to carry out iodination of thyroglobulin, one of the steps in thyroid hormone biosynthesis.

11.6 Functional Partners of Nox Isoforms

In phagocytic cells, gp91[phox] is the core catalytic component of a multi-component enzyme complex. However, p22[phox], p47[phox], and p67[phox] are also essential for superoxide production, as is evident in chronic granulomatous disease, where defects or the absence of any one of these components result in oxidase deficiencies. p47[phox], a classic adaptor protein, recruits p67[phox] into the complex, whereas p67[phox] and Rac appear to regulate catalysis directly. An essential role for Rac in oxidase activation was well established *in vitro* (Abo, A., Pick, E., Hall, A., Totty, N., Teahan, C. G., and Segal, A. W. (1991) *Nature* **353**, 668–670) and was later confirmed in an oxidase-deficient patient who expressed mutant Rac2 (Ambruso, D. R., Knall, C., Abell, A. N., Panepinto, J., Kurkchubasche, A., Thurman, G., Gonzalez-Aller, C., Hiester, A., deBoer, M., Harbeck, R. J., Oyer, R., Johnson, G. L., and Roos, D. (2000) *Proc. Natl. Acad. Sci. U. S. A.* **97**, 4654–4659) and in mice deficient in Rac2.

The molecular architectures of the non-phagocytic oxidases are a subject of intense interest, as emerging evidence suggests that some of the closest homologues of gp91^{phox} also function as multicomponent oxidases. Interestingly, **co-expression of p47^{phox} and p67^{phox} augments superoxide production in cells expressing Nox1** (Banfi, B., Clark, R.A., Steger, K., and Krause, K. H. (2003) *J. Biol. Chem.* **278,** 3510–3513).

The **mRNA for Noxo1 is detected at high levels within colon crypts,** where Nox1 is also expressed (Banfi, B., Clark, R.A., Steger, K., and Krause, K. H. (2003) *J. Biol. Chem.* **278,** 3510–3513).

Together, these findings illustrate that the colon oxidase has close structural and functional similarities to the phagocytic enzyme.

Homologous multicomponent Nox family oxidases of phagocytes and colon epithelium. *Left,* the phagocyte oxidase assembles on newly forming phagosomes, following recruitment of Rac and phosphorylated cytosolic Phox proteins. *Right,* the Nox1-based oxidase of colon cells comprises some of the same or related cofactors.

Distinct roles for Noxa1 as a regulator of other Nox/Duox isoforms are possible because its expression is detected in several tissues, notably thyroid and salivary glands, kidney, and pancreas (Takeya, R., Ueno, N., Kami, K., Taura, M., Kohjima, M., Izaki, T., Nunoi, H., and Sumimoto, H. (2003) *J. Biol. Chem.* **278,** 25234–25246).

The widespread expression of p22^{phox} may also be indicative of its involvement with other Nox isoforms, particularly Nox4 because this transcript is **abundant in kidney** (Sumimoto, H., Nozaki, M., Sasaki, H., Takeshige, K., Sakaki, Y., and Minakami, S. (1989) *Biochem. Biophys. Res. Commun.* **165,** 902–906).

An association of p22^{phox} with Duox isoforms is unlikely, however, because **p22phox-deficient chronic granulomatous disease patients have no problems in thyroid function**. Furthermore,

genes homologous to p22^{phox} are not detected in the genome of
C. elegans, which encodes Duox genes.[3] Rac is another widely
expressed candidate modulator of the novel Nox enzymes. Some
of the earliest suggestions that NADPH oxidases function in non-
myeloid cells were based on observation in cells overexpressing
mutant Racs; however, there is little evidence confirming that Rac
proteins directly regulate the novel Nox enzymes (Park, H. S., Lee,
S. H., Park, D., Lee, J. S., Ryu, S. H., Lee, W. J., Rhee, S. G., and Bae, Y.
S. (2004) *Mol. Cell. Biol.* **24**, 4384–4394). The best direct evidence
linking Rac to the non-phagocytic Nox enzymes relates to recent
demonstrations of Rac binding to Nox a1; thus, the Nox enzymes
regulated by Nox a1, or its homologue p67^{phox}, are prime candidates
for modulation by Rac.

11.7 Conclusion

**With the recent discovery of new Nox/Duox family
members it clear that ROS production in many non-
phagocytic cells can originate from multiple, related
enzymatic sources.** Novel signaling roles for these enzymes
have been proposed in a variety of tissues where they are
detected at low levels. However, **their high levels at other
sites, particularly terminally differentiated epithelial
cells, suggest that they have other dedicated functions in
addition to host defense, such as in hormone biosynthesis,
fertilization, oxygen sensing, and extracellular matrix
cross-linking.** It is likely that ROS-based innate host defense
processes are not restricted to phagocytes and that **epithelial
cells can also use this weapon against invading microbes,
particularly along mucosal surfaces**. Current challenges
are to characterize better the molecular composition of these
novel oxidases and to define their precise physiological roles.
With recognition of these exciting new functions come the
possibilities that these enzymes also have roles in a variety of
disease processes related to inappropriate overproduction or
underproduction of ROS.

Some of the following was abstracted, excerpted or modified from: **Chronic Granulomatous Disease and Other Disorders of Phagocyte Function. Mary C. Dinauer.** Hematology 2005.

The analysis of specific gene defects in disorders of phagocyte function has shed light on important aspects of the **innate immune response**. Each disorder has distinctive features in the clinical presentation and characteristic microbial pathogens. Chronic granulomatous disease has been extensively studied both in patient series and in mouse models. New insights continue to be obtained regarding the role of the nicotinamide dinucleotide phosphate (NADPH) oxidase and related enzymes in host defense and other aspects of the inflammatory response, as well as optimal management of this disorder. Also briefly summarized are updates on newly described leukocyte adhesion defects and on inherited susceptibility to mycobacterial infection due to defects in interleukin (IL)-12 and interferon-gamma pathways.

Phagocytic leukocytes are an essential component of the innate immune system that has evolved to **respond rapidly to the presence of invading bacteria, fungi, and parasites**. Hence, patients with defects in phagocyte function typically present in infancy or childhood with recurrent, unusual, and/or difficult to clear bacterial infections. **Infections commonly seen include those of skin or mucosa, lung, lymph node, deep tissue abscesses, or childhood periodontitis.** Bacterial sepsis is an unusual initial symptom and usually reflects dissemination from an infected site. Many of these disorders have distinctive clinical and microbiologic features related to the particular functional defect.

Recent findings have confirmed the speculation that NADPH oxidase of much lower activity has widespread tissue distribution than that of the WBC, showing clearly that a low-activity NADPH oxidase is present in a variety of nonphagocytic cells, most of which are derived from the embryonic mesoderm, and that this oxidase is a source of second messengers. **This is a most important**

221

observation because it increases the role of O_2^- H_2O_2 and $^1O_2$ beyond the bounds of phagocytes and distributes their role through out tissues and organs of the body ((Babior, B.M. **NADPH oxidase: An update.** Blood 1999; 93(5): 1464-1476).

An **NADPH oxidase** similar to the one found in phagocytes has been reported to occur in **all three layers of the aorta** (endothelial cells, aortic smooth-muscle cells and fibroblasts from aortic adventitia), all of which produce O_2^-. It was postulated that the O_2^- generated by the aorta was functioning as a blood pressure regulator by consuming nitric oxide, a well known hypotensive agent with which it reacts at a diffusion-limited rate.

In joint tissues, O_2^- production has been detected in **synoviocytes** (both type A and type B) and in **chondrocytes**.

There is evidence that NADPH oxidase serve as components of oxygen sensors in various tissues. Erythropoietin production in some hepatoma lines appears to be regulated by O_2^- and $p22^{PHOX}$, the alpha-subunit of cytochrome b_{558} has been detected immunologically in **renal peritubular fibroblasts and in cells of the liver**, both of which may be sources of erythropoietin. In **the lung**, pulmonary neuroepithelial bodies have been proposed as airway oxygen sensors.

Inhibition of O_2^- and H_2O_2 production by diphenylamine iodonium is generally regarded as presumptive evidence for an NADPH oxidase. Furthermore, the K+ current in these cells increased when the cells were exposed to H_2O_2. **These results suggest that the cells contain an NADPH oxidase whose output is a function of the ambient oxygen tension and whose dismutated product (i.e., H_2O_2) regulates the flow of current through the K+ channel, the latter representing the signal by which the oxygen tension is communicated to the rest of the organism.**

12.0 CHRONIC GRANULOMATOUS DISEASE

Chronic granulomatous disease (CGD) is caused by defects in the phagocyte nicotinamide dinucleotide phosphate (NADPH) oxidase (also referred to as the **respiratory burst oxidase**) (Dinauer M. The phagocyte system and disorders of granulopoiesis and granulocyte function. In: Nathan D, Orkin S, Ginsburg D, Look A, eds. Nathan and Oski's Hematology of Infancy and Childhood. Vol. I (ed 6th). Philadelphia: W.B. Saunders Company; 2003:923–1010).

Superoxide generated during the phagocyte respiratory burst is the precursor to numerous microbicidal oxidants, including hydrogen peroxide and myeloperoxidase-catalyzed formation of hypochlorous acid. Respiratory burst-derived oxidants are an important component of the innate immune response, and their absence results in recurrent, often life-threatening bacterial and fungal infections and is also associated with formation of inflammatory granulomas, a distinctive feature of CGD.

NADPH oxidase and molecular genetics of CGD

The NADPH oxidase is a phagosomal and plasma membrane-associated enzyme complex that is **dormant in resting neutrophils** and rapidly assembled when cells are activated by a variety of inflammatory stimuli (Dinauer M. The phagocyte system and disorders of granulopoiesis and granulocyte function. In: Nathan D, Orkin S, Ginsburg D, Look A, eds. Nathan and Oski's Hematology of Infancy and Childhood. Vol. I (ed 6th). Philadelphia: W.B. Saunders Company; 2003:923–1010) (Nauseef WM. Assembly of the phagocyte NADPH oxidase. Histochem Cell Biol. 2004;122:277–291). Four polypeptide subunits are essential for NADPH oxidase activity and mutations in the corresponding genes are responsible for the four different genetic subgroups of CGD. The oxidase subunits are referred to by their apparent molecular mass (kDa) and have been given the designation **phox, for phagocyte oxidase**. Overall, CGD has a minimum estimated incidence of between 1/200,000 and 1/250,000 live births (Winkelstein JA, Marino MC, Johnston RB, Jr., et al. Chronic granulomatous disease. Report on a national registry of 368 patients. Medicine (Baltimore). 2000;79:155–169).

Approximately two-thirds of CGD cases result from defects in the X-linked gene encoding the gp91^{phox} subunit of flavocytochrome b_{558}, a membrane-bound heterodimer that is the redox center of the oxidase. When neutrophils or macrophages are exposed to inflammatory or phagocytic stimuli, p47^{phox} and p67^{phox} rapidly move to the membrane to activate flavocytochrome b_{558} **and induce superoxide formation**.

NADPH oxidase, proteases and microbial killing

The generation of respiratory burst oxidants is essential for normal killing within the phagosome, acting in concert with proteases, defensins, and other compounds released into the phagosome by fusion of different granule populations. Activation of the NADPH oxidase also results in changes in intraphagosomal pH that facilitate microbial killing (Harrison RE, Touret N, Grinstein S. Microbial killing: oxidants, proteases and ions. Curr Biol. 2002;12:R357–359).

The importance of granule compounds for intact innate immunity is well illustrated by the rare neutrophil function defect, **specific granule deficiency**. In this disorder, which is due in at least some cases to mutations in the myeloid transcription factor C/EBPε, patients lack primary granule defensins, gelatinase, and all secondary granule proteins, and consequently suffer from a variety of bacterial infections. Of note, studies in **knock-out mice genetically deficient in neutrophil elastase show enhanced susceptibility to gram-negative organisms such as Klebsiella** and *Escherichia coli,* and mice deficient in cathepsin **G** and/ or elastase appear to be more susceptible to *Aspergillus.*

A large body of evidence supports the view that respiratory burst oxidants have direct microbicidal effects (Fang FC. Antimicrobial reactive oxygen and nitrogen species: concepts and controversies. Nat Rev Microbiol. 2004;2:820–832) (Rada BK, Geiszt M, Kaldi K, Timar C, Ligeti E. Dual role of phagocytic NADPH oxidase in bacterial killing. Blood. 2004;104:2947–2953).

12.1 Clinical Features of CGD

The clinical manifestations of CGD typically begin in **infancy** or **early childhood**. CGD patients are particularly susceptible to *Staphylococcus aureus, Aspergillus* species, *Nocardia* species, and a variety of gram-negative enteric bacilli including *Serratia marcescens, Salmonella* species and *Burkholderia cepacia.* **Many of these organisms contain catalase, which prevents CGD phagocytes from utilizing microbe-generated hydrogen peroxide to promote killing of ingested organisms.**

Frequent sites of infection include skin and its draining lymph nodes, lungs, bone and gastrointestinal tract, including *Staphylococcal* liver abscesses, which are almost unique to CGD (Dinauer M. The phagocyte system and disorders of granulopoiesis and granulocyte function. In: Nathan D, Orkin S, Ginsburg D, Look A, eds. Nathan and Oski's Hematology of Infancy and Childhood. Vol. 1 (ed 6th). Philadelphia: W.B. Saunders Company; 2003:923–1010) (Winkelstein JA, Marino MC, Johnston RB, Jr., et al. Chronic granulomatous disease. Report on a national registry of 368 patients. Medicine (Baltimore). 2000;79:155–169).

In contrast to infections with bacteria and *Nocardia, Aspergillus* species infections can often be indolent with absence of fever or leukocytosis, and few if any symptoms (Segal BH, DeCarlo ES, Kwon-Chung KJ, Malech HL, Gallin JI, Holland SM. Aspergillus nidulans infection in chronic granulomatous disease. Medicine (Baltimore). 1998;77:345–354). Although *S aureus* **is the most frequently isolated organism** overall, the most common causes of death reported in a recent series were pneumonia and/or sepsis due to *Aspergillus* or *B cepacia*.

Many CGD patients also **develop chronic inflammatory granulomas**, which are a distinctive hallmark of this disorder. Symptomatic disease can include colitis/enteritis or granulomatous obstruction of either the gastric outlet or urinary tract. A recent analysis of 140 patients with CGD followed at the National Institutes of Health revealed inflammatory involvement of the gastrointestinal tract in 32.8% of patients, 89% of whom had X-linked inheritance (Marciano BE, Rosenzweig SD, Kleiner DE, et al. Gastrointestinal involvement in chronic granulomatous disease. Pediatrics. 2004;114:462–468).

In some cases, **granuloma formation** is a response to active infection, but in many cases **it is believed to reflect a dysregulated inflammatory response and/or inefficient degradation of inflammatory mediators and debris in the absence of respiratory burst-derived oxidants** (Morgenstern D, Gifford M, Li L, Doerschuk C, Dinauer M. Absence of respiratory burst in x-linked chronic granulomatous disease mice leads to abnormalities in both host defense and inflammatory response to *Aspergillus fumigatus*. J Exp Med. 1997;185:207–218) (Segal BH, Kuhns DB, Ding L, Gallin JI, Holland SM. Thioglycollate peritonitis in mice lacking C5, 5-lipoxygenase, or p47(*phox*): complement, leukotrienes, and reactive oxidants in acute inflammation. J Leukoc Biol. 2002;71:410–416).

Production of oxidants appears to be an important trigger of neutrophil apoptosis at sites of inflammation, which is also important for resolution of the inflammatory response. Recent studies have shown that **apoptosis is delayed in CGD neutrophils** (Hiraoka W, Vazquez N, Nieves-Neira W, Chanock S,

Pommier Y. Role of oxygen radicals generated by NADPH oxidase in apoptosis induced in human leukemia cells. J of Clinical Investigation. 1998;102:1961–1968) (Brown JR, Goldblatt D, Buddle J, Morton L, Thrasher AJ. Diminished production of anti-inflammatory mediators during neutrophil apoptosis and macrophage phagocytosis in chronic granulomatous disease (CGD). J Leukoc Biol. 2003;73:591–599) (Kobayashi SD, Voyich JM, Braughton KR, et al. Gene expression profiling provides insight into the pathophysiology of chronic granulomatous disease. J Immunol. 2004;172:636–643.).

However, despite the fact that more than 90% of patients with non-p47^{phox}-deficient forms of **CGD have undetectable levels of O$_2^-$ production,** there is a surprising clinical heterogeneity. At one end of the spectrum are patients who develop severe and recurrent bacterial and fungal infections beginning during infancy. At the other end of the spectrum are patients who are well for many years and then unexpectedly develop a serious infection typical of CGD. **Polymorphisms in oxygen-independent antimicrobial systems or other components regulating the innate immune response are likely to play an important role in modifying disease severity.** These remain to be fully defined, although specific polymorphisms in the myeloperoxidase, mannose binding lectin, and FcγRIIa genes are associated with a higher risk for granulomatous or autoimmune/rheumatologic complications in CGD.

Mouse Models of CGD

Gene targeting has been used to develop mouse models for both X-linked (gp91^{phox}-/-) and an autosomal recessive (p47^{phox}-/-) form of CGD. CGD mice have abnormalities in both host defense and inflammation that are similar to their human counterpart, **confirming the importance of the respiratory burst in innate immunity.** CGD mice exhibit a marked increase in susceptibility to the **opportunistic pathogens, _B cepacia_ and _Aspergillus_ species, two organisms that are particularly**

227

problematic in CGD patients. Other organisms showing increased virulence in CGD patients and, similarly, in CGD mice include *S aureus, Salmonella typhimurium, Mycobacterium tuberculosis*, and Candida. **The generation of reactive nitrogen intermediates via inducible nitric oxide synthase (NOS2) is a second oxygen-dependent phagocyte antimicrobial system that plays an important role in host defense** (Fang FC. Antimicrobial reactive oxygen and nitrogen species: concepts and controversies. Nat Rev Microbiol. 2004;2:820–832).

Mice with a double deficiency in both the NADPH oxidase (gp91[phox]-/-) and NOS2 have a high rate of spontaneous infection with commensal organisms, mostly enteric bacteria, whereas mice with a single enzyme deficiency rarely exhibit spontaneous infections when raised in specific pathogen-free conditions. **Superoxide production from xanthine oxidase**, which is expressed in endothelial cells and other tissues, may be another source of antioxidants that can function as a back-up to the phagocyte NADPH oxidase (Fang FC. Antimicrobial reactive oxygen and nitrogen species: concepts and controversies. Nat Rev Microbiol. 2004;2:820–832).

Both gp91[phox]- and p47[phox]-deficient CGD mice also have abnormalities in the inflammatory response. These include a marked increase in exudate neutrophils compared to wild-type mice in response to peritoneal instillation of thioglycollate, which may be related to impaired degradation of leukotriene B4. gp91[phox]-/- mice exhibit an exaggerated acute inflammatory response after instillation of sterilized hyphae into the lungs or upon intradermal injection, which evolves into a chronic granulomatous infiltrate. In models of experimental arthritis, both gp91[phox]- and p47[phox]-deficient CGD mice had more severe joint inflammation that developed into a granulomatous synovitis (van de Loo FA, Bennink MB, Arntz OJ, et al. Deficiency of NADPH oxidase components p47phox and gp91phox caused granulomatous synovitis and increased connective tissue destruction in experimental arthritis models. Am J Pathol.

2003;163:1525–1537). **These studies support the concept that respiratory burst products play an important role in inflammation outside of their function in microbial killing.**

Whether absence of phagocyte NADPH oxidase activity has a protective effect in diseases with an inflammatory component has also been investigated using knockout CGD mice. Decreased injury has been reported in some models including stroke due to transient occlusion of the carotid artery, **whereas protection against atherosclerotic lesions has generally not been observed** (Dinauer M, Lekstrom-Himes J, Dale D. Inherited neutrophil disorders: molecular basis and new therapies. Hematology. 2000:303–318). **I believe that this invalidates the theory of oxidation by oxygen free radicals of LDL as being causative of artherosclerosis.**

12.2 Treatment of CGD

The use **of prophylactic antibiotics and interferon-γ (IFN-γ),** coupled with aggressive treatment of acute infections and prolonged courses of antimicrobial treatment, has markedly improved the clinical course of patients with CGD. Trimethoprim/ sulfamethoxazole (or, in sulfa-allergic patients, dicloxacillin) is ordinarily used for antibiotic prophylaxis. Prophylactic IFN-γ is another mainstay of current management, **although its use is not accompanied by any measurable improvement in phagocyte NADPH oxidase activity in the majority of CGD patients.** The clinical benefit of IFN-γ is probably related to enhanced phagocyte function and killing by non-oxidative mechanisms and perhaps the NOS2 and xanthine oxidase pathways. A large, multicenter trial initially established that recipients of IFN-γ had 70% fewer and less severe infections (The International Chronic Granulomatous Disease Cooperative Study Group. A controlled trial of interferon gamma to prevent infection in chronic granulomatous disease. N Engl J Med. 1991;324:509–516). A recent update reinforced these findings, reporting only 0.30 serious bacterial infections and 0.12 serious fungal infections observed per patient-year, in patients observed for up to 9 years, with a total observation period of 328.4 patient-years. The most common side effects were fever and flu-like symptoms. Importantly, **there was no increase in the incidence of chronic inflammatory complications of CGD in patients receiving IFN-γ.** A new study showed that itraconazole is an effective agent for prophylaxis for fungal infections in CGD, as evaluated in a randomized, double blind, placebo-controlled study conducted by the National Institutes of Health (Gallin JI, Alling DW, Malech HL, et al. Itraconazole to prevent fungal infections in chronic granulomatous disease. N Engl J Med. 2003;348:2416–2422). Hence, **for all patients with CGD, regardless of genetic subgroup, the current recommendation is to use prophylaxis with trimethoprim/ sulfamethoxazole, itraconazole, and IFN-γ.**

Corticosteroids are used to treat clinically significant granulomatous complications of CGD, although with caution, given the underlying microbial killing defect.

The prognosis of CGD has improved dramatically in the past two decades with the advent of prophylactic antimicrobials and IFN-γ. **(RMH Note: I believe that this is due to the generation of EMODs secondary to interferon.)** The overall mortality rate in the study on long-term IFN-γ therapy cited above was 1.5% per patient-year, and may be even lower in newly diagnosed children managed with optimal care, including the use of anti-fungal prophylaxis.

Allogeneic bone marrow transplantation can be used to treat CGD and has been employed successfully. However, because of the risks associated with this procedure and the frequent lack of an HLA-matched sibling, conventional marrow transplantation has generally been considered only for those patients who have frequent and severe infections despite aggressive medical management. A "mini-transplant" regimen was used successfully in a small number of children, **but graft-versus-host disease was a significant problem in the adult patients in this study**.

CGD is also a candidate disease for gene therapy targeted at hematopoietic stem cells (HSCs). Observations on female carriers of X-linked CGD, variant X-linked CGD patients with residual enzyme activity, and preclinical studies in murine CGD models suggest that **complete correction of respiratory burst activity in ~10% of circulating neutrophils would lead to clinically relevant improvements in host defense, particularly against Aspergillus (**Barese CN, Goebel WS, Dinauer MC. Gene therapy for chronic granulomatous disease. Expert Opin Biol Ther. 2004;4:1423–1434**)**. However, **correction of > 20% of neutrophils will likely provide broadest protection against bacterial infection and granulomatous complications**. The relative level of superoxide within individual neutrophils may also be an important factor, and only partial correction of cellular NADPH oxidase activity may not restore full antimicrobial activity.

The majority of preclinical studies in CGD to date have used gamma-retroviral vectors, although lentiviral vectors have attracted increasing attention. Lentiviral vectors can transduce quiescent cells, which is an advantage for future use in human hematopoietic stem cells. "Self-inactivating" lentiviral vectors with deleted viral enhancer sequences may also provide safety advantages over gamma-retroviral vectors, because the former tend to insert into the body of the gene rather than near gene promoters, with less chance of activating expression of neighboring genes.

A new trial being conducted in Europe for X-linked CGD patients utilizes moderate dose busulfan as conditioning prior to infusion of $CD34^+$ cells transduced with a gamma-retroviral vector for $gp91^{phox}$ expression. In the two patients reported thus far, both adults, higher than expected numbers of oxidase-positive granulocytes were seen post-transplant, which then increased in the months following reinfusion, reaching over 35% in one patient and ~15% in the second. Both patients are currently well, with normal peripheral blood counts, and chronic infections associated with CGD have resolved. Analysis of peripheral blood granulocyte DNA showed that the majority of proviral insertions were non-random, and the authors postulated that vector-mediated activation of genes at the insertion sites contributed to the increase in oxidase-positive neutrophils. A recent study using the mouse transplant model also suggested that retroviral integration might trigger non-malignant expansion in murine hematopoiesis due to transcriptional activation of neighboring genes.

13.0 CATALASE (CAT)

Decomposition of H_2O_2 by the catalytic activity of catalase follows the fashion of a **first-order reaction**, and its **rate is dependent on the concentration of H_2O_2**. In fact, **catalase belongs to the group of enzymes that catalyze reactions at a rate near kinetic perfection**; the reaction rate is only limited by the rate at which the enzyme collides with the substrate.

Homozygous CAT knockout mice, which are completely deficient in catalase expression, develop normally and show no gross abnormalities. This fact should allay any misgivings regarding the harmful nature of H_2O_2. (Y-S Ho, Y Xiong, W Ma, A Spector, and D S Ho. Mice Lacking Catalase Develop Normally but Show Differential Sensitivity to Oxidant Tissue Injury. J. Biol. Chem., Vol. 279, Issue 31, 32804-32812, July 30, 2004).

Slices of liver and lung and lenses from **the knockout mice exhibited a retarded rate in decomposing extracellular hydrogen peroxide compared with those of wild-type mice.** However, **mice deficient in catalase were not more vulnerable to hyperoxia-induced lung injury; nor did their lenses show any increased susceptibility to oxidative stress generated by photochemical reaction, suggesting that the antioxidant function of catalase in these two models of oxidant injury is negligible.**

This further supports my Unified Theory, in that, EMODs are not basically toxic and it is their absence, which "allows" development of cataracts, cancer and atherosclerosis. This acatalasemia study shows that excess H_2O_2 is not causative of cataracts, ischemia/reperfusion injury or any of the other diseases attributed to EMODs, since these animals live normal lives.

Mouse L cells and rat aortic smooth muscle cells **overexpressing catalase display heightened oxidant sensitivity and retarded growth with increased cell death.**

Japanese acatalasemic patients are phenotypically normal with the exception of an increased tendency in development of progressive oral gangrene.

13.1 Catalase Regenerates Oxygen

Catalase is ubiquitously present in all prokaryotes and eukaryotes. With the exception of erythrocytes, it is predominantly located in peroxisomes of all types of mammalian cells where H_2O_2 is generated by various oxidases (Bosch, V. D. H., Schutgens, R. B. H., Wanders, R. J. A., and Tager, J. M. (1992) Annu. Rev. Biochem. 61, 157-197). However, a certain amount of catalase has also been found in mitochondria of rat heart (Radi, R., Turrens, J. F., Chang, L. Y., Bush, K. M., Crapo, J. D., and Freeman, B. A. (1991) J. Biol. Chem. 266, 22028-22034).

Since H_2O_2 serves as a substrate for Fenton reaction to generate the highly reactive hydroxyl radical, catalase is believed to play a role in cellular antioxidant defense mechanisms by limiting the accumulation of H_2O_2. **However, I believe that catalase also functions to regenerate O_2 during the decomposition of H_2O_2 and simultaneously avoids the formation of the hydroxyl radicals.**

The role of catalase in defending cells and tissues against oxidative stress has been studied extensively. However, as can now be seen, catalase is not needed to defend the cell against H_2O_2 injury. This may be due to a lack of actual damaging effects of H_2O_2 or to the fact that other H_2O_2 decomposing enzymes, such as GSH-Px, can accommodate H_2O_2 destruction.

No catalase-mediated protection for the heart against adriamycin toxicity is evident in certain lines of transgenic mice in which catalase is extensively overexpressed (Kang, Y. J., Chen, Y., and Epstein, P. N. (1996) J. Biol. Chem. 271, 12610-12616). Furthermore, mouse L cells and rat aortic smooth muscle cells **overexpressing catalase display heightened oxidant sensitivity and retarded growth with increased cell death,** respectively, compared with the corresponding parental cells (Brown, M. R., Miller, F. J., Jr., Li, W. G., Ellingson, A. N., Mozena, J. D., Chatterjee, P., Engelhardt, J. F., Zwacka, R. M., Oberley, L. W., Fang, X., Spector, A. A., and Weintraub, N. L. (1999) Circ. Res. 85, 524-533). **I interpret this to mean that removal of too much H_2O_2 is a bad thing.**

13.2 Catalase Deficiency in Humans (Normal Development)

Catalase deficiency in humans was first documented by Dr. Takahara in 1946 (Takahara, S., and Miyamoto, H. (1948) Jpn. J. Otol. 51, 163-164). **Japanese acatalasemic patients are phenotypically normal with the exception of an increased tendency in development of progressive oral gangrene,** presumably as a result of tissue damage from H_2O_2 produced by peroxide-generating bacteria such as streptococci and pneumococci as well as by the phagocytic cells at the sites of bacterial infection (Eaton, J. W., and Ma, M. (1995) in *The Metabolic and Molecular Bases of Inherited Disease* (Scriver, C. R., Beaudet, A. L., Sly, W. S., and Valle, D., eds) pp. 2371-2383, McGraw-Hill Inc., New York).

13.3 Catalase Deficiency in Mice (Normal Development)

The tissues of acatalasaemic mice apparently express normal levels of catalase mRNA compared with those of

wild-type mice. However, the severity of catalase deficiency in these mice varies from tissue to tissue.

In addition, **although tissues of catalase knockout mice show a retarded rate in consuming extracellular H_2O_2, the mice are not more susceptible to hyperoxia-induced lung injury and lens damage from oxidative stress** generated by photochemical reaction compared with wild-type mice.

Although catalase is among the first isolated and characterized enzymes, its role in vivo under normal physiological conditions and in the pathogenesis of oxidant-mediated diseases remains poorly understood. These **acatalasaemic mice are phenotypically normal and, unlike human patients, have no clinical manifestations of acatalasemia**.

Every collision between H_2O_2 and catalase is productive. This understanding suggests that **removal of H_2O_2 by catalase is extremely efficient at relatively high concentrations of H_2O_2**, and the rate is proportional to the levels of H_2O_2 and catalase in the cells. Complete disposal of H_2O_2 **requires** the interaction of two molecules of H_2O_2 with a single heme group in the active site of catalase. **The chance for this reaction to occur is greatly limited at very low concentrations of H_2O_2 in the cells.**

13.4 Catalase Can Produce Peroxidations of Alcohols

In the absence of a second reactive H_2O_2, compound I can oxidize alcohols such as methanol and ethanol by the peroxidation reaction, suggesting that the peroxidative activity of catalase may prevail at relatively low concentrations of H_2O_2. However, this reaction may also be limited by the cellular concentrations of alcohols. Thus, **it is generally believed that Gpx, which exhibits a low K_m for H_2O_2 (8.8-22.6 µM at 2 mM of GSH), plays a major role in** removing H_2O_2 at relatively low concentrations of H_2O_2 in the cells, whereas catalase is more effective at high concentrations of H_2O_2 (Makino, N., Mochizuki, Y., Bannai, S., and Sugita, Y. (1994) J. Biol. Chem. 269, 1020-1025). **I believe that this is extremely important information, in that CAT can act oxidatively and can produce peroxidations. Yet, it is touted as a great antioxidant enzyme.**

13.5 Lipid Peroxides Serves as a Source of H_2O_2

Investigators describe the stable overexpression of human catalase in smooth muscle cells and the **resistance of these cells to cytotoxicity induced not only by the addition of H_2O_2** but also by the addition of 13-hydroperoxyoctadecadienoic acid (13-HPODE). **The results pose an intriguing possibility of the generation of H_2O_2 from a peroxidized fatty acid.** Accordingly, **incubation of cells with both 13-HPODE and 13-hydroxyoctadecadienoic acid resulted in the generation of intracellular H_2O_2.** To explain the observed results by which catalase could overcome the effects of 13-HPODE, **they proposed that oxidized fatty acids are degraded in the cellular peroxisomes, resulting in the generation of H_2O_2.** In other words, the cellular effects of peroxidized fatty acids could be attributed to the generation of H_2O_2 or **lipid peroxides can serve as another plentiful source for the generation of H_2O_2.**

Catalase (EC 1.11.1.6 [EC] ; H_2O_2 oxidoreductase) is a **heme-**containing homotetrameric protein (for a review, see Ref. 1). Catalase can decompose hydrogen peroxide (H_2O_2) in reactions catalyzed by two different modes of enzymatic activity: the catalatic mode of activity ($2H_2O_2 \rightarrow O_2 + 2H_2O$) and the peroxidatic mode of activity ($H_2O_2 + AH_2 \rightarrow A + 2H_2O$). Although several substrates such as methanol and **ethanol** can be oxidized by the peroxidation reaction, the physiological significance of this catalase function is not understood.

I believe that this is as important as the realization that SOD is a prooxidant and that GPx can react with singlet oxygen and H_2O_2 in a prooxidant manner and produce HOCl.

The studies by Mueller and colleagues showed that **catalase is responsible for removing more than 90% of H_2O_2 in erythrocytes even at very low concentration of H_2O_2, 10^{-7} M,** suggesting that catalase may still play a major role in decomposing H_2O_2 at certain physiological concentrations of H_2O_2 in tissues (10^{-10} to 10^{-7} M) (Mueller, S., Riedel, H.-D., and Stremmel, W. (1997) Blood 90, 4973-4978).

Studies on the decay of extracellular H_2O_2 by lung and liver slices of $Cat^{+/+}$, $Cat^{+/-}$, and $Cat^{-/-}$ mice provide some insights into the function of catalase in the disposal of H_2O_2. The rates of H_2O_2 degradation by lung and liver slices at a high concentration (300 µM) of H_2O_2 are proportional to the tissue levels of catalase. However, at lower concentrations of H_2O_2 (10 and 40 µM) lung slices of $Cat^{+/-}$ and $Cat^{-/-}$ mice remove H_2O_2 at the same rate, which is slower than that of $Cat^{+/+}$ mice. It seems **that in tissues expressing low levels of catalase, such as the lungs, the low concentrations of H_2O_2 limit its availability to the enzyme.**

Thus, **H_2O_2 is predominantly degraded by other enzymatic (such as Gpx and peroxiredoxins) and nonenzymatic (such as GSH) antioxidant systems,** and the residual catalase activity in $Cat^{+/-}$ mice does not significantly contribute to the detoxification process.

Since brain exhibits the least catalase activity in all tissues studied, the levels of H_2O_2 in cells and tissues under oxidative stress as a result of different pathological conditions are not understood and may not exceed 10 µM.

H_2O_2 may be degraded predominately by Gpx and peroxiredoxins using the reducing equivalents of GSH and thioredoxin, respectively, in low H_2O_2 concentrations. Since recycling of oxidized GSH and thioredoxin consumes NADPH, **the cellular levels of NADPH and its synthesis may represent the rate-limiting factors for H_2O_2 consumption by catalase-deficient tissues.**

Red blood cells are believed to be constantly under oxidative stress due to high oxygen tension and generation of EMODs by autoxidation of oxyhemoglobin. Hence, according to the free radical theory, the enzymes CuZn-SOD, catalase, and Gpx1, which are highly expressed in these cells, are considered to be protective.

However, **mice deficient in either catalase or Gpx1 show a normal hematological profile,** suggesting that the role of these two enzymes in limiting alleged EMOD-induced damage in erythrocytes under normal physiological conditions is negligible.

Studies show **that mice deficient in peroxiredoxin I or II (Prdx1 or Prdx2, respectively) develop hemolytic anemia** in association with extensive protein oxidation in erythrocytes (Neumann, C. A., Krause, D. S., Carman, C. V., Das, S., Dubey, D. P., Abraham, J. L., Bronson, R. T., Fujiwara, Y., Orkin, S. H., and Van Etten, R. A. (2003) Nature 424, 561-565). Whether Prdx1 and Prdx2 serve as the primary enzymes for removing H_2O_2 or function to protect specific target proteins through protein-protein interactions in erythrocytes remains to be investigated.

Interestingly, catalase-deficient tissues also exhibit a reasonable H_2O_2 removal capacity, presumably from other cellular enzymatic and nonenzymatic antioxidant systems. **(RMH Note: I believe that H_2O_2 has the ability of self-regulation by acting with other EMODs and by thus producing other oxygen species.)** Since catalase competes with these cellular H_2O_2-removing systems in disposal of H_2O_2, **its function in antioxidant defense may vary from tissue to tissue and depend on the levels of its expression and the cellular concentrations of H_2O_2.**

13.6 H_2O_2 Modulates Vascular Smooth Muscle Cell Survivability and Proliferation

The role of EMODs, such as superoxide anions ($O_2 \cdot$) and hydrogen peroxide (H_2O_2),in modulating vascular smooth muscle cell proliferation and viability is controversial. To investigate the role of endogenously produced H_2O_2, rat aortic smooth muscle cells were infected with adenoviral vectors containing cDNA for human catalase (AdCat) or a control gene, ß-galactosidase (AdLacZ). These findings indicate that **overexpression of catalase inhibited smooth muscle proliferation while increasing the rate of apoptosis**, possibly through a COX-2–dependent mechanism. These results suggest that **endogenously produced H_2O_2 importantly modulates survival and proliferation of vascular smooth muscle cells** (M R Brown, F J Miller, Jr, et al. Overexpression of Human Catalase Inhibits Proliferation and Promotes Apoptosis in Vascular Smooth Muscle Cells. *Circulation Research.* 1999;85:524-533).

It has been reported that EMODs, such as superoxide anions ($O_2 \cdot$) and hydrogen peroxide (H_2O_2), are capable of stimulating vascular smooth muscle cell proliferation. **These oxidants were shown to be rapidly produced by smooth muscle cells after exposure to platelet-derived growth factor or angiotensin II, factors that stimulate smooth muscle cell growth** (Sundaresan M, Yu XZ, Victor JF, Irani K, Finkel T. Requirement for generation of H_2O_2 for platelet-derived growth factor signal transduction. Science. 1995;270:297–299).

13.7 Mn-SOD and Vascular Physiology

Although **the levels of Mn-SOD in blood vessels are relatively small,** Mn-SOD may exert important functional effects in cerebral circulation, because **endothelium expresses high levels of Mn-SOD** (Suzuki K, Tatsumi H, Satoh S, Senda T, Nakata T, Fujii J, Taniguchi N. Manganese-superoxide dismutase in endothelial cells:

localization and mechanism of induction. Am J Physiol. 1993; 265: H1173–1178) **and levels of Mn-SOD are higher in cerebral arteries than in extracranial arteries** (Napoli C, Witztum JL, de Nigris F, Palumbo G, D'Armiento FP, Palinski W. Intracranial arteries of human fetuses are more resistant to hypercholesterolemia-induced fatty streak formation than extracranial arteries. Circulation. 1999; 99: 2003–2010).

The mitochondrial content of cerebral endothelium is greater than that in other cells (Oldendorf WH, Cornfield ME, Brown WJ. The large apparent work capability of the blood-brain barrier: a study of the mitochondrial content of capillary endothelial cells in brain and other tissues of the rat. Ann Neurol. 1977; 1: 409–417), and high levels of Mn-SOD may be required to limit oxidative stress in the metabolically active cerebral endothelium (the blood-brain barrier). Actually, **I believe that the high levels of H_2O_2 produced by SOD are needed for normal cerebral function.**

Recent studies of **Mn-SOD heterozygous–deficient mice (Mn-SOD$^{+/-}$)** on an apolipoprotein E–deficient background indicate that Mn-SOD protects against vascular mitochondrial DNA damage and development of atherosclerosis in aorta. With regard to the microcirculation, our preliminary studies indicate that **endothelial function is impaired in cerebral arterioles from Mn-SOD$^{+/-}$ mice** (Didion and Faraci, unpublished data, 2002).

Treatment of cholesterol-fed rabbits with SOD conjugated to polyethylene glycol increased vascular SOD activity and improved ·NO-mediated arterial relaxation (Mugge A, Elwell JH, Peterson TE, Hofmeyer TG, Heistad DD, and Harrison DG. Chronic treatment with polyethylene-glycolated superoxide dismutase partially restores endothelium-dependent vascular relaxations in cholesterol-fed rabbits. Circ Res 69: 1293–1300, 1991). **I believe that this is the effect of increased levels of H_2O_2 from SOD. Thus, H_2O_2 improves vascular NO function indirectly.**

I believe that arteriosclerosis is similar to cancer, in that, it is always with us and it is allowed to manifest itself in times of **EMODs** deficiency states, in which there can be aggregation of circulating particulates. Only when the plaque-dissolving **EMODs** are in a deficiency state, will the plaques be allowed to aggregate and form blockages. Also, it should be kept in mind that **all layers of the arterial wall are capable of and are constantly producing EMODs.** I believe that this normal steady state of **EMODs** production keeps arteriosclerotic buildup from occurring. **This is analogous to the increased levels of EMODs produced by PDT, which can dissolve clots in situ. As long as the body is producing adequate EMODs levels by the arterial wall, clots will be dissolved and oxidized cholesterol particulates will not aggregate and they will be excreted. A deficiency state of RONS (EMODs) will allow for plaque formation.**

There is a **reversibility of arteriosclerosis which has been seen in smokers, after they stop smoking.** This is also another example of **spontaneous regression.** This illustrates my belief that arteriosclerosis is potentially always present and it is only through the activity of our **internal oxidative-cure system (NOHB)** that it is kept in abeyance. During times of deficiency levels of **EMODs**, plaque is allowed to manifest itself as arterial blockages.

Excessive production of EMODs in the vasculature **allegedly** contributes to cardiovascular pathogenesis. Among biologically relevant and abundant reactive oxygen species, **superoxide (O_2^-) and hydrogen peroxide (H_2O_2) appear most important in redox signaling.** O_2^- predominantly induces endothelial dysfunction by rapidly inactivating nitric oxide (NO^-). H_2O_2 influences different aspects of endothelial cell function via complex mechanisms (Hua Cai. NAD(P)H Oxidase–Dependent Self-Propagation of Hydrogen Peroxide and Vascular Disease. *Circulation Research.* 2005;96:818).

Please keep in mind that, even though EMODs have repeatedly been accused of being causative of

atherogenesis, it has been shown that supplementation with antioxidant vitamins does not lower serum lipid and lipoproteins or blood pressure (Hodis, H. N., Mack, W. J., LaBree, L., Mahrer, P. R., Sevanian, A., Liu, C. R., Liu, C. H., Hwang, J., Selzer, R. H. & Azen, S. P. (2002) *Circulation* 106, 1453-1459) (Collins, R., Armitage, J., Parish, S., Sleight, P. & Peto, R. (2002) *Lancet* 360, 23-33) (Brown, B. G., Zhao, X. Q., Chait, A., Fisher, L. D., Cheung, M. C., Morse, J. S., Dowdy, A. A., Marino, E. K., Bolson, E. L., Alaupovic, P., *et al.* (2001) *N. Engl. J. Med.* 345, 1583-1592) (Gruppo Italiano per lo Studio della Sopravvivenza nell'Infarto miocardico (1999) *Lancet* 354, 447-455) (Waters, D. D., Alderman, E. L., Hsia, J., Howard, B. V., Cobb, F. R., Rogers, W. J., Ouyang, P., Thompson, P., Tardif, J. C., Higginson, L., *et al.* (2002) *J. Am. Med. Assoc.* 288, 2432-2440) (Fang, J. C., Kinlay, S., Beltrame, J., Hikiti, H., Wainstein, M., Behrendt, D., Suh, J., Frei, B., Mudge, G. H., Selwyn, A. P., *et al.* (2002) *Lancet* 359, 1108-1113).

Moreover, a recent study, conducted in more than 20,000 subjects, found that vitamin E, vitamin C, and β-carotene supplementation resulted in small but significant increases in plasma Tchol (serum total cholesterol), LDL-C (low density lipoprotein-cholesterol), and TG (triglyceride) concentrations (Collins, R., Armitage, J., Parish, S., Sleight, P. & Peto, R. (2002) *Lancet* 360, 23-33).

In another study, no significant differences were found in serum lipid, lipoprotein, and CRP (C reactive protein) concentrations, BP (blood pressure), or IMT (intima-media thickness) between supplemented and not-supplemented subjects (L Fontana, T E. Meyer, S Klein and J O. Holloszy. Long-term calorie restriction is highly effective in reducing the risk for atherosclerosis in humans. PNAS. April 27, 2004, vol. 101, no. 17, pp. 6659-6663).

I discuss the role of H_2O_2 and EMODs in great detail in my book entitled, "The Medical and Scientific Significance of Oxygen Free Radical Metabolism" in section 3.5.10.

Please do not forget the Baylor studies which showed that H_2O_2 would mobilize vascular wall lipids and dissolve plaque.

14.0 PEROXIDASES

LOOH are metabolized principally through peroxidase-mediated reduction to the corresponding alcohols.

Peroxidases, besides their main function in H_2O_2 elimination, **can also catalyze O_2^- and H_2O_2 formation** by a complex reaction in which NADH is oxidized using trace amounts of H_2O_2 first produced by the non-enzymatic breakdown of NADH. Next, the NAD radical formed reduces O_2 to O_2^-, some of which dismutates to H_2O_2 and O_2 (Lamb, C., and Dixon, R.A. The oxidative burst in plant disease resistance. Ann Rev Plant Phys and Plant Mole Biol 1997; 48: 251-275). **Thus, peroxidases and catalases play an important role in the fine regulation of EMOD concentration in the cell through activation and deactivation of H_2O_2** (Elstner, E.F. Metabolism of activated oxygen species. In: Davies DD, ed. Biochemistry of plants. 1987 Vol. 11 London: Academic press, 253-315).

Peroxidases, besides their main function in H_2O_2 elimination, **can also catalyze O_2^- and H_2O_2 formation** by a complex reaction in which NADH is oxidized using trace amounts of H_2O_2 first produced by the non-enzymatic breakdown of NADH. Next, the NAD radical formed reduces O_2 to O_2^-, some of which dismutates to H_2O_2 and O_2 (Lamb, C., and Dixon, R.A. The oxidative burst in plant disease resistance. Ann Rev Plant Phys and Plant Mole Biol 1997; 48: 251-275). **Thus, peroxidases and catalases play an important role in the fine regulation of EMOD concentration in the cell through activation and deactivation of H_2O_2** (Elstner, E.F. Metabolism of activated oxygen species. In: Davies DD, ed. Biochemistry of plants. 1987 Vol. 11 London: Academic press, 253-315). Lipoxygenase (LOX, linoleate:oxygen oxidoreductase, EC.1.13.11.12) reaction is another possible source of ROS and other radicals. It catalyses the hydroperoxidation of polyunsaturated fatty acids (PUFA) (Rosahl, S. Lipoxygenases in plants - their role in development and stress response. Zeitschrift fur Naturforschung. 1996 51c: 123-138). The hydroperoxyderivatives of PUFA can undergo autocatalytic degradation, producing radicals and thus initiating the chain reaction of lipid peroxidation (LP). **In addition, LOX-mediated formation of singlet oxygen (Kanofsky, J.R., et al. 1986) or superoxide has been shown.** Lipoxygenases represent another potential enzymatic source **of singlet oxygen.**

Numerous enzymes (peroxidases) use hydrogen peroxide as a substrate in oxidation reactions involving the synthesis of complex organic molecules, such as thyroxine peroxidase and glutathione peroxidase. (RMH Note: I must point out that the **peroxidases are not out to destroy hydrogen peroxide.** In fact, **they need H_2O_2 as a substrate such that they can complete the reactions which they catalyze.**)

Catalase directly decomposes H_2O_2 to water and molecular oxygen, whereas peroxidases eliminate H_2O_2 by using it to oxidize another substrate.

I find it extremely interesting that the 3 big antioxidant enzymes, i.e., SOD, CAT and GPx, generate H_2O_2, O_2 and organic peroxides, respectively. Thus, I ask, "Does that sound like ANTI-oxidants?" **I believe that an argument could be made that they are producing conditions favorable for oxidation or they are acting as "co-oxidants." SOD, CAT and GPx, generate H_2O_2, O_2 and organic alcohols, respectively. Actually, at low peroxide concentrations, catalase will peroxidize alcohols.**

Peroxidases:

Thyroperoxidase
Cytochrome c peroxidase
Eosinophil peroxidase
Myeloperoxidase

Thylperoxidase
Glutathione peroxidase
Prostaglandin synthase
Horseradish peroxidase the enzyme is purified from horseradish
but it is also found in turnips and potatoes.
Human salivary peroxidase
Chloroperoxidase

14.1 Lipoxygenase (LOX)

Lipoxygenase (LOX, linoleate:oxygen oxidoreductase,
EC.1.13.11.12) reaction is another possible source of **EMODs**
and other radicals. **It catalyses the hydroperoxidation of
polyunsaturated fatty acids (PUFA)** (Rosahl, S. Lipoxygenases
in plants - their role in development and stress response. Zeitschrift
fur Naturforschung. 1996 51c: 123-138). The hydroperoxyderivatives
of PUFA can undergo autocatalytic degradation, producing radicals
and thus initiating the chain reaction of lipid peroxidation (LP).
**In addition, LOX-mediated formation of singlet oxygen
(Kanofsky, J.R., et al. 1986) or superoxide has been shown**.
Lipoxygenases represent another potential enzymatic source of
singlet oxygen, H_2O_2 and a variety of EMODs. Theoretically,
polyunsaturated fatty acids, which are found predominantly in
cellular membranes, are especially vulnerable to attack by EMODs
in vitro because of the high concentration of allylic hydrogens in
their structure. Yet, **organs such as the brain do not undergo
chain reactions of PUFAs.** However, others have found **that
lipid peroxides may be metabolized by peroxisomes and
generate H_2O_2.**

14.2 Thyroid Cancer

In thyroid, SOD catalyses the removal reaction of superoxide anion
with production of **hydrogen peroxide, which is used as a
substrate by thyroid peroxidase (TPO) for thyroid hormone
synthesis.** Very little is known about the tissue antioxidant defense

in thyroid cancers. **CAT activities have been reported to be significantly higher in follicular carcinomas,** compared with those in normal thyroid tissues (Sadani GR, Nadkarni GD. Role of tissue antioxidant defense in thyroid cancers. Cancer Lett 1996;109:231–5). **I interpret this to mean that the high level of CAT breaks down H_2O_2 such that an EMOD deficiency state is created, which allows for the development of cancer.** In another study, **Cu/Zn-SOD activities were reported to be significantly lower in follicular adenomas and papillary carcinomas** compared with those of normal thyroid tissues (Mano T, Shinohara R, Iwase K, Kotake M, Hamada M, Uchimura K, et al. Changes in free radical scavengers and lipid peroxide in thyroid glands of various thyroid disorders. Horm Metab Res 1997;29:351–4).

Mn-SOD activities were significantly higher in differentiated tumors compared with those of normal thyroid tissues (Nishida S, Akai F, Iwasaki H, Hosokawa K, Kusunoki T, Suzuki K, et al. Manganese superoxide dismutase content and localization in human thyroid tumors. J Pathol 1993;169:341–5).

Anaplastic carcinoma cells are likely to have no or weak resistance against EMODs, because the expression levels of most of the enzymes that are engaged in the defense mechanism were decreased. Hydrogen peroxide especially, which shows strong cytotoxity, can be easily accumulated in anaplastic cells, since the expression of **GPx and CAT enzymes that catalyze hydrogen peroxide was greatly decreased. Please keep in mind that many of these tumors are under hypoxic conditions, thus, very few EMODs are likely produced in vivo.**

It is assumed that decreased expression of CAT mRNA is critical for anaplastic carcinoma cells even though the expression of Mn-SOD mRNA is maintained, because the expression of mRNAs of two other enzymes, TPO and GPx, that catalyze hydrogen peroxide is much decreased. Therefore, Hasegawa et al concludes that a **molecular-based treatment, which facilitates the production** of excessive oxygen radicals inside the anaplastic carcinoma cells, may be one of the promising methods for the treatment of this most aggressive and lethal carcinoma (Y Hasegawa, T Takano, A Miyauchi, F Matsuzuka, H Yoshida, K Kuma and N Amino. Decreased Expression of Catalase mRNA in Thyroid Anaplastic Carcinoma. *Japanese Journal of Clinical Oncology* 33:6-9 (2003). **I have been saying for years that high levels of EMODs will kill cancer and that a high prooxidative state is a very good thing.**

14.3 EMOD Killing of Cancer Cells

It has been postulated that **when EMOD stress reaches a certain threshold, an apoptotic program is triggered to kill the cancer cells.** This hypothesis is supported by the observations that **the anticancer agent 2-methoxyestradiol (2-ME) inhibits the eliminating enzyme SOD and causes an accumulation of superoxide radicals in cancer cells, leading to a preferential killing of the malignant cells and an enhancement of photodynamic therapy** (Huang, P., Feng, L., Oldham, E. A., Keating, M. J., and Plunkett, W. (2000) *Nature* 407, 390–395) (Wood, L., Leese, M. R., Leblond, B., Woo, L. W., Ganeshapillai, D., Purohit, A., Reed, M. J., Potter, B. V., and Packham, G. (2001) *Anticancer Drug Des.* 16, 209–215) (Golab, J., Nowis, D., Skrzycki, M., Czeczot, H., Baranczyk-Kuzma, A., Wilczynski, G. M., Makowski, M., Mroz, P., Kozar, K., Kaminski, R., Jalili, A., Kopec', M., Grzela, T., and Jakobisiak, M. (2003) *J. Biol. Chem.* 278, 407–414).

I have been saying all along that excess EMODs will kill cancer cells, just as has been seen in PDT and in my singlet oxygen cancer therapy system.

14.4 Prostate Cancer

I believe that this data supports my UTOPIA theory, in that it shows that testosterone deficiency, through

castration, increases **EMODs and this is the best treatment for prostate cancer, which has resulted in cases of long term total remission of the cancer.** Administration of testosterone to the castrated group resulted in decreases in **EMODs, which would "allow" for continued growth of prostate cancer. Additionally, antioxidant enzymes are restored by testosterone administration, which would result in a further deficiency state of EMODs and a more favorable environment for cancer survival and growth.** (Tam NN, Gao Y, Leung YK, Ho SM. Androgenic regulation of oxidative stress in the rat prostate: involvement of NAD(P)H oxidases and antioxidant defense machinery during prostatic involution and regrowth. Am J Pathol. 2003 Dec;163(6):2513-22).

Remember, people with normal hormone levels have more cancer than people who are deficient. The most effective treatment for advanced prostate cancer is castration—or the chemical equivalent with testosterone blockers. The prostate is highly dependent on testosterone. Even when prostate cancer is far advanced and has spread to bones, **castration will often bring a near total remission lasting several years. I believe that this hormone data is strong support for my Unified Theory.**

This study provided the first evidence that **androgen regulates redox status in vivo** in the rat VP. This corroborates findings from a single previously published in vitro study that reported induction of EMODs in a prostate cancer cell line by androgen (Ripple MO, Henry WF, Rago RP, Wilding G: Prooxidant-antioxidant shift induced by androgen treatment of human prostate carcinoma cells. J Natl Cancer Inst 1997, 89:40-48). **Castration clearly induced an elevated pro-oxidant state. Testosterone replacement in castrated rats was only partially effective in reducing EMOD levels** in the VP of the castrates. The extent of oxidative damage in VPs of testosterone-treated castrates was still higher than that of intact rats.

They focused on the metabolic pathways responsible for EMOD anabolism and catabolism. Steady-state mRNA levels of all three NAD(P)H oxidases, Nox1, gp91^{phox} (Nox2), and Nox4, **were significantly up-regulated** in the rat VP **after castration.** Concomitantly, expression of several key EMODs detoxification enzymes/scavengers, SOD2, Gpx1, Txn, and Prdx5 declined whereas transcripts levels of catalase, GR, GGTP, and GS remained unchanged in the VPs of castrated rats.

Because **Noxs are responsible for generating superoxide** and SOD2 responsible for its removal, whereas Gpx1, Txn, and Prdx5 are intimately linked to the removal of H_2O_2, alterations in the expression of these genes, collectively, are expected to result in accumulation of EMODs, leading to a **higher pro-oxidant state in the VPs of castrated rats.** This is **all consistent with my Unified Theory**, in that deficiency levels "allow" cancer manifestation and increased levels of **EMODs** kill cancer. In these studies, **the body responds to castration by increasing EMODs production and by decreasing antioxidant enzymes.**

Testosterone replacement in castrated rats caused a complete restoration of expression of SOD2, Gpx1, Txn, and Prdx5 mRNA to levels found in intact rats. However, expression of the Nox genes, although much reduced when compared with levels in castrates, were still significantly higher than those found in intact rats. Interestingly, although levels of mRNA expression of catalase, GR, GGTP, and GS were not changed by castration, they were significantly elevated when androgen was replaced in castrated rats.

Evidence has demonstrated that **EMODs**, using H_2O_2, **evokes apoptosis and proliferation.** In culture, proliferating cells exhibit a broad spectrum of responses to graded levels of oxidants. **A very low level of H_2O_2 (3 to 15 μmol/L) causes a significant mitogenic response; whereas, higher levels of H_2O_2 (120 to 400 μmol/L) results in a growth-arrested state, whereas a**

further increase of H_2O_2 to I mmol/L triggers apoptosis.
Extrapolated from cell culture data, these findings thus support
the hypothesis that different levels of **EMODs** may contribute to
cell death, as well as to cell growth, in vivo. Specifically, 8-OHdG
and 4-HNE protein adducts were found to be highly expressed in
the regressing VP epithelia, with the frequent association of these
markers with apoptotic cells, **suggesting a possible causal
relationship between EMODs and apoptosis.**

EMOD-mediated apoptosis has been demonstrated in a variety
of biological systems, including brain-derived neurotrophic factor-
or zinc-induced neuronal cell death, **anti-cancer drug-induced
apoptosis** (Mizutani H, Tada-Oikawa S, Hiraku Y, Oikawa S,
Kojima M, Kawanishi S: Mechanism of apoptosis induced by a new
topoisomerase inhibitor through the generation of **hydrogen
peroxide.** J Biol Chem 2002, 277:30684-30689), **and hyperoxia-**
or vanadium-induced pulmonary apoptosis (Wang L, Medan D,
Mercer R, Overmiller D, Leornard S, Castranova V, Shi X, Ding M,
Huang C, Rojanasakul Y: Vanadium-induced apoptosis and pulmonary
inflammation in mice: role of reactive oxygen species. J Cell Physiol
2003, 195:99-107).

14.5 EMODs, Hormones and Cancer

After the testosterone-treatment of castrated rats, they observed
evidence of continued elevation of **EMODs** at moderate levels
in the regenerating VP, suggesting a plausible role for low levels of
EMODs in the regulation of cell proliferation, differentiation, and/or
tissue remodeling in the gland.

Castration and androgen replacement had minimal effects on the
levels of **EMODs** markers in the ducts but distinctly regulated
those in the acini. These findings indicate differential regulation
of **EMODs** in ducts versus that in acini by circulating androgen.
Previous studies have reported that prostatic ducts are markedly
different from acini with regard to morphology, hormonal

responsiveness, proliferation, apoptosis, stromal/epithelial cell ratio, and composition of the extracellular matrix. Thus, constitutively high levels of **EMODs** found in the ductal regions may explain the reported **high susceptibility of tumor development from prostatic ducts in hormone-treated Noble rats** (Bosland MC, Ford H, Horton L: Induction at high incidence of ductal prostate adenocarcinomas in NBL/Cr and Sprague-Dawley Hsd:SD rats treated with a combination of testosterone and estradiol-17 beta or diethylstilbestrol. Carcinogenesis 1995, 16:1311-1317) (Tam NN, Chung SS, Lee DT, Wong YC: Aberrant expression of hepatocyte growth factor and its receptor, c-Met, during sex hormone-induced prostatic carcinogenesis in the Noble rat. Carcinogenesis 2000, 21:2183-2191). It is currently unknown why ductal epithelia express such a high level of OS constitutively.

This data suggest that **normal physiological levels of androgen maintain a homeostasis between cellular pro-oxidant and antioxidant contents**, as well as a balance between cell death and proliferation in the prostate. **When normal androgenic status is disrupted, such as under the condition of castration-induced deprivation, EMODs are increased in the prostate via up-regulation of Nox-dependent EMOD anabolism and down-regulation of a number of key antioxidant enzymes/ EMOD scavengers.**

All of these factors help to increase EMODs, which will control neoplastic growth, and thus, it has been found that castration is the best treatment for prostatic cancer. This data strongly supports my Unified theory.

This data may relate to the results from the Finasteride Prostate Cancer Prevention Trial, which demonstrated that **androgen-blockade at the cellular level lowers prostate cancer risk** but increases the prevalence of high-grade cancers (Thompson IM, Goodman PJ, Tangen CM, Lucia MS, Miller GJ, Ford LG, Lieber MM, Cespedes RD, Atkins JN, Lippman SM, Carlin SM, Ryan A, Szczepanek

CM, Crowley JJ, Coltman CA, Jr: The influence of finasteride on the development of prostate cancer. N Engl J Med 2003, 349:215-224).

Expression of antioxidant enzymes can be altered by hormones such as:

-ANG II
-tumor necrosis factor (TNF)-a
-and interleukin (IL)-1β, thus profoundly affecting **EMODs** levels. **The tight regulation of both production and removal of EMODs makes fluctuations in their levels transient,** another requirement for second messengers. **EMODs** may also act as an **intracellular "rheostat,"** closely modulating the activity of a discrete set of biochemical reactions.

Ang II stimulated $O_2^{-\cdot}$ is converted to H_2O_2 as early as 1 minute after addition of the Ang II hormone (Zafari, A. M., Ushio-Fukai, M. Akers, M., Yin, Q., Shah, A. Harrison, D. G., Taylor, W. R. and Griendling K. K. Novel role of NADH/NADPH oxidase-derived hydrogen peroxide in angiotensin II-induced hypertrophy of rat vascular smooth muscle cells. Hypertension. 1998; 32; 488-495)

14.6 GPx (Glutathione Peroxidase)

The main role of glutathione peroxidase is to remove lipid peroxides. Like SOD, seleno-dependent glutathione peroxidase behaves in two different ways in the presence of oxidative stress: first the enzyme is over expressed and then, **if the oxidative stress persists, it is destroyed.** A reduced GPx activity may reflect too little selenium in the diet. **I find it curious that both SOD and GPx are destroyed, even though they act as catalysts.**

Glutathione peroxidases are widely distributed in animal tissues and can act on peroxides other than H_2O_2. Most importantly with regard to oxidative modification in the artery wall, **they can catalyze GSH-dependent reduction of LOOH to the corresponding alcohol**

(LOH). Phospholipid hydroperoxide glutathione peroxidase (PHGPx) is the only enzyme known to reduce complex lipid hydroperoxides in lipoproteins (Maiorino M, Thomas JP, Girotti AW, and Ursini F. Reactivity of phospholipid hydroperoxide glutathione peroxidase with membrane and lipoprotein lipid hydroperoxides. *Free Radic Res Commun* 12–13: 131–135, 1991)

Stimulated neutrophils undergo a burst of respiration in which oxygen is reduced to superoxide. About 40 years ago Sbarra and Karnovsky demonstrated that neutrophils undergo a marked respiratory burst when they phagocytize bacteria. This was cyanide insensitive, so not part of mitochondrial respiration. It was shown that oxygen was converted to hydrogen peroxide. At that stage it was thought that hydrogen peroxide was responsible for killing bacteria. Then Klebanoff showed that neutrophils use myeloperoxidase to oxidize chloride to hypochlorous acid (HOCl). (Oxygen Society Annual Meeting, RTP, NC Nov 16-19, 2001 Tony Kettle, pages 1-8).

HOCl is a highly toxic oxidant that kills almost all pathogens. The story seemed complete. Neutrophils were reducing oxygen to **hydrogen peroxide**, which was used by the peroxidase to produce the ultimate anti-microbial agent **chlorine bleach**. However, bleach was largely ignored as fashion took control of science. Just after McCord and Fridovich discovered superoxide dismutase, **Babior demonstrated that superoxide is the primary product of the neutrophil respiratory burst**. He and others, notably Segal, showed that the cells contain an NADPH-oxidase that reduces molecular oxygen to superoxide. Superoxide was the molecule of fascination at the time and it was believed that it was the bactericidal product of neutrophils. Then came a period of distraction. Also the case for myeloperoxidase and bleach was not helped because **myeloperoxidase-deficiency was found to be relatively common (1:3000) and generally not to have major consequences.** However, some individuals, particularly those with diabetes often get severe infections.

Prof Randolph Michael Howes MD, PhD

Superoxide was found to be poor at killing bacteria. Its controversial
toxicity was then explained in terms of the Fenton reaction
and production of hydroxyl radicals. Much effort was put into
demonstrating that neutrophils could produce hydroxyl radicals.
Indeed many studies showed that hydroxyl radicals were formed
but most indicated that hydroxyl radical production was not
very significant and involved myeloperoxidase in some way. This
controversy is still waged tody. A situation developed where
oxidants were trying to be imposed on the neutrophil. Although
hydroxyl radicals and superoxide were receiving attention because
of their general importance in biology, **it is not known if they
are major players as far as toxic neutrophil oxidants are
concerned.**

**One investigator stated, "If only researchers had stopped
and wondered why neutrophils and pus have a green hue."**

**When Weiss showed that 25% of extracellular hydrogen
peroxide was converted to HOCl it became clear
that chlorine bleach is a major oxidant generated by
neutrophils. Subsequently, Hurst showed that at least 10%
of the oxygen consumed by neutrophils was converted
to HOCl that reacted inside phagosomes. These two
results clearly confirmed Klebanoff's earlier assertion that
myeloperoxidase plays a central part in neutrophil oxidant
production.**

Myeloperoxidase is a fascinating green enzyme. The heme
groups act independently and have equal reactivity with hydrogen
peroxide and reducing substrates. **Myeloperoxidase** undergoes a
complex array of redox transformations that enable it to produce
HOCl, degrade hydrogen peroxide to oxygen and water, convert
tyrosine and other phenols and anilines to reactive free radicals, and
hydroxylate aromatic substrates via a cytochrome P450 type activity.
It also reacts rapidly with superoxide in reactions that modulate
production of HOCl.

I believe that this is fascinating in that peroxidases have been touted as great antioxidants; whereas in reality, they are generating the powerful oxidant, HOCl. Therefore, peroxidases are **NOT** great antioxidants.

15.0 GPX CAN BLOCK OR CAUSE APOPTOSIS

Oxidative injuries including apoptosis can be induced by reactive oxygen species (ROS) and reactive nitrogen species (RNS) in aerobic metabolism. We determined impacts of a selenium-dependent glutathione peroxidase-1 (GPX1) on apoptosis induced by diquat (DQ), a ROS (superoxide) generator, and peroxynitrite (PN), a potent RNS. Hepatocytes were isolated from GPX1 knockout (GPX1 $-/-$) or wild-type (WT) mice, and treated with 0.5 mM DQ or 0.1-0.8 mM PN for up to 12 h. Loss of cell viability, high levels of apoptotic cells, and severe DNA fragmentation were produced by DQ in only GPX1 $-/-$ cells and by PN in only WT cells. These two groups of cells shared similar cytochrome c release, caspase-3 activation, and p21$^{WAFI/CIPI}$ cleavage. Higher levels of protein nitration were induced by PN in WT than GPX1 $-/-$ cells. Much less and/or slower cellular GSH depletion was caused by DQ or PN in GPX1 $-/-$ than in WT cells, and corresponding GSSG accumulation occurred only in the latter. In conclusion, it is most striking that, **although GPX1 protects against apoptosis induced by superoxide-generator DQ, the enzyme actually promotes apoptosis induced by PN in murine hepatocytes.** Indeed, GSH is a physiological substrate for GPX1 in coping with ROS in these cells (**Yangxin Fu, Helmut Sies, and Xin Gen Lei.** Opposite Roles of Selenium-dependent Glutathione Peroxidase-1 in Superoxide Generator Diquat- and Peroxynitrite-induced Apoptosis and Signaling. J. Biol. Chem., Vol. 276, Issue 46, 43004-43009, November 16, 2001). **Again, we see the difficulty of making generalities about antioxidant enzymes. GPx, which normally blocks EMOD-induced apoptosis, now causes apoptosis.**

Glutathione peroxidases detoxify hydrogen peroxide and fatty acid-derived hydroperoxides. This is the antioxidant role of these enzymes. However, **recent research indicates that reactive oxygen species play important roles in signal transduction** processes. Therefore, by affecting the concentrations of reactive oxygen species in cells, the glutathione peroxidases may also be considered to play regulatory roles in signal transduction.

15.1 GPx4

Among the glutathione peroxidases, Gpx4 is unique in several ways. First, **in addition to the common substrates (hydrogen peroxide and alkyl peroxides) reduced by all glutathione peroxidases,** Gpx4 reduces hydroperoxide groups on phospholipids, lipoproteins, and cholesterol esters.

Second, unlike the other glutathione peroxidases, which are tetrameric enzymes, Gpx4 is a monomeric enzyme and is rich in hydrophobic amino acid residues. Because of its small size and large hydrophobic surface, Gpx4 can interact with complex lipids in membranes and thereby detoxify membrane lipid hydroperoxides. The other pathway for removing membrane lipid peroxides from membranes is through the coupled actions of phospholipase A_2 (PLA_2) and Gpx1: PLA_2 first excises the fatty acid hydroperoxide from the phospholipid hydroperoxide in the membrane, and **then Gpx1 reduces the fatty acid hydroperoxide to alcohol and water.** From kinetic modeling, the Gpx4 pathway is estimated to be far more efficient at removing phospholipid hydroperoxides than the PLA_2-Gpx1 pathway, because **the affinity of Gpx4 to membrane lipid peroxides is more than 10^4-fold greater than PLA_2.**

I believe that this may be the source of alcohol, which can be peroxidized by catalase (CAT).

Therefore, Gpx4 is considered to be the primary enzymatic defense system against oxidative damage to cellular membranes. Contrary to the predictions of the free radical theory, **a recent report showed that overexpression of Gpx4 induced the expression of COX-2 in colon carcinoma cells** (Barriere, G., Rabinovitch-Chable, H., Cook-Moreau, J., Faucher, K., Rigaud, M., and Sturtz, F. (2004) Anticancer Res. 24, 1387–1392).

Gpx4 is ubiquitously expressed; however, its activity makes up only a fraction of the total cellular glutathione peroxidase activity in most tissues. The exception is the **testes, where Gpx4 activity makes up the majority of the glutathione peroxidase activity.** Despite its relative low cellular abundance, Gpx4 was shown to play a critical role in the antioxidant defense system in our study using mice deficient in Gpx4. **The Gpx4 null mutation (Gpx4$^{-/-}$) is embryonically lethal; Gpx4$^{-/-}$ embryos die** at embryonic stage E7.5 to E8.5. In addition, embryonic fibroblasts derived from mice heterozygous for the Gpx4 gene (Gpx4$^{+/-}$) have increased lipid peroxidation, more cell death after exposure to oxidizing agents, and experienced growth retardation under high oxygen.

Among the glutathione peroxidase genes, knockout mice have been generated for the Gpx1, Gpx2, and Gpx4 genes. **The phenotype of Gpx4 null mutation is much more severe than the phenotypes reported for null mutations in the other glutathione peroxidases.**

15.2 Animals Null for CAT and Gpx1 and Gpx2 Develop Normally

Mice null for the Gpx1 and Gpx2 genes appear normal under normal housing conditions, although they tend to be more sensitive to oxidative stress. More recently, knockout mice for catalase were generated, and these mice null for catalase appear normal as well (Ho, Y. S., Xiong, Y., Ma, W., Spector, A., and Ho, D. S. (2004) J. Biol. Chem. 279, 32804–32812).

Animals Null for CAT and Gpx1 and Gpx2 Develop Normally

I believe that it is of utmost importance to consider the fact that animals null for CAT and Gpx1 and Gpx2 appear to develop normally and live normal lives. This must

weaken the argument that EMODs are extremely toxic and causative of up to 200 pathophysiologies.

Based on observations of the phenotypes of knockout mice null for Gpx1, Gpx2, and catalase, which detoxify hydrogen peroxide and alkyl peroxides (for the glutathione peroxidases) but not the complex lipid hydroperoxides found in membranes, **the embryonic lethal phenotype of Gpx4 knockout mouse points to the critical importance of Gpx4 in repairing membrane lipid hydroperoxides.**

The overexpression of Gpx4 in RBL2H3 and 104C1 cells has been shown to reduce EMODs -induced toxicity (Yagi, K., Komura, S., Kojima, H., Sun, Q., Nagata, N., Ohishi, N., and Nishikimi, M. (1996) Biochem. Biophys. Res. Commun. 219, 486–491).

There is no information on the effect of overexpressing Gpx4 in tissues of whole animals.

Chloroperoxidases, generate singlet oxygen from H_2O_2 and chloride *in vitro*, and singlet oxygen is produced in **neutrophils, which contain abundant H_2O_2 and chloroperoxidases** (Steinbeck, M. J., Khan, A. U., and Karnovsky, M. J. (1992) *J. Biol. Chem.* **267**, 13425-13433). **Singlet oxygen is a greater oxidant than H_2O_2, thus, chloroperoxidases are not great antioxidant enzymes because they are actually capable of generating a stronger oxidant than H_2O_2, namely $^1O_2$.**

16.0 MYELOPEROXIDASE

$O_2^{.-}$ that exits from, or is produced outside of, vascular cells can be converted by extracellular SOD (ECSOD) to H_2O_2. In addition, $O_2^{.-}$ produced within the cell is converted by Cu/Zn SOD and Mn SOD to H_2O_2, which can readily cross cellular membranes. H_2O_2 present in the extracellular space can be, in turn, converted to the highly reactive species HOCl by the enzyme **myeloperoxidase**.

Atherosclerotic plaques exhibit evidence for HOCl generation and HOCl-mediated oxidation (Hazell LJ, Arnold L, Flowers D, Waeg G, Malle E, and Stocker R. Presence of hypochlorite-modified proteins in human atherosclerotic lesions. *J Clin Invest* 97: 1535–1544, 1996) (Hazell LJ, Baernthaler G, and Stocker R. Correlation between intima-to-media ratio, apolipoprotein B-100, myeloperoxidase and hypochlorite-oxidized proteins in human atherosclerosis. *Free Radic Biol Med* 31: 1254–1262, 2001), all the more important considering that **HOCl induces growth arrest and apoptosis of vascular cells.**

In patients with coronary artery disease low red blood cell peroxidase 1 activity or increased plasma levels of myeloperoxidase (Brennan ML, Penn MS, Van Lente F, Nambi V, Shishehbor MH, Aviles RJ, Goormastic M, Pepoy ML, McErlean ES, Topol EJ, Nissen SE, and Hazen SL. Prognostic value of myeloperoxidase in patients with chest pain. *N Engl J Med* 349: 1595–1604, 2003) **are associated with increased risk of events.**

Myeloperoxidase exists in atherosclerotic lesions and vascular disease, and HOCl is the major product at physiological concentrations of chloride ions (Harrison JE and Schultz J. Studies on the chlorinating activity of myeloperoxidase. *J Biol Chem* 251: 1371–1374, 1976). **Hypochlorous acid can oxidize a large variety of biological molecules, particularly proteins and amino acids.**

16.1 Clinical Manifestation

Neutrophilic polymorphonuclear leukocytes (**neutrophils**) are highly specialized for their primary function, the phagocytosis and destruction of microorganisms. When coated with opsonins (generally complement and/or antibody), microorganisms bind to specific receptors on the surface of the phagocyte and invagination of the cell membrane occurs with the incorporation of the microorganism into an intracellular phagosome. There follows a **burst of oxygen consumption, and much, if not all, of the extra oxygen consumed is converted to highly reactive oxygen species**. In addition, the cytoplasmic granules discharge their contents into the phagosome, and death of the ingested microorganism soon follows. **Among the antimicrobial systems formed in the phagosome is one consisting of myeloperoxidase (MPO), released into the phagosome during the degranulation process, hydrogen peroxide (H_2O_2) formed by the respiratory burst and a halide, particularly chloride. The initial product of the MPO- H_2O_2-chloride system is hypochlorous acid, and subsequent formation of chlorine, chloramines, hydroxyl radicals, singlet oxygen, and ozone has been proposed.** These same toxic agents can be released to the outside of the cell, where they may attack normal tissue and thus contribute to the pathogenesis of disease. **It is concluded that the MPO system plays an important role in the microbicidal activity of phagocytes** (Myeloperoxidase: friend and foe. Klebanoff SJ. J Leukoc Biol. 2005 May;77(5):598-625. Epub 2005 Feb 2). **I believe that short diffusion distances will limit the toxicity of most of these oxygen products.**

Investigators demonstrated the ability of human **PMNs to act as effector cells against mammalian tumor cells** in vitro using a relatively low ratio of effector to target cells and two cytotoxicity assays: S 1Cr release and loss of oncogenicity. Cytotoxicity depends on the presence of intact PMN, phagocytosable particles, and a halide cofactor. **Studies employing inhibitors and leukocytes from patients with neutrophil dysfunction syndromes clearly implicate MPO and H$_2$O$_2$ in mediating this cytotoxic effect.** Since the **blood monocyte** also contains MPO and forms **H$_2$O$_2$** during phagocytosis, the MPO-mediated cytotoxicity system may also be operative with this cell type. **I believe that this data bolsters the tumoricidal activity of EMODs and solidifies the role of H$_2$O$_2$.**

While the data presented point out the cytotoxic potential of PMN via the MPO-**H$_2$O$_2$**-halide system, the effects observed are **not target cell specific.** In particular there is **currently no evidence for increased susceptibility of tumor cells** to peroxidase-mediated damage and toxic effects of the isolated peroxidase system on normal mammalian cells have been effectively demonstrated. Attachment of **antibody molecules** to the tumor cell surface would also provide a mechanism for immunologically specific release of peroxidase system components. **Secretion of enzymes including MPO and metabolic stimulation also occur when neutrophils come in contact with antigen-antibody complexes on a nonphagocytosable membrane surface.** Evidence has been presented for in vivo attachment of immunoglobulins to the surface of tumor cells and a report of **in vitro killing of antibody-coated malignant cells by human neutrophils has recently appeared.** The demonstration of peroxidase-mediated cytotoxicity for mammalian tumor cells using both cell-free systems and intact human PMNs raises the possibility that the neutrophil is involved via the peroxidase system in the host defense against neoplastic disease.

A cytotoxic effect of human neutrophils on mammalian tumor cells is demonstrated. Cytotoxicity depends on the presence of intact neutrophils, phagocytosable particles, and a halide cofactor and is inhibited by azide, cyanide, and catalase. **Neutrophils from patients with myeloperoxidase (MPO) deficiency or defective H$_2$O$_2$ production are not cytotoxic,** but activity is restored by addition of purified MPO **or H₂O₂** respectively. The findings support a mechanism involving the phagocytosis-induced extracellular release of MPO and **H₂O₂** and their reaction with a halide cofactor to damage the target cells (Neutrophil-mediated tumor cell cytotoxicity: role of the peroxidase system. Clark RA, Klebanoff SJ J Exp Med. 1975 Jun 1;141(6):1442-7). **I believe that this data clearly demonstrates the need for EMODs and H₂O₂ for tumoricidal activity.**

Endothelial cells are known to transcytose myeloperoxidase leading to enzyme deposition in the subendothelial space and the facilitation of extracellular matrix protein tyrosine nitration (Baldus S, Eiserich JP, Mani A, Castro L, Figueroa M, Chumley P, Ma W, Tousson A, White CR, Bullard DC, Brennan ML, Lusis AJ, Moore KP, and Freeman BA. Endothelial transcytosis of myeloperoxidase confers specificity to vascular ECM proteins as targets of tyrosine nitration. *J Clin Invest* 108: 1759–1770, 2001).

**As goes oxygen,
so goes the undulating waves of biota life forms,
clinging to our planet's fragile surface.
Life flourished during the oxygen-rich Triassic times
and die-offs paralleled spans of atmospheric hypoxia.
Oxygen is the brain's mate and the heart's mistress.
It is the lover to all aerobic cells.
The thought of anoxia is
"simply out of this world."**
R. M. Howes M.D., Ph.D.
12/23/05

16.2 Myeloperoxidase Deficiency Increases Infections, arteriosclerosis and Cancer

I had predicted that a true (not partial) MPO deficiency would result in an increase in malignancies due to deficiencies of EMODs.

Myeloperoxidase (MPO), an iron-containing heme protein localized in the azurophilic granules of neutrophil granulocytes and in the lysosomes of monocytes, **is involved in the killing of several micro-organisms and foreign cells, including bacteria, fungi, viruses, red cells, and malignant and nonmalignant nucleated cells.** Despite the primary role of the oxygen-dependent MPO system in the destruction of certain phagocytosed microbes, **subjects with total or partial MPO** deficiency generally **do not** have an **increased frequency of infections**, probably because other MPO-independent mechanism(s) for microbicidal activity compensate for the lack of MPO. **Infectious diseases, especially with species of Candida, have been observed predominantly in MPO-deficient patients who also have diabetes mellitus,** but the frequency of such cases is very low, less than 5% of reported MPO-deficient subjects. Evidence from a number of investigators indicates **that individuals with total MPO deficiency show a high incidence of malignant tumors.** Since MPO-deficient PMNs exhibit in vitro a depressed lytic action against malignant human cells, it can be speculated that the neutrophil MPO system plays a central role in the tumor surveillance of the host. However, any definitive conclusion on the association between MPO deficiency and the occurrence of cancers needs to be confirmed in further clinical studies. **Clinical manifestations of this disorder depend on the nature of the defect**; an acquired abnormality associated with other hematological or nonhematological diseases has been occasionally described, but the primary deficiency is the form more commonly reported. (Abstract: Clinical manifestation of myeloperoxidase deficiency. Lanza F. J Mol Med. 1998 Sep;76(10):676-81).

Thirty six unrelated individuals with neutrophil MPO deficiency, (10 totally MPO deficient) were found on screening a population of **148,000 subjects**. A further 2 subjects with total and 22 with partial MPO deficiency were identified through family studies. The assessment of neutrophil function, i.e., peroxidase activity, superoxide anion generation, microbicidal activity towards fungi and bacteria, and locomotor behaviour, was carried out in 10 subjects with total and 4 with partial MPO deficiency. We found that the enzyme defect is associated with a marked impairment in the killing of both S. aureus and C. albicans, without affecting microbicidal activity against S. faecalis. **There appears to be a high incidence of malignancy in patients with complete MPO deficiency**, suggesting a relationship between a defective MPO system and neutrophil-mediated tumor cell cytotoxicity. (Abstract: Does a relationship exist between neutrophil myeloperoxidase deficiency and the occurrence of neoplasms? Lanza F, Fietta A, Spisani S, Castoldi GL, Traniello S. J Clin Lab Immunol. 1987 Apr;22(4):175-80).

See, I told you so!

Activity of N-acetyl-beta-D-glucosaminidase, beta-glucuronidase, and acid phosphatase and **myeloperoxidase** was determined **in neutrophils and lymphocytes of patients with cancer of the larynx and precancerous states of the larynx as well as--for comparative reasons--in patients with malignant tumors of female generation organs, breast carcinoma, cancer of the stomach and endometriosis**. The main result of investigations performed was in fact that **intracellular deficiency of beta-glucuronidase** within the neutrophils characterizes patients with cancer and precancerous states of the larynx. **Patients with cancer of the larynx show additionally a deficiency of**

neutrophil myeloperoxidase. Deficiency of N-acetyl-beta-D-glucosaminidase occurs, in contrast, in patients with malignancies of female generation organ. **Activity of myeloperoxidase in neutrophils from patients with gastric carcinoma is slightly elevated.** (Abstract: Enzymatic deficiencies of the immune system cells in patients with cancer of the larynx and other malignancies. Gierek T, Lisiewicz J, Moszczynski P, Pilch J, Namyslowski G. Auris Nasus Larynx. 1985;12(1):47-51).

In 74 cases of **acute myeloid leukaemia (AML)** the relation between pretreatment **myeloperoxidase (MPO)** activity in polymorphonuclear leucocytes (PMN) and the incidence of infection in the preremission phase of the disease was investigated retrospectively. 36 patients had abnormal numbers (greater than 4%) of MPO-deficient PMN and 38 had normal numbers. In the first group more patients experienced fever attacks, more showed an infectious focus and an aetiological cause was demonstrated more frequently than among patients in the second group. This difference was statistically significant (P less than 0.01). Furthermore, the patients in the first group experienced **more fever attacks, showed more infectious focus and had infectious microorganisms** demonstrated in more febrile episodes than patients in the second group (P less than 0.01). The differences were not explained by differences in the incidences of neutropenia or other parameters investigated. It is concluded that **decreased MPO activity in PMN from AML patients may contribute to the increased susceptibility to infections** and that in the preremission phase of the disease it may account for approximately 15% of the infections. (Abstract: Myeloperoxidase-deficient polymorphonuclear leucocytes (III): Relation to incidence of infection in acute myeloid leukaemia. Nielsen HK, Bendix-Hansen K. Scand J Haematol. 1984 Jul;33(1):75-9).

Neutrophil myeloperoxidase (MPO) activity was analysed semi-quantitatively both by (i) MPO-scoring of polymorphonuclear leucocytes (PMN) and (ii) counting the MPO-deficient PMN (PMN lacking MPO) in 164 subjects (60 cases of leukaemia and 104 normal humans). **The scoring method showed that 10 out of 21 (48%) cases of acute myeloid leukaemia (AML), 2 out of 10 (20%) cases of chronic myeloid leukaemia (CML), 0 out of 29 cases of lymphoid leukaemia (ALL + CLL), and 1 out of 104 normal humans had decreased MPO scores.** These figures correlated well with the more simple counting of PMN lacking MPO in the same groups: 8 out of 21 (37%) cases of AML, 6 out of 10 (60%) cases of CML and 0 out of 29 cases of lymphoid leukaemia showing more than 4% PMN lacking MPO. In cases of otherwise unclassifiable acute leukaemia, a decreased MPO score and an increased number of MPO-deficient PMN suggests the diagnosis of AML and not ALL. **Counting the number of PMN lacking MPO was found to be a time-saving and even more reliable method than the semiquantitative scoring of MPO activity in PMN.** (Abstract: Myeloperoxidase-deficient polymorphonuclear leucocytes. (I) Incidence in untreated myeloid leukaemia, lymphoid leukaemia and normal humans.

Bendix-Hansen K, Kaspersen Nielsen H. Scand J Haematol. 1983 May;30(5):415-9).

Phagocytosis and lysis of C. pseudotropicalis by peripheral blood monocytes from Hodgkin's and non-Hodgkin's lymphoma were analysed. In Hodgkin's disease, there was a decrease in the phagocytic activity of blood monocytes; moreover, the candidacidal activity was significantly decreased as compared with normal controls. Although monocytes from non-Hodgkin's patients presented normal phagocytic function, the ability to kill C. pseudotropicalis was impaired. In both groups of lymphomas, the data showed that the abnormal findings were not related to treatment. These results indicate that **monocytes from Hodgkin's and non-Hodgkin's lymphoma posses a deficiency in killing C. pseudotropicalis, which could be due to an intrinsic macrophage defect in the myeloperoxidase-independent mechanisms and which may be responsible for**

the predisposition of these patients to candida infections.
(Abstract: Defective function of peripheral blood monocytes in
patients with Hodgkin's and non-Hodgkin's lymphomas. Estevez ME,
Sen L, Bachmann AE, Pavlovsky A. Cancer. 1980 Jul 15;46(2):299-302).

**A complete lack of myeloperoxidase (MPO) was
demonstrated in a boy suffering from acute myeloic
leukemia during the acute phase of the disease and
after a remission was achieved.** A partial defect of MPO was
demonstrated in the patient's father, no further abnormalities were
seen in other members of the family. The fine structure of the
patient's neutrophils and monocytes appeared normal, no activity of
MPO was demonstrated on the fine structural level. In the father's
neutrophils transitional forms between cells exhibiting a normal
MPO activity and those without activity were demonstrated. The
neutrophil bactericidal activity was strongly inhibited in the patient
and decreased in his father. Normal values were found in: NBT
test, chemotaxis, serum-dependent phagocytosis, number of B and
T lymphocytes, serum immunoglobulins, and complement. **This
indicates a possible connection between MPO deficiency
and leukemia.** (Abstract: Familial peroxidase-deficiency and acute
myeloid leukemia (author's transl) Hunh D, Belohradsky BH, Haas R.
Acta Haematol. 1978;59(3):129-43).

A group of 100 totally or **subtotally** myeloperoxidase (MPO)-
deficient individuals was compared to a reference population of
118 probands selected at random. Data for a protective effect of
the deficiency against cardiovascular damage are presented. On
the other hand, **a significantly higher occurrence of severe
infections and chronic inflammatory processes was noted
among the deficient patients.** An increased incidence of cancer
among the MPO-deficient individuals was not demonstrated.
(Consequences of total and subtotal myeloperoxidase deficiency:
risk or benefit ? Kutter D, Devaquet P, Vanderstocken G, Paulus JM,
Marchal V, Gothot A. Acta Haematol. 2000;104(1):10-5). **I believe
that a most important observation is that infections**

Prof Randolph Michael Howes MD,PhD

increased with decreased oxidant production with MPO, but so did chronic inflammation. Inflammation has always been blamed on excess EMODs but it may be due to a deficiency of EMODs, which I have been arguing for many years. Also, please remember that inflammation is always associated with hypoxia, which again argues for my Unified theory.

Peripheral blood leukocytes and the sera from 10 healthy women and 12 patients with **invasive carcinoma of the cervix** (stages I to IV), showed **no differences in their capacity to inhibit the replication of an invasive strain of Escherichia coli.** The serum from only one patient was unable to arrest the bacterial growth. **The quantitation of myeloperoxidase in the polymorphonuclear leukocytes from 21 patients (stages I to III) and 11 healthy women showed, however, a lower activity in the group of patients (P = 0.001).** Most patients also showed lymphocytopenia, neutrophilia, and eosinophilia but normal counts of total leukocytes. (Abstract: Phagocytic activity of circulating polymorphonuclear leukocytes from patients with carcinoma of the uterine cervix. Garcia-Gonzalez JE, Rojas-Espinosa O, Aguilar-Santelises M. Rev Latinoam Microbiol. 1992 Apr-Jun;34(2):135-41). **I believe that this indicates that patients with carcinoma of the cervix, have lower levels of myeloperoxidase.**

It is **hypothesized that dietary iodine deficiency is associated with the development of mammary pathology and cancer.** A review of the literature on this correlation and of the author's own work on the antioxidant function of iodide in iodide-concentrating extrathyroidal cells is reported. Mammary gland is embryogenetically derived from primitive iodide-concentrating ectoderm, and alveolar and ductular cells of the breast specialize in uptake and secretion of iodine in milk in order to supply offsprings with this important trace-element. **Breast and thyroid share an important iodide-concentrating ability and an efficient peroxidase activity, which transfers electrons from iodide**

to the oxygen of hydrogen peroxide, forming iodoproteins
and iodolipids, and so protects the cells from peroxidative damage.
The mammary gland has only a temporary ability to
concentrate iodides, almost exclusively during pregnancy
and lactation, which are considered protective conditions against
breast cancer. I believe that, just as with the thyroid, the
breast needs H$_2$O$_2$ to perform its function.

Myeloperoxidase (MPO) is a glycoprotein released by activated
polymorphonuclear neutrophils, which takes part in the defense
of the organism through production of hypochlorous acid
(HOCl), a potent oxidant. Apart from its implications
for host defense, the expression of MPO restricted to
myeloid precursors makes MPO mRNA a good marker of
acute myeloid leukemia. In addition, during the last few years,
involvement of MPO has been described in numerous diseases
such as atherosclerosis, lung cancer, Alzheimer's disease and
multiple sclerosis. Both strong oxidative activity and MPO genetic
polymorphism have been involved. (Abstract: Is there a role for iodine in
breast diseases? Venturi S. Breast. 2001 Oct;10(5):379-82.)

Molecular ground state dioxygen is converted to superoxide by
NADPH oxidase and NADH oxidase. Superoxide is converted
to hydrogen peroxide by superoxide dismutate at a rate
that is 100 times faster than spontaneous non-enzymatic
conversion. Oxidative mechanisms can be mediated by
myeloperoxidase (MPO) or may be independent from MPO.
(Growing significance of myeloperoxidase in non-infectious diseases.
Hoy A, Leininger-Muller B, Kutter D, Siest G, Visvikis S. Clin Chem
Lab Med. 2002 Jan;40(1):2-8).

Also, mice deficient in myeloperoxidase have somewhat
increased atherosclerosis (Brennan ML, Anderson MM, Shih
DM, Qu XD, Wang X, Mehta AC, Lim LL, Shi W, Hazen SL, Jacob JS,
Crowley JR, Heinecke JW, and Lusis AJ. Increased atherosclerosis in
myeloperoxidase-deficient mice. J Clin Invest 107: 419–430, 2001).

17 SUPEROXIDE GENERATION

Superoxide is formed upon one-electron reduction of oxygen mediated by enzymes such as NADPH oxidase or xanthine oxidase or from the respiratory chain. The half-life of O_2^- in tissues is dependent on the presence of the enzyme superoxide dismutase in different cellular compartments. Some believe that **most superoxide is rapidly converted to hydrogen peroxide and that very little superoxide anion, per se, actually exists**. In my opinion, this is a most important consideration and it provides for high steady states of hydrogen peroxide. However, high levels of **H_2O_2 inactivates SOD.**

Oxyhemoglobin slowly releases O_2^- to form methemoglobin, which can not bind and transport O_2. This occurs in 1 in 1000 cycles of O_2 binding and release but it is estimated that **3% of hemoglobin releases O_2^- RMH Note: This represents another huge source of O_2^-, H_2O_2 and $^1O_2$.**

The stationary stage concentration of O_2^- is maintained by SOD at 10^{-11} M in cytosol and 10^{-10} M in mitochondrial matrix.

17.0 O_2^- Produced Daily

The mitochondria are one of the main sites of **superoxide production and can be enhanced by increasing the O_2 concentration or when the respiratory chain becomes fully reduced as happens in ischemia.**

Under normal conditions, the amount of O_2^- generated by a mitochondrion has been estimated to be as high as 10^7 O_2^- radicals per day. This equates to 416,666.6/ hour or 6,944/minute or 116/second. If we multiply this times an average of 200 mitochondria per cell, we get 23,000/ sec/cell or if we multiply this times 75 trillion cells, we get 2.3 X 10^{16} superoxide anions produced by the body every second of every day.

It takes enormous volumes of O_2 and RONS to keep us going. Shockingly, a 70 kilogram/154 lb. adult with a 1% "leak" would produce annually 1.7 kilograms of $O_2^{\cdot-}$ (presumably and/or H_2O_2 or .OH) and a 5% leak would generate an astonishing 8.5 kilograms of $O_2^{\cdot-}$ in a year. In other words, **at a 5% leak of $O_2^{\cdot-}$, an average adult would produce more than his entire body weight in $O_2^{\cdot-}$ in 6 years.** If he lived to be **a healthy 83 year old, he would have produced over 10 times his body weight in oxygen free radicals (705 kg of $O_2^{\cdot-}$)** and many individuals appear to do this and are just fine. So, I ask my question again, "How toxic are RONS?" They do not sound very toxic to me.

According to the director of the Linus Pauling Institute, Dr. Frei Balz, **under normal metabolic conditions, each cell in our body is exposed to about 10^{10} molecules of superoxide each day.** For a person weighing 150 pounds, this amounts to about 4 pounds of superoxide per year, a substantial amount! Once formed, superoxide is converted to other **EMODs**. For a 200 pound man this equates to formation of 5.3 pounds of $O_2^{\cdot-}$ per year. That means that in 37.7 years, this person would have formed an amount of $O_2^{\cdot-}$ equal to his body weight and **at 75 years of age, he would have formed 2 times his body weight of $O_2^{\cdot-}$.** Please remember that $O_2^{\cdot-}$ is immediately converted into H_2O_2 and **one would have a corresponding amount of H_2O_2 formed in the same time frame.**

If $O_2^{\cdot-}$ were stable, O_2 cellular utilization would produce 5 μmol l^{-1} intracellular $O_2^{\cdot-}$ per second (O_2 toxicity, Fridovich).

One rat liver mitochondrion produces 3×10^7 superoxide radicals per day.
Figures vary according to the reference cited.

The stationary stage concentration of $O_2^{\cdot-}$ is maintained by SOD at 10^{-11} M in cytosol and 10^{-10} M in mitochondrial matrix.

3% of total hemoglobin forms $O_2^{\cdot-}$ (Free Radical Vet Paper).

O$_2^-$ can be formed enzymatically by flavoprotein dehdydrogenases and more importantly **non-enzymatically** by autoxidation of ferridoxins, hydroquinones, thiols and reduced hemoproteins (Fridovich).

The following enzymes are capable of producing large amounts of **oxygen free radicals**:

Xanthine oxidase
Prostaglandin synthase
Lipoxygenase
Aldehyde oxidase
Amino acid oxidase
Myeloperoxidase (uses H$_2$O$_2$ to oxidize chloride ions to form HOCl)

Superoxide is Produced Enzymatically By

- NADPH oxidases (phagocytosis)
- Mitochondrial cytochrome c oxidase (cell respiration)
- Liver Cytochrome P 450 (oxidation of xenobiotics)
- Xanthine oxidase (ischemic reperfusion)
- Prostaglandin synthetase
- Lipoxygenase
- Aldehyde oxidase
- Amino acid oxidase
- Myeloperoxidase (uses H$_2$O$_2$ to oxidize chloride ions to form HOCl)

Cell membrane NADPH-oxidase is activated to produce O$_2^-$ by:

Immunologic-coated bacteria
Immune complexes
Complement 5a
Leukotrienes

NADPH-oxidase is the main source of superoxide radicals in human phagocytes, producing up to 15 fmol per cell per minute for the explicit purpose of destroying the biological activity of foreign organisms.

- Based on O_2^{-} generation in vitro in the mitochondria and microsomes of rat lungs and livers, **the formation rate of ROS is estimated to be 50 nmol/g of tissue per min or about 10^{11} radicals/cell/day** (Free Radicals in Aging, Yu).

In cultured mouse embryos, **ethanol induces:**

superoxide generation

Superoxide anion is generated at the ubiquinone site in complex III, where it acts as a prooxidant.

O_2^{-} that exits from, or is produced outside of, vascular cells can be converted by extracellular SOD (ECSOD) to H_2O_2. In addition, O_2^{-} produced within the cell is converted by Cu/Zn SOD and Mn SOD to H_2O_2

Most superoxide is rapidly converted to hydrogen peroxide and very little superoxide anion, per se, actually exists.

O_2^{-} is a very transient intermediate, and H_2O_2 production by mitochondria is catalyzed by mitochondrial SOD (Kerwin, J.F., Jr., Lancaster, J.R., Jr. and Feldman, P.L. Nitric oxide: A new paradigm for second messengers. J Med Chem 1995; 38: 249-253).

$$QH^{\cdot} + O_2 \text{ --- } Q + H^+ + O_2^{-}$$

$$SOD$$

$$2H+ + 2O_2^{-} \rightarrow\rightarrow\rightarrow H_2O_2 + O_2$$

Interestingly, **this is one of the few situations in biology in which SOD has been demonstrated to cause an increase in H_2O_2 generation**.

Focusing on isolated mitochondria, and considering the succinate dehydrogenase-ubiquinone segment as the most important source of ROS (60-80%), then the rate of RONS production is modulated by the steady-state concentrations of ubisemiquinone and oxygen.

At a 5% leak of $O_2^{·-}$, an average adult would produce more than his entire body weight in $O_2^{·-}$ in 6 years.

Please keep in mind that $O_2^{·-}$, in aqueous solutions, is a reductant, not an oxidant. In fact, an ideal place for $O_2^{·-}$ to give up its spare electron is to lose it to iron.

An enzyme, NADPH oxidase, is found on the surfaces of macrophages and neutrophils and is stimulated by invading pathogens to produce $O_2^{·-}$.

It has been estimated that an individual produces approximately **1 kg of oxygen radicals per year**, the consequence of which is approximately 100,000 oxidative "attacks" on mitochondrial DNA per cell each day.

Humans consume ~250 g of oxygen every day, and of this ~3-5% is converted to $O_2^{·-}$ and other reactive species.

It was experimentally proven that high doses of beta-carotene produced superoxide radicals.

Potential cellular sources of $O_2^{·-}$ in blood vessels include **infiltrating phagocytic cells**, which contain the high-capacity $O_2^{·-}$ generating flavoenzyme NADPH oxidase, as well as **vascular endothelial cells, smooth muscle cells** (SMC) and **fibroblasts**.

Non-phagocytic NAD(P)H oxidase is a major source of EMODs in cultured vascular cells.

Xanthine oxidase, nitric oxide synthase, cytochrome *P-450* and the mitochondrial electron transport chain may be important sources of EMODs.

Cellular antioxidant regulation does not completely remove endogenously generated H_2O_2. Rather these processes **appear to permit levels of H_2O_2 that are sufficient to exert modulatory actions.**

Superoxide can be nonenzymatically converted into H_2O_2 and $^1O_2$.

70-90% of O_2 uptake during the respiratory burst goes to O_2^- formation but this goes to produce singlet oxygen. Shift of oxygen to this system reduces electron transport and lactic acid accumulates and is transported to the lysosome. **Acid pH aids in the production of singlet oxygen.** However, the respiratory burst within the phagocytic vacuoles is accompanied by a surge in the intra-vacuolar pH—from 6 to nearly 8. A large influx of potassium ions through the vacuolar membrane occurs and offsets the anionic charge. That happens in spite of the release of predominantly acidic granular contents since protons are consumed in neutralizing the excess of basic superoxide ions and other radicals. (Di A, Krupa B, Bindokas VP, et al. Quantal release of free radicals during exocytosis of phagosomes. Nature Cell Biol. 2002;4:279- 285).

Superoxide anion and hydrogen peroxide are constantly being produced by:

> Mitochondrial respiratory chain
> Electron transport chain
> > Endoplasmic reticulum
> > Nuclear membranes

17.1 Antioxidant Enzyme Defenses

Enzyme antioxidants

Superoxide dismutase
Catalase
Glutathione peroxidase
Glutathione S-transferases
Phospholipid-hydroperoxide glutathione peroxidase
Ascorbate peroxidase
Monodehydroascorbate reductase
Dehydroascorbate reductase
Glutathione reductase

Enzymatic antioxidants principally include SOD, catalase, glutathione peroxidases, glutathione reductase and transferases, thiol-disulfide oxidoreductases, and peroxiredoxins. Many of these enzymatic antioxidants are **present in normal arteries,** most likely within vascular wall cells as **extracellular fluid is largely devoid of enzymatic antioxidants** (Stocker R and Frei B. Endogenous antioxidant defenses in human blood plasma. In: *Oxidative Stress: Oxidants and Antioxidants,* edited by Sies H. London: Academic, 1991, p. 213–243).

In this monograph I will consider primarily CAT, SOD and GPX. To date, Catalase and GPx have been viewed as the major enzymes responsible for removal of cytotoxic H_2O_2. However, catalase is largely or entirely located in peroxisomes and GPx is present mainly in mitochondria and nuclei. The fact that GPx is located in the nucleus indicates the nuclear presence of H_2O_2; otherwise, why would GPx be there?

Superoxide in aqueous media undergoes a spontaneous second order reaction with itself, a dismutation reaction that yields one molecule each of H_2O_2 and oxygen in a

relatively slow reaction at pH 7.4 (the second order rate constant is of the order of 10 to the 4.5^{th} power), when compared with the rate at which superoxide or $HO_2.-$ can abstract an H-atom from such key biological targets as catecholamines or the allylic CH in lipid where the second order rate constant exceeds 10^7.

Although the dismutation would be spontaneous at physiological pH at high superoxide concentrations, **the concentration of superoxide approaches 10 μM (physiological)** as the self reaction slows down considerably and its lifetime becomes extended by many seconds. Consequently, nature has evolved a class of superoxide dismutase (SOD2), enzymes to remove this potentially deleterious free radical byproduct of oxygen metabolism. **These enzymes can react rapidly with superoxide (rates approaching or exceeding 10^9 power) and dismutate the radical to the nonradical products, O_2 and H_2O_2, faster than superoxide can react with other potential biological targets.** The short half-life should not be misinterpreted as mitigating the potential reactivity of O_2^- because the half-life is actually quite long in relation to the **phenomenal diffusion coefficient of the radical.** Given that superoxide can interact with a variety of biological target molecules, the reaction with the enzyme literally can shunt the superoxide production into H_2O_2 and oxygen.

17.2 SOD is a Prooxidant Enzyme

Howes Evolves a New Concept: SOD is <u>NOT an Antioxidant</u>

It has occurred to me that superoxide dismutases only convert O_2^- to H_2O_2 and this serves as another huge intra-mitochondrial source for H_2O_2 production. MnSOD is an intra-mitochondrial "antioxidant enzyme." As I will discuss in detail later, SOD can be viewed as <u>NOT being an antioxidant</u> enzyme merely because it reduces O_2^-, when in actuality, it is creating a more potent oxidant in

the process. **SOD is a reducing or antioxidant enzyme in name only. The one electron reduction potential of $O_2{}^{\cdot-}$ is -330 mV and the reduction potential is +320 mV for H_2O_2, respectively. Thus, in actuality, SOD is a prooxidant enzyme! I believe that my new realization is of utmost importance for the correct interpretation of redox studies and data.**

The enzyme superoxide dismutase ensures elimination of the superoxide anion, the first toxic species to be formed from oxygen. SOD thus carries out first-line defense against oxidative stress. To function correctly, the enzyme requires **oligoelements such as copper and zinc (Cu-Zn SOD present in the cytosol) or manganese (Mn SOD** present in the mitochondrion. There also exists an extracellular SOD.

Low SOD levels may reflect low levels of oligoelements, but there is no absolute correlation between the former and the latter. In the presence of oxidative stress, SOD shows two different behaviors. First, in response to a moderate level of oxidative stress (due, e.g., to physical exercise), **the organism over expresses SOD** (Levine SA and Kidd PM. Antioxidant adaptation. Its role in free radical pathology. San Leandro, California. Eds A. Biocurrents division, Allergy Research Group, 1996.). Then, **if the stress persists and involves massive production of toxic EMODs, SOD is destroyed and its concentration drops. Paradoxically, a too-high SOD concentration can be dangerous, because it leads to overproduction of hydrogen peroxide (paradoxical effect of antioxidants). Actually, I firmly believe that the purpose of SOD is to produce H_2O_2, because it is an excellent second messenger in a vast and increasing number of crucial biochemical events.**

Superoxide is redox ambivalent. The relative levels of SOD, catalase, and glutathione peroxidase are important. For instance, an increase in SOD would deplete the cell of superoxide but would increase H_2O_2 production.

Curiously, SOD is one of the most important enzymes in the front line of defense against oxidative stress. According to Dr. Cutler, **SOD is also a factor that controls organisms' life-spans** (J.M. Tolmasoff, T. Ono and R.G. Cutler, Proc. Natl. Acad. Sci. USA, 77, 2777 (1980). I do not believe that we know what controls lifespans or we would be using it now (unless you are a fruit fly).

The large body of literature has not yet definitely demonstrated a causal relationship between free radicals, antioxidant enzymes, and cancer in humans. Powerful evidence of a causal relationship is that, in various model systems, ROS cause cancer (in vitro). Moreover, antioxidants, and **SOD in particular, inhibit malignant transformation**. (Larry Oberley, Ph.D. Free radicals biology: A molecular approach to suppressing cancer cell growth. Currents: Summer 2001, Volume 2, Number 3). **I believe that SOD inhibits mutagenesis because it is a highly efficient generator of H_2O_2.** It has been shown that **malignant blood cells differentiate and stop proliferating in the presence of liposomal SOD**. Implicit in this evidence is that the loss of SOD activity may in some way be causal to malignant transformation.

Oberley demonstrated that the **transfection of MnSOD cDNA into cultured human melanoma cells resulted in the loss of the malignant phenotype by at least five-fold.** The most important observation was that in the nude mouse assay, 18 out of 18 sites injected with parental melanoma cell line developed tumors, while **none of the 16 sites injected with melanoma cells expressing high levels of MnSOD developed tumors. . Again, I believe that this demonstrates the cytotoxicity of H_2O_2 for cancer cells.**

Further, Oberley also have found that **MnSOD in combination with certain chemicals can have an anticancer effect via cell killing**, in contrast to the non-cytotoxic tumor suppression effect of MnSOD alone. The rationale behind this combination comes from the enzymatic action of MnSOD protein: it dismutes superoxide radicals into hydrogen peroxide. If hydrogen peroxide removal is inhibited, cancer cells will die due to hydrogen peroxide-mediated cell damage. Thus, we have treated rat glioma cells with a derivative of nitrosourea (BCNU), a clinically used anticancer drug that inhibits the enzyme that mediates the removal of hydrogen peroxide from the cell. We found that **the higher the MnSOD levels in these cells, the higher the killing rate.** Using another inhibitor of hydrogen peroxide removal, buthionine sulfoximine (BSO), in combination with MnSOD, the killing rate reached 100 percent. **I believe that all of this is consistent with the cytotoxic activity of H_2O_2, which is produced by SOD.**

I have been saying all along that SOD serves as a plentiful source of H_2O_2 and it is, thus, an excellent prooxidant and tumoricidal agent.

The rapid dismutation of O_2^- to H_2O_2 is (spontaneous, 10^5 [mol/L]$^{-1}$ · s^{-1}, SOD-catalyzed, 10^9 [mol/L]$^{-1}$ × s^{-1}).

O_2^- inactivates catalase and glutathione peroxidase and epinephrine oxidation. **(RMH Note: Thus, O_2^- blocks the breakdown of H_2O_2.)**

O_2^- at physiological pH has a pK of 4.8 and it can readily pass through membranes on the anion channels.

The influence of an antioxidant vitamin supplement on immune cell response to prolonged exercise was determined using a randomized, double-blind, placebo-controlled, cross-over study. Twelve healthy endurance subjects (n = 6 male, n = 6 female; mean +/- SD for age, 30.1 +/- 6.2 yr; height, 1.76 +/- 7 m; body mass, 72.2 +/- 10.2 kg; VO_2max, 63.7 +/- 12 ml x kg(-1) x min(-1)) participated in the study. Following a 3-week period during which subjects ingested a multivitamin and -mineral complex sufficient to meet the recommended daily allowance, they took either a placebo or an antioxidant vitamin supplement (containing 18 mg beta-carotene, 900 mg vitamin C, and 90 mg vitamin E) for 7 days prior to a 2-h treadmill run at 65% VO_2 max. Blood samples were drawn prior to and immediately following exercise. These were analyzed for neutrophil oxidative burst activity, cortisol and glucose concentrations, and white blood cell counts, as well as serum anti-oxidant vitamin concentrations. **Plasma vitamin C, vitamin E, and beta-carotene concentrations significantly increased following 7-day supplementation ($p < .05$).** In comparison to the placebo group, **neutrophil oxidative burst was significantly higher following exercise ($p < .05$) in the antioxidant vitamin group,** but no differences were found in any other parameter following the 7-day supplementation period. Although the impact of exercise on neutrophil function is multifactorial, our data suggest that antioxidant supplementation may be of benefit to endurance athletes for the maintenance of this particular function of the innate immune system following the 7-day supplementation period (Antioxidant supplementation enhances neutrophil oxidative burst in trained runners following prolonged exercise. Robson PJ, Bouic PJ, Myburgh KH. Int J Sport Nutr Exerc Metab. 2003 Sep;13(3):369-81). **I believe that this study invalidates the free radi-crap theory, in that it shows that antioxidants actually increase the generation of EMODs during the respiratory burst. Since the respiratory burst is associated with up to a 200% increase in O_2 consumption and EMOD production, the antioxidant vitamins predictabily should have blocked this production of EMODs. It did not and it, in fact, increased them.**

Studies have demonstrated that the **tumor suppressor PTEN** (phosphatase and tensin homolog deleted from chromosome 10), the antagonist of the phosphosphoinositol-3-kinase (PI3K) signaling cascade, is **susceptible to H_2O_2-dependent oxidative inactivation.**

Overexpression of PTEN prevented the H_2O_2-dependent increase in vascular endothelial growth factor promoter activity and immunoreactive protein, whereas a mutant PTEN (G129R), lacking phosphatase activity, did not. Furthermore, mitochondrial generation of H_2O_2 by Sod2 promoted endothelial cell sprouting in a three-dimensional *in vitro* angiogenesis assay that was attenuated by catalase coexpression or the PI3K inhibitor LY2949002. **Sod2 overexpression resulted in increased** *in vivo* **blood vessel formation that was H_2O_2-dependent** as assessed by the chicken chorioallantoic membrane assay. The findings of Connor, et al, provide the first evidence for the involvement of mitochondrial H_2O_2 in regulating PTEN function and the angiogenic switch, **indicating that SOD2 can serve as an alternative physiological source of the potent signaling molecule, H_2O_2** . (KM. Connor, S Subbaram, KJ. Regan, KK. Nelson, JE. Mazurkiewicz, PJ. Bartholomew, AE. Aplin, YT Tai, J Aguirre-Ghiso, SC. Flores, and J A Melendez. Mitochondrial H_2O_2 Regulates the Angiogenic Phenotype via PTEN Oxidation. J. Biol. Chem., Vol. 280, Issue 17, 16916-16924, April 29, 2005)

EC-SOD is an extracellular form of the enzyme. It also contains copper-zinc and is a notable exception in that **significant amounts of this antioxidant enzyme are present in the normal arterial wall outside cells** (Strålin P, Karlsson K, Johansson BO, and Marklund SL. The interstitium of the human arterial wall contains very large amounts of extracellular superoxide dismutase. *Arterioscler Thromb Vasc Biol* 15: 2032–2036, 1995).

In **the presence of bicarbonate, Cu, Zn-SOD also has peroxidase activity towards H_2O_2** (Hink HU, Santanam N, Dikalov S, McCann L, Nguyen AD, Parthasarathy S, Harrison DG, and Fukai T. Peroxidase properties of extracellular superoxide dismutase: role of uric acid in modulating in vivo activity. *Arterioscler Thromb Vasc Biol* 22: 1402–1408, 2002), **that results in the oxidation of cosubstrates and may inactivate the enzyme distinct from that seen with H_2O_2 at high pH.** Thus, I favor an acidic cellular milieu.

17.3 MnSOD Deficiency is Lethal in Mice

Previous studies have shown that the lack of MnSOD gene in Escherichia coli and yeast leads to hypersensitivity and oxidative stress. Homozygous mutant **mice lacking MnSOD died within the first 10 days after birth and showed dilated cardiomyopathy, accumulation of lipid in liver and skeletal muscle, and metabolic acidosis**. Furthermore, mice lacking MnSOD showed degenerative injury of the central nervous system, particularly in the basal ganglia and brain stem associated with damaged mitochondria (Takada Y, Hachiya M, Park SH, Osawa Y, Ozawa T, Akashi M. (2002) The Role of reactive oxygen species in cells overexpressing manganese superoxide dismutase: mechanism for induction of radioresistance. Mol Cancer Res. 1:137-46). **I believe that this lack of MnSOD, which is the only mitochondrial enzyme to convert $O_2^{\cdot-}$ to H_2O_2, shows that the cells desperately need adequate levels of H_2O_2. I consider this further support for my Unified Theory.**

17.4 Cancer Cells are Low in MnSOD

Cancer cells are nearly always low in MnSOD (Oberley LW. (2001) Anticancer therapy by overexpression of superoxide dismutase. Antioxid Redox Signal. 3:46-472). I believe that this creates the low levels of RONS (MnSOD is not present to form H_2O_2) and this "allows" for cancer growth.

17.5 Overexpression of CuZnSOD Inhibits Tumor Cell Growth

One study demonstrated that overexpression of CuZnSOD can inhibit tumor cell growth (Zhang Y, Zhao WL, Zhang HJ, Doman FE, Oberley LW. (2002) Overexpression of copper zinc superoxide dismutase suppresses human glioma cell growth. Cancer Res. 62:1205-1212). **Again, H_2O_2 is generated to increased levels such that it demonstrates antineoplastic properties,**

in accordance with my Unified theory. To the contrary, in tumor cells, the activity of CuZnSOD is usually low (Oberley LW. (2001) Anticancer therapy by overexpression of superoxide dismutase. Antioxid Redox Signal. 3:46-472).

Catalase is not essential for some cells under normal conditions and further argues that excess levels of hydrogen peroxide are not very toxic. This is verified by the fact that most acatalasemia patients get along quite well.

One study double overexpressed MnSOD and GPx1 into PU1 18-9 cells (Li SJ, Yan T, Yang JQ, Oberley TD, Oberley LW. (2000) The role of cellular glutathione peroxidase redox regulation in suppression of tumor cell growth by manganese superoxide dismutase. Cancer Res. 60:3927-3939). **They found that overexpression of GPx1 rescues the growth suppression by MnSOD. This evidence indicates that GPx1 is a major antioxidant enzyme that protects cells against lethal oxidative stress.**

I believe that these results are because the GSH-Px breaks down the H$_2$O$_2$ formed by the overexpressed MnSOD, and consequently, the repressed growth is blocked by deficiency levels of EMODs.

17.6 SOD Increases H$_2$O$_2$

Thus, theoretically, in vivo, the presence of highly active **SOD enzymes will lead to an increase in the local concentration of H$_2$O$_2$.**

The foregoing collection of data presents an overwhelming number of ways in which O$_2^-$ is produced in the cell. Surely, not all of these are the result of evolutionary mistakes and **it seems plausible to me that even enzymes, such as superoxide dismutase, may have evolved to more efficiently produce H$_2$O$_2$.**

Basically, all cells continuously form O$_2$· and submitochondrial particles generate O$_2$· at a rate of 4-7 nmol/min^{-1}/mg protein^{-1} (Chance, B., Sies, H. and Boveris, A. Hydroperoxide metabolism in mammalian organs. Physiol Rev 59: 527-605, 1979).

Again, I feel that this is a most important aspect of superoxide chemistry, in that it provides an adequate and continual supply of life-sustaining hydrogen peroxide. This also means that it can be viewed as a prooxidant enzyme and not an antioxidant enzyme. I feel that my take on this position is bolstered by the fact that nature has developed the peroxisome expressly for the purpose of hydrogen peroxide production (during fatty acid oxidation). Hydrogen peroxide is a non-radical and is readily diffusible throughout the cell. In fact, I look at the production of **superoxide anion as an innate pathway for hydrogen peroxide production,** which allows for an adequate source of **singlet oxygen** production following reaction with hypochlorous acid or otherwise. **This constant supply of singlet oxygen can then serve the body in its many capacities as an anti-inflammatory, anti-bacterial, anti-fungal, anti-virucidal and anti-cancer agent. Thus, I believe that H$_2$O$_2$ and ^{1}O$_2$ may be two of the most beautifully designed molecular structures in the aerobic cell and in the human body.**

Mutations occurring at the SOD1 gene are associated with reduced SOD activities and amyotrophic lateral sclerosis (Kohno S, Takahashi Y, Miyajima H, Serizawa M, Mizoguchi K. A novel mutation (Cys6Gly) in the Cu/Zn superoxide dismutase gene associated with rapidly progressive familial amyotrophic lateral sclerosis. *Neurosci Lett.* 1999;276:135–137). **I believe that these diseases are due to a lack of EMODs and especially H$_2$O$_2$.**

As mentioned previously, it takes enormous volumes of O$_2$ and RONS to keep us going. Shockingly, a 70 kilogram/154 lb. adult with a 1% "leak" would produce annually 1.7 kilograms of O$_2$· (presumably and/or H_2O_2 or .OH) and a 5% leak would generate an astonishing 8.5 kilograms of O_2^- in a year. In other words, **at a 5% leak of O_2^-, an average adult would produce more than his entire body weight in O_2^- in 6 years.** If he lived to be **a healthy 83 year old, he would have produced over 10 times his body weight in oxygen free radicals (705 kg of O_2^-)** and many individuals appear to do this and are just fine. So, I ask my question again, "How toxic are RONS?" They do not sound very toxic to me.

17.7 Mn-SOD

Although **the levels of Mn-SOD in blood vessels are relatively small,** Mn-SOD may exert important functional effects in cerebral circulation, because **endothelium expresses high levels of Mn-SOD** (Suzuki K, Tatsumi H, Satoh S, Senda T, Nakata T, Fujii J, Taniguchi N. Manganese-superoxide dismutase in endothelial cells: localization and mechanism of induction. Am J Physiol. 1993; 265: H1173–1178) **and levels of Mn-SOD are higher in cerebral arteries than in extracranial arteries** (Napoli C, Witztum JL, de Nigris F, Palumbo G, D'Armiento FP, Palinski W. Intracranial arteries of human fetuses are more resistant to hypercholesterolemia-induced fatty streak formation than extracranial arteries. Circulation. 1999; 99: 2003–2010).

The mitochondrial content of cerebral endothelium is greater than that in other cells (Oldendorf WH, Cornfield ME, Brown WJ. The large apparent work capability of the blood-brain barrier: a study of the mitochondrial content of capillary endothelial cells in brain and other tissues of the rat. Ann Neurol. 1977; 1: 409–417), and high levels of Mn-SOD may be required to limit oxidative stress in the metabolically active cerebral endothelium (the blood-brain barrier). Actually, **I believe that the high levels of H_2O_2 produced by SOD are needed for normal cerebral function.**

Recent studies of **Mn-SOD heterozygous–deficient mice (Mn-SOD$^{+/-}$)** on an apolipoprotein E–deficient background indicate that

Mn-SOD protects against vascular mitochondrial DNA damage and development of atherosclerosis in aorta. With regard to the microcirculation, our preliminary studies indicate that **endothelial function is impaired in cerebral arterioles from Mn-SOD$^{+/-}$ mice** (Didion and Faraci, unpublished data, 2002).

Please keep in mind that SOD generates H$_2$O$_2$.

17.8 EC-SOD

Based on its subcellular localization and because **EC-SOD is a major component of total SOD activity in blood vessels, it** has been hypothesized that EC-SOD would protect NO as it diffuses through the vessel wall. The first study that addressed this hypothesis using **EC-SOD–deficient mice reported a surprisingly modest role for EC-SOD with regard to endothelial function in the cerebral microcirculation** (Demchenko IT, Oury TD, Crapo JD, Piantadosi CA. Regulation of the brain's vascular responses to oxygen. Circ Res. 2002; 91: 1031–1037).

17.9 Autoxidation

Autoxidation produces superoxide anion (O$_2^{\cdot-}$).

Autoxidation of epinephrine and glutathione generate O$_2^{\cdot-}$ and H$_2$O$_2$.

Some of the molecules that undergo autoxidation are the following:

> **catecholamines,**
> **hemoglobin,**
> **myoglobin,**
> **reduced cytochrome C**
> **Thiol**

Cu+
Fe++
Epinephrine
glutathione

Autoxidation of any of these molecules results in RONS, **primarily superoxide.**

Autoxidation of many molecules results in EMODs, **primarily superoxide.** Copper or ferrous ions (Fe II) can also autoxidize to produce **superoxide** and ferric (Fe III) iron.

Autoxidation of epinephrine and glutathione generate O_2^{-} and H_2O_2.

Sugars, glucose, mannose and deoxy sugars auto-oxidize to produce H_2O_2 (Lam).

H_2O_2 production during glucose autoxidation is low, but measurable.

18.0 H$_2$O$_2$ PRODUCTION BY BACTERIA

18.1 H$_2$O$_2$ as Protection for Bacteria

Streptococcal species other than group A streptococci (GAS; Streptococcus pyogenes) can cause a wide range of diseases in animals and humans, including nonsymptomatic commensal-like carriage, skin infections, septicemia, arthritis, endocarditis, otitis media, pneumonia, and meningitis (Jedrzejas, M. J. 2001. Pneumococcal virulence factors: structure and function. Microbiol. Mol. Biol. Rev. 65:187-207). Pneumococci, viridans streptococci, some GCS, and GGS produced similar amounts of H$_2$O$_2$ and showed similar killing kinetics as equimolar amounts of pure H$_2$O$_2$. **Killing by all strains depended completely upon the amount of H$_2$O$_2$ produced and could be prevented with catalase.** None of the GBS produced H$_2$O$_2$; therefore, they did not affect the viability of C. elegans. **There was no correlation between human pathogenicity of the strains and their killing capacity for C. elegans** in the assays just described. Pathogenic bacteria like S. pneumoniae show the same killing effects as oral commensals like S. mitis and S. oralis. The mortality of C. elegans reflected solely the H$_2$O$_2$ production of the bacterial strains.

18.2 Streptococcal Production of H$_2$O$_2$

Streptococcal production of H$_2$O$_2$ has several effects in humans. It inhibits a variety of competing organisms in the upper respiratory tract (Pericone, C. D., K. Overweg, P. W. Hermans, and J. N. Weiser. 2000. Inhibitory and bactericidal effects of hydrogen peroxide production by Streptococcus pneumoniae on other inhabitants of the upper respiratory tract. Infect. Immun. 68:3990-3997) **and causes direct oxidative damage to brain ependymal cells** (Hirst, R. A., K. S. Sikand, A. Rutman, T. J. Mitchell, P. W. Andrew, and C. O'Callaghan. 2000. Relative roles of pneumolysin and hydrogen peroxide from Streptococcus pneumoniae in inhibition

of ependymal ciliary beat frequency. Infect. Immun. 68:1557-1562),
ciliated nasal epithelium (Feldman, C., R. Anderson, R. Cockeran,
T. Mitchell, P. Cole, and R. Wilson. 2002. The effects of pneumolysin
and hydrogen peroxide, alone and in combination, on human
ciliated epithelium in vitro. Respir. Med. 96:580-585), **and alveolar
epithelial cells** (Duane, P. G., J. B. Rubins, H. R. Weisel, and E. N.
Janoff. 1993. Identification of hydrogen peroxide as a *Streptococcus
pneumoniae* toxin for rat alveolar epithelial cells. Infect. Immun.
61:4392-4397). **It is an important virulence factor in, e.g.,
pneumococcal colonization and host cell damage and
induces apoptosis in brain cells** (Braun, J. S., J. E. Sublett, D. Freyer,
T. J. Mitchell, J. L. Cleveland, E. I. Tuomanen, and J. R. Weber. 2002.
Pneumococcal pneumolysin and H_2O_2 mediate brain cell apoptosis
during meningitis. J. Clin. Investig. 109:19-27). **I am not at all
surprised that other species utilize prooxidant protection.
It works well for us and for them.**

18.3 Enterococcus H_2O_2 Production

**Enterococci are gram-positive bacteria that usually reside
in the gastrointestinal tract as commensal organisms,**
but they are also capable of causing severe infections (**Gilmore,
M. S., P. S. Coburn, S. R. Nallapareddy, and B. E. Murray.**
2002. Enterococcal virulence, p. 301-354. *In* M. S. Gilmore, D. B.
Clewell, P. Courvalin, G. M. Dunny, B. E. Murray, and L. B. Rice (ed.),
The enterococci: pathogenesis, molecular biology, and antibiotic
resistance. ASM Press, Washington, D.C.). **Enterococci are the
third leading source of nosocomial infections,** causing
endocarditis, peritonitis, bacteremia, and urinary tract infections.
Two enterococcal species are responsible for almost all of these
infections. According to a 1997 survey, the majority (85 to 90%)
of enterococcal infections are caused by Enterococcus faecalis,
and the remaining infections are due to Enterococcus faecium. The
mechanism underlying E. faecium pathogenesis is obscure.

Researchers identified conditions in which E. faecium kills C. elegans, and presented evidence that **the killing is due to the production by E. faecium of hydrogen peroxide** (T. I. Moy, E. Mylonakis, S. B. Calderwood, and F. M. Ausubel. Cytotoxicity of Hydrogen Peroxide Produced by Enterococcus faecium. Infection and Immunity, August 2004, p. 4512-4520, Vol. 72, No. 8).

Mycobacterium tuberculosis can survive and grow inside macrophages, likely due to production of cell wall glycolysis that remove ROS (**some bacteria have catalase to break down hydrogen peroxide**) and these types of organisms that survive inside phagocytes produce persistent diseases.

Please remember that just as we use H_2O_2 for prooxidant protection from pathogens and neoplasia, pathogens can also use H_2O_2 for their own protection.

19.0 HYPOXIA AND TUMORS

Tissue hypoxia results from an inadequate supply of oxygen (O₂) that compromises biologic functions and EMOD production. Evidence from experimental and clinical studies increasingly points to a fundamental role for hypoxia in solid tumors. Hypoxia in tumors is primarily a pathophysiologic consequence of structurally and functionally disturbed microcirculation and the deterioration of diffusion conditions. **I believe that hypoxia provides the fertile soil for the growth of neoplastic cells in that it is an area of EMOD deficiency.**

Clinical studies have shown that **metastatic spread is associated with hypoxia in the primary tumor.** (Hypoxia Promotes Lymph Node Metastasis in Human Melanoma Xenografts by Up-Regulating the Urokinase-Type Plasminogen Activator Receptor. Einar K. Rofstad, Heidi Rasmussen, Kanthi Galappathi, Berit Mathiesen, Kristin Nilsen and Bjørn A. Graff. Cancer Research 62, 1847-1853, March 15, 2002) (**Tumor Hypoxia: Definitions and Current Clinical, Biologic, and Molecular Aspects.** Michael Höckel, Peter Vaupel. Journal of the National Cancer Institute, Vol. 93, No. 4, 266-276, February 21, 2001).

Most human tumors develop regions of chronically or transiently hypoxic cells during growth (Vaupel P., Kallinowski F., Okunieff P. Blood flow, oxygen and nutrient supply, and metabolic microenvironment of human tumors: a review. Cancer Res., 49: 6449-6465, 1989). Hypoxic tumor regions may show increased expression of many genes because of hypoxia-induced activation of DNA transcription factors. Hypoxia may also lead to increased gene expression in tumor tissue by inducing amplifications, rearrangements, translocations, and genomic instability. Several of the gene products that are induced or up-regulated under hypoxic conditions may play an important role in the metastatic process. Therefore, it has been suggested that **hypoxia may promote the development of metastatic disease in human cancer**

(Rofstad E. K. Microenvironment-induced cancer metastasis. Int. J. Radiat. Biol., 76: 589-605, 2000; Höckel M., Vaupel P. Tumor hypoxia: definitions and current clinical, biologic, and molecular aspects. J. Natl. Cancer Inst. (Bethesda), 93: 266-276, 2001). **I believe that hypoxia allows for the progression and metastasis of cancer.**

This suggestion is supported by recent clinical studies that have shown that **invasive growth and metastatic spread are associated with tumor hypoxia** (Höckel M., Schlenger K., Arai B., Mitze M., Schäffer U., Vaupel P. Association between tumor hypoxia and malignant progression in advanced cancer of the uterine cervix. Cancer Res., 56: 4509-4515, 1996; Brizel D. M., Scully S. P., Harrelson J. M., Layfield L. J., Bean J. M., Prosnitz L. R., Dewhirst M. W. Tumor oxygenation predicts for the likelihood of distant metastases in human soft tissue sarcoma. Cancer Res., 56: 941-943, 1996; Rofstad E. K., Sundfør K., Lyng H., Tropé C. G. Hypoxia-induced treatment failure in advanced squamous cell carcinoma of the uterine cervix is primarily due to hypoxia-induced radiation resistance rather than hypoxia-induced metastasis. Br. J. Cancer, 83: 354-359, 2000).

Human cervical carcinomas with a median pO_2 < 10 mm Hg were found to have larger tumor extensions, more frequent parametrical infiltration, and more extensive lymph-vascular space involvement than those with a median pO_2 > 10 mm Hg (Höckel M., Schlenger K., Arai B., Mitze M., Schäffer U., Vaupel P. Association between tumor hypoxia and malignant progression in advanced cancer of the uterine cervix. Cancer Res., 56: 4509-4515, 1996).

Pretreatment median pO_2 was shown to be lower in soft tissue sarcomas that gave rise to pulmonary metastases after treatment than in those that did not metastasize (Brizel D. M., Scully S. P., Harrelson J. M., Layfield L. J., Bean J. M., Prosnitz L. R., Dewhirst M. W. Tumor oxygenation predicts for the likelihood of distant metastases in human soft tissue sarcoma. Cancer Res., 56: 941-943, 1996).

The primary tumors of cervical carcinoma patients with regional lymph node metastases at presentation were found to have higher hypoxic fractions, *i.e.,* **higher fractional volumes with pO$_2$ < 5 mm Hg, than those of the patients without metastases** (Rofstad E. K., Sundfør K., Lyng H., Tropé C. G. Hypoxia-induced treatment failure in advanced squamous cell carcinoma of the uterine cervix is primarily due to hypoxia-induced radiation resistance rather than hypoxia-induced metastasis. Br. J. Cancer, *83:* 354-359, 2000). However, these clinical studies do not necessarily implicate that hypoxia promotes metastasis. An alternative interpretation is that the **most aggressive tumors develop in the most extensive hypoxic regions, where EMODs are low.**

Some recent studies of experimental tumors are also consistent with the suggestion that **hypoxia may promote cancer metastasis**. Studies of the KHT-C fibrosarcoma have indicated that mice with tumors having high hypoxic fractions may show a slightly higher number of lung microcolonies than those with tumors having low hypoxic fractions. However, **studies of experimental tumors giving conclusive evidence that hypoxia may promote the development of macroscopic spontaneous metastases have not been reported thus far**. In fact, experiments attempting to establish correlations between hypoxia and spontaneous metastasis in the KHT-C and SCC-VII tumors have given negative results (De Jaeger K., Kavanagh M-C., Hill R. P. Relationship of hypoxia to metastatic ability in rodent tumours. Br. J. Cancer, *84:* 1280-1285, 2001; De Jaeger K., Merlo F. M., Kavanagh M-C., Fyles A. W., Hedley D., Hill R. P. Heterogeneity of tumor oxygenation: relationship to tumor necrosis, tumor size, and metastasis. Int. J. Radiat. Oncol. Biol. Phys., *42:* 717-721, 1998).

Tumor hypoxia appears to be strongly associated with tumor propagation, malignant progression, and resistance to therapy, and it has thus become a central issue in tumor physiology and cancer treatment. Biochemists and clinicians (as

Prof Randolph Michael Howes MD,PhD

well as physiologists) define hypoxia differently; biochemists define it as O_2-limited electron transport, and physiologists and clinicians define it as a state of reduced O_2 availability or decreased O_2 partial pressure that restricts or even abolishes functions of organs, tissues, or cells. **I believe that the decreased electron transport results in deficiency levels of EMODs, which "allows" for the manifestation of cancer.**

Hypoxia is a common feature of solid tumors that occurs across a wide variety of malignancies. Hypoxia and anemia (which contributes to tumor hypoxia) can lead to ionizing radiation and chemotherapy resistance by depriving tumor cells of the oxygen essential for the cytotoxic activities of these agents. **Hypoxia may also reduce tumor sensitivity to radiation therapy and chemotherapy (**Hypoxia and Anemia: Factors in Decreased Sensitivity to Radiation Therapy and Chemotherapy? Louis Harrison, Kimberly Blackwell. *Oncologist* 9: 31-40)**.** Investigations of the prognostic significance of pretreatment tumor oxygenation status have shown that **hypoxia (oxygen tension [pO_2] value ≤ 10 mmHg) is associated with lower overall and disease-free survival, greater recurrence, and less locoregional control in head and neck carcinoma, cervical carcinoma, and soft-tissue sarcoma.**

Tumour hypoxia is associated with adverse clinical outcomes and reduced patient survival. Hypoxia may be a factor in activation of extracellular matrix-degrading proteases, and some studies have **correlated primary tumour hypoxia with likelihood of tumour cell dissemination. Exposure to hypoxia either induces or selects for cells that are hyperglycolytic, and this in turn produces local acidosis which is also a common feature of solid tumors** (Raghunand, N, Gatenby, R A, Gillies, R J (2003). Microenvironmental and cellular consequences of altered blood flow in tumours. *Br J Radiol* 76: S11-S22).

Tumor hypoxia has been linked to acquired treatment resistance, tumor progression, and poor prognosis. Because anemia is a major causative factor for the development of hypoxia. **In breast cancers, even mild anemia (grade I anemia) is a major causative factor for the development of hypoxia or anoxia** (Vaupel, P., Mayer, A., Briest, S., Hockel, M. (2003). Oxygenation Gain Factor: A Novel Parameter Characterizing the Association between Hemoglobin Level and the Oxygenation Status of Breast Cancers. *Cancer Res* 63: 7634-7637**).**

Tumor hypoxia is a therapeutic concern since it can reduce the effectiveness of radiotherapy, some O_2-dependent cytotoxic agents, and photodynamic therapy (Tumor Hypoxia: Causative Factors, Compensatory Mechanisms, and Cellular Response. P. Vaupel and L. Harrison. Oncologist, November 1, 2004; 9(suppl_5): 4 – 9**).**

20.0 THE BEST FOR LAST: PEROXIDE KILLS CANCER

Having discussed many areas of hydrogen peroxide reactivity, it is with great pleasure that I now discuss the specific role of H_2O_2 in apoptosis and cancer killing.

It is now becoming apparent that cellular suicide or apoptosis is initiated by EMODs, especially H_2O_2. Scientific investigators state it as follows: "Efficient apoptotic signaling is a function of a permissive intracellular milieu created by a decrease in the ratio of superoxide to hydrogen peroxide and cytosolic acidification."

Most of the past studies seem to imply that **the mitochondrial burst of H_2O_2 is likely to be a downstream effector mechanism for the execution signal. Hydrogen peroxide (H_2O_2) is considered to be a mediator of apoptotic cell death** (Apoptosis induced by hydrogen peroxide is mediated by decreased superoxide anion concentration and reduction of intracellular milieu. Clement MV, Ponton A, Pervaiz S. FEBS Lett. 1998 Nov 27;440(1-2):13-8).

A growing body of evidence seems to **favor the involvement of intracellular reactive oxygen species at some point during apoptotic execution** (Fleury C, Mignotte B, Vayssiere JL Mitochondrial reactive oxygen species in cell death signaling. Biochimie 2002;84:131-41) (Mansat-de Mas V, Bezombes C, Quillet-Mary A, et al Implication of radical oxygen species in ceramide generation, c-Jun N-terminal kinase activation and apoptosis induced by daunorubicin. Mol Pharmacol 1999;56:867-74) (Simizu S, Umezawa K, Takada M, Arber N, Imoto M Induction of hydrogen peroxide production and Bax expression by caspase-3(-like) proteases in tyrosine kinase inhibitor-induced apoptosis in human small cell lung carcinoma cells. Exp Cell Res 1998;238:197-203) (Hirpara JL, Clement MV, Pervaiz S Intracellular acidification triggered by mitochondrial-derived hydrogen peroxide is an effector mechanism for drug-induced apoptosis in tumor cells. J Biol Chem 2001;276:514-21) (Clement MV, Ponton A, Pervaiz S Apoptosis induced by hydrogen peroxide is mediated by decreased superoxide anion concentration and reduction of intracellular milieu. FEBS Lett 1998;440:13-8).

The effector components **of apoptotic death signaling** and their intricate networking have been unraveled during the past couple of decades (Green D., Kroemer G. The central executioners of apoptosis: caspases or mitochondria?. Trends Cell Biol., 8: 267-271, 1998) (Brenner C., Kroemer G. Apoptosis. Mitochondria—the death signal integrators. Science (Wash. DC), 289: 1150-1151, 2000) (Reed J. C., Kroemer G. Mechanisms of mitochondrial membrane permeabilization. Cell Death Differ., 7: 1145 2000).

Thus, it is now well established that depending on the level of activation of the initiator caspase, such as **caspase-8**, the death signal can recruit directly downstream effector caspases or engage the mitochondria with the resultant release of death amplification factors, such as cytochrome c, apoptosis inducing factor, and Smac/ DIABLO (Scaffidi C., Fulda S., Srinivasan A., Friesen C., Li F., Tomaselli K. J., Debatin K. M., Krammer P. H., Peter M. E. Two CD95 (APO-1/ Fas) signaling pathways. EMBO J., 17: 1675-1687, 1998) (Kroemer G., Reed J. C. Mitochondrial control of cell death. Nat. Med., 6: 513-519, 2000).

Even death signaling by anticancer drugs generally relies on positive input from the mitochondria, as is evidenced by the resistance of tumor cells overexpressing the death-inhibitory protein Bcl-2 that is localized to the membranes of mitochondria, endoplasmic reticulum, and nucleus (Tsujimoto Y., Shimizu S. VDAC regulation by the Bcl-2 family of proteins. Cell Death Differ., 7: 1174- 1181, 2000) (Korsmeyer S. J. BCL-2 gene family and the regulation of programmed cell death. Cancer Res., 59: 1693-1700S, 1999) (Harris M. H., Thompson C. B. The role of the Bcl-2 family in the regulation of outer mitochondrial membrane permeability. Cell Death Differ, 7: 1182-1191, 2000).

The critical role of cellular redox status in the regulation of death signaling has been demonstrated (Clement M.V., Pervaiz S. Reactive oxygen intermediates regulate cellular response to apoptotic stimuli: an hypothesis. Free Radic. Res., 30: 247-252, 1999) (Clement M.V., Pervaiz S. Intracellular superoxide and hydrogen peroxide concentrations: a critical balance that determines survival or death. Redox. Rep., 6: 211-214, 2001) (Pervaiz S., Clement M. V. Hydrogen peroxide-induced apoptosis: oxidative or reductive stress?. Methods Enzymol., 352: 150-159, 2002) (Pervaiz S., Clement M.V. A permissive apoptotic environment: function of a decrease in intracellular superoxide anion and cytosolic acidification. Biochem. Biophys. Res. Commun., 290: 1145-1150, 2002).

These observations become more important considering the critical role of the mitochondria during apoptosis and the fact that **mitochondria have been implicated directly or indirectly as the prime source of reactive oxygen species during drug-induced apoptosis** (Fleury C, Mignotte B, Vayssiere JL Mitochondrial reactive oxygen species in cell death signaling. Biochimie 2002;84:131-41) (Childs AC, Phaneuf SL, Dirks AJ, Phillips T, Leeuwenburgh C Doxorubicin treatment in vivo causes cytochrome C release and cardiomyocyte apoptosis, as well as increased mitochondrial efficiency, superoxide dismutase activity, and Bcl-2:Bax ratio. Cancer Res 2002;62:4592-8) (Quillet-Mary A, Jaffrezou JP, Mansat V, Bordier C, Naval J, Laurent G Implication of mitochondrial hydrogen peroxide generation in ceramide-induced apoptosis. J Biol Chem 1997;272:21388-95). As the mitochondria are a major source of intracellular reactive oxygen species, **it is tempting to speculate that reactive oxygen species, such as H_2O_2, may function both upstream and downstream of the mitochondria. Tumor cells lacking Bax (Bax–/–) are resistant to the effect of some anti-cancer drugs** (Zhang L, Yu

J, Park BH, Kinzler KW,Vogelstein B Role of BAX in the apoptotic response to anticancer agents. Science 2000;290:989-92).

Analysis of subcellular distribution of Bax (in HCT116, HL60, and CEM cells) revealed that **Bax redistributed to the mitochondrial fraction from the cytosol on exposure to H_2O_2, which could be significantly blocked by the H_2O_2 scavenger catalase.**

Investigators exploited the ability of certain anticancer drugs to increase intracellular production of reactive oxygen species, specifically H_2O_2 (Hirpara JL, Clement MV, Pervaiz S Intracellular acidification triggered by mitochondrial-derived hydrogen peroxide is an effector mechanism for drug-induced apoptosis in tumor cells. J Biol Chem 2001;276:514-21). Indeed, exposure of HCT116 Bax+/− or HL60 cells to a novel anticancer compound C1 resulted in an increase in intracellular H_2O_2 and translocation of Bax to the mitochondria. This translocation of Bax was **inhibited by catalase,** thus **establishing the critical role of intracellular H_2O_2 in mitochondrial recruitment during drug-induced apoptosis of tumor cells.**

Recruitment of Bax to the mitochondria during apoptotic signaling has been linked to the activation of upstream caspase 8 and caspase 8-mediated cleavage of the proapoptotic protein Bid. This is particularly true on ligation of death receptors, such as CD95 (Apo1/Fas). Incidentally, **H_2O_2 and anticancer drugs have been shown to up-regulate the expression of the CD95 receptor or its ligand (CD95L) in some systems** (Hug H, Strand S, Grambihler A, et al Reactive oxygen intermediates are involved in the induction of CD95 ligand mRNA expression by cytostatic drugs in hepatoma cells. J Biol Chem 1997;272:28191-3) (Suhara T, Fukuo K, Sugimoto T, et al Hydrogen peroxide induces up-regulation of Fas in human endothelial cells. J Immunol 1998;160:4042-7).

These data indicate that Bax translocation triggered in tumor cells during drug (C1)-induced apoptosis was a direct result of intracellular H₂O₂ production, independent of the upstream caspase 8 or ceramide pathways.

Investigators showed that **intracellular increase in H₂O₂ was a critical effector mechanism during drug-induced apoptosis of human tumor cells** (Hirpara JL, Clement MV, Pervaiz S Intracellular acidification triggered by mitochondrial-derived hydrogen peroxide is an effector mechanism for drug-induced apoptosis in tumor cells. J Biol Chem 2001;276:514-21). This increase in H₂O₂ was responsible for early cytosolic acidification, thus creating an environment conducive for caspase activation.

Even though an overwhelming accumulation of intracellular reactive oxygen species can create an oxidatively stressed environment leading to necrosis, **a slight increase is a stimulus for cellular proliferation** (Burdon R. H., Gill V., Rice-Evans C. Cell proliferation and oxidative stress. Free Radic. Res. Commun., 7: 149-159, 1989) (Burdon R. H. Superoxide and hydrogen peroxide in relation to mammalian cell proliferation. Free Radic. Biol. Med., 18: 775-794, 1995).

Pro-oxidant intracellular milieu is a hallmark of many tumor cells and is believed to endow tumor cells with a survival advantage over their normal counterparts (Cerutti P.A. Prooxidant states and tumor promotion. Science (Wash. DC), 227: 375-381, 1985) (Burdon R. H., Gill V., Rice-Evans C. Oxidative stress and tumour cell proliferation. Free Radic. Res. Commun., 11: 65-76, 1990). **However, I believe that it is this very feature which allows us to have selectivity for cancer cell killing.**

It has been shown previously that **maintaining a slightly elevated intracellular O₂⁻ promotes cellular proliferation** (Burdon R. H. Superoxide and hydrogen peroxide in relation to mammalian cell proliferation. Free Radic. Biol. Med., 18: 775-794, 1995) (Burdon R.

H. Control of cell proliferation by reactive oxygen species. Biochem. Soc. Trans., *24:* 1028-1032, 1996) and inhibits apoptotic signaling (Pervaiz S., Ramalingam J. K., Hirpara J. L., Clement M.V. Superoxide anion inhibits drug-induced tumor cell death. FEBS Lett., *459:* 343-348, 1999) (Fadeel B., Ahlin A., Henter J. I., Orrenius S., Hampton M. B. Involvement of caspases in neutrophil apoptosis: regulation by reactive oxygen species. Blood, *92:* 4808-4818, 1998).

Also, it has demonstrated that **a slightly elevated intracellular concentration of superoxide (O_2^-) inhibited apoptotic signaling,** irrespective of the trigger (Clement M.V., Stamenkovic I. Superoxide anion is a natural inhibitor of FAS-mediated cell death. EMBO J., *15:* 216-225, 1996) (Pervaiz S., Ramalingam J. K., Hirpara J. L., Clement M.V. Superoxide anion inhibits drug-induced tumor cell death. FEBS Lett., *459:* 343-348, 1999).

Many investigators have demonstrated the critical role of intracellular H_2O_2 in rendering the cytosolic milieu permissive for efficient apoptotic execution (Hampton M. B., Orrenius S. Dual regulation of caspase activity by hydrogen peroxide: implications for apoptosis. FEBS Lett., *414:* 552-556, 1997) (Clement M.V., Ponton A., Pervaiz S. Apoptosis induced by hydrogen peroxide is mediated by decreased superoxide anion concentration and reduction of intracellular milieu. FEBS Lett., *440:* 13-18, 1998) (Hirpara J. L., Clement M.V., Pervaiz S. Intracellular acidification triggered by mitochondrial-derived hydrogen peroxide is an effector mechanism for drug-induced apoptosis in tumor cells. J. Biol. Chem., *276:* 514-521, 2001). **I believe that this is as clear as it can get. H_2O_2 is essential for cellular killing.**

It has been hypothesized that a critical balance between intracellular H_2O_2 and O_2^- dictates the response of tumor cells to apoptotic stimuli, and any stimulus/signal that inhibits the ability of intracellular H_2O_2, triggered on drug exposure, to reduce the intracellular environment could potentially favor the acquisition of the resistant phenotype. **I believe that this is saying that blocking H₂O₂ can favor the development of neoplastic cells.**

20.1 Resveratrol (RSV)

A **phytoalexin, resveratrol (RSV)** is found in grapes and wines and known for its diverse biological activities, including **antioxidant property** (Bhat K. P. L., Kosmeder J. W., 2nd, Pezzuto J. M. Biological effects of resveratrol. Antioxid. Redox. Signal, *3:* 1041-1064, 2001) (Soleas G. J., Diamandis E. P., Goldberg D. M. The world of resveratrol. Adv. Exp. Med. Biol., *492:* 159-182, 2001) (Pervaiz S. Resveratrol: from grapevines to mammalian biology. FASEB J., *17:* 1975-1985, 2003). **RSV has been shown to induce or inhibit cellular proliferation and death signaling** (Mizutani K., Ikeda K., Kawai Y., Yamori Y. Resveratrol stimulates the proliferation and differentiation of osteoblastic MC3T3–E1 cells. Biochem. Biophys. Res. Commun., *253:* 859-863, 1998) (Jang M., Cai L., Udeani G. O., Slowing K. V., Thomas C. F., Beecher C. W., Fong H. H., Farnsworth N. R., Kinghorn A. D., Mehta R. G., Moon R. C., Pezzuto J. M. Cancer chemopreventive activity of resveratrol, a natural product derived from grapes. Science (Wash. DC), *275:* 218-220, 1997) (Huang C., Ma W. Y., Goranson A., Dong Z. Resveratrol suppresses cell transformation and induces apoptosis through a p53-dependent pathway. Carcinogenesis (Lond.), *20:* 237-242, 1999) (She Q. B., Ma W. Y., Wang M., Kaji A., Ho C. T., Dong Z. Inhibition of cell transformation by resveratrol and its derivatives: differential effects and mechanisms involved. Oncogene, *22:* 2143-2150, 2003).

However, some **data provide strong evidence that contrary to its proapoptotic activity at ≥25 µM, low micromolar concentrations (4–8 µM) inhibit apoptotic signaling** (Ahmad N., Adhami V. M., Afaq F., Feyes D. K., Mukhtar H. Resveratrol causes WAF-1/p21-mediated G(1)-phase arrest of cell cycle and induction of apoptosis in human epidermoid carcinoma A431 cells. Clin. Cancer Res., *7:* 1466-1473, 2001) (She Q. B., Bode A. M., Ma W.Y., Chen N. Y., Dong Z. Resveratrol-induced activation of p53 and apoptosis is mediated by extracellular-signal-regulated protein kinases and p38 kinase. Cancer Res., *61:* 1604-1610, 2001). This effect on up-regulation of the death receptor ligand is not observed at concentrations of RSV <16 µM, hence the inability to trigger apoptosis in these cells (data not shown). Contrarily, **at these concentrations, RSV inhibits apoptotic signaling upstream of the mitochondria, thus blocking the recruitment of mitochondrial-derived amplification factors, such as cytochrome c.**

Evidence has been provided that **RSV has a potent effect on the intracellular redox status,** a critical determinant of the efficacy of the death signal (Clement M.V., Pervaiz S. Reactive oxygen intermediates regulate cellular response to apoptotic stimuli: an hypothesis. Free Radic. Res., *30:* 247-252, 1999) (Fadeel B., Ahlin A., Henter J. I., Orrenius S., Hampton M. B. Involvement of caspases in neutrophil apoptosis: regulation by reactive oxygen species. Blood, *92:* 4808-4818, 1998) (Hampton M. B., Orrenius S. Redox regulation of apoptotic cell death. Biofactors, *8:* 1-5, 1998). **I believe that the prooxidant activity of RSV can be utilized in stacking of oxidative therapies. A pro-oxidant intracellular milieu is an invariable finding in cancer cells** and has been shown to endow cancer cells with a survival advantage over their normal counterparts (Cerutti P.A. Prooxidant states and tumor promotion. Science (Wash. DC), *227:* 375-381, 1985).

Some investigators have found paradoxical findings providing evidence for a **pro-oxidant effect of RSV** at concentrations that do not trigger apoptosis (Zini R., Morin C., Bertelli A., Bertelli A. A., Tillement J. P. Resveratrol-induced limitation of dysfunction of mitochondria isolated from rat brain in an anoxia-reoxygenation model. Life Sci., *71:* 3091-3108, 2002).

Such **pro-oxidant activity of polyphenolics,** such as RSV, has been reported recently in different systems (Martinez R., Quintana K., Navarro R., Martin C., Hernandez M. L., Aurrekoetxea I., Ruiz-Sanz J. I., Lacort M., Ruiz-Larrea M. B.

Pro-oxidant and antioxidant potential of catecholestrogens against ferrylmyoglobin-induced oxidative stress. Biochim. Biophys. Acta, *1583*: 167-175, 2002) (Tinhofer I., Bernhard D., Senfter M., Anether G., Loeffler M., Kroemer G., Kofler R., Csordas A., Greil R. Resveratrol, a tumor-suppressive compound from grapes, induces apoptosis via a novel mitochondrial pathway controlled by Bcl-2. FASEB J., *15*: 1613-1615, 2001). Results implicate **the membrane NADPH oxidase complex as a potential source of O$_2^-$ on incubation with low doses of RSV. Inhibition of the NADPH oxidase complex** not only restored death signaling but also resulted in reverting the negative effect of RSV on drug-induced intracellular H$_2$O$_2$ production. This fits in well with the hypothesis that **a balance between intracellular O$_2^-$ and H$_2$O$_2$ could be a critical factor in the response of cells to apoptotic triggers, with a tilt toward the former favoring survival and a predominance of the latter facilitating death execution** (Clement M.V., Pervaiz S. Intracellular superoxide and hydrogen peroxide concentrations: a critical balance that determines survival or death. Redox. Rep., *6*: 211-214, 2001).

Therefore, **the use of RSV in combination with drugs such as C2, vincristine, or daunorubicin could be a dangerous mixture because the slight pro-oxidant effect may provide tumor cells with not only a survival advantage but also impede death signals. This could present an ideal environment for the propagation and proliferation of tumor cells.**

Furthermore, these data strongly support and **underscore the critical role of H$_2$O$_2$ in creating a permissive intracellular milieu for efficient drug-induced execution of tumor cells** (LY294002 and LY303511 Sensitize Tumor Cells to Drug-Induced Apoptosis via Intracellular Hydrogen Peroxide Production Independent of the Phosphoinositide 3-Kinase-Akt Pathway. Tze Wei Poh and Shazib Pervaiz. Cancer Research 65, 6264-6274, July 15, 2005**).

Data has been presented which not only implicates mitochondrial H$_2$O$_2$ production as a critical effector mechanism during drug-induced apoptosis but also demonstratse the ability of an increase in intracellular O$_2^-$ to prevent H$_2$O$_2$ production and thereby impede the recruitment of the mitochondrial death pathway.

Investigators have shown that **hydrogen peroxide (H$_2$O$_2$)-mediated cytosolic acidification is an effector mechanism during drug-induced apoptosis of tumor cells** (Hydrogen Peroxide-Mediated Cytosolic Acidification Is a Signal for Mitochondrial Translocation of Bax during Drug-Induced Apoptosis of Tumor Cells. Kashif A. Ahmad, Kartini B. Iskandar, Jayshree L. Hirpara, Marie-Veronique Clement and Shazib Pervaiz *Cancer Research* 64, 7867-7878, November 1, 2004). These findings provide a novel mechanism for mitochondrial translocation of Bax and **directly implicate H$_2$O$_2$-mediated cytosolic acidification in the recruitment of the mitochondrial pathway during drug-induced apoptosis of tumor cells.**

20.2 Cytosolic Acidification

Cytosolic acidification is an early event in apoptosis and provides an intracellular milieu permissive for efficient death execution. In this regard, **exposure of cells to H$_2$O$_2$ or drugs that trigger intracellular increase in H$_2$O$_2$ results in a significant drop in cytosolic pH** (Hirpara JL, Clement MV, Pervaiz S Intracellular acidification triggered by mitochondrial-derived hydrogen peroxide is an effector mechanism for drug-induced apoptosis in tumor cells. J Biol Chem 2001;276:514-21).

Accordingly, **signals that inhibit apoptotic acidification impede death signaling** as demonstrated in our recent study (Ahmad KA, Clement MV, Hanif IM, Pervaiz S. Resveratrol inhibits drug-induced apoptosis in human leukemia cells by creating an intracellular milieu nonpermissive for death execution. Cancer Res

2004;64:1452-9). Investigators **results provided strong evidence that the link between H_2O_2 and Bax translocation could be the drop in cytosolic pH brought about by exposure of cells to exogenous H_2O_2 or endogenous production of H_2O_2 on drug exposure. I believe that this indicates the central role of H_2O_2 in cancer cell killing or apoptotic execution.**

Investigators demonstrated the ability of commonly used chemotherapeutic drugs vincristine and daunorubicin to trigger an early increase in intracellular H_2O_2 (Ahmad KA, Clement MV, Hanif IM, Pervaiz S Resveratrol inhibits drug-induced apoptosis in human leukemia cells by creating an intracellular milieu non-permissive for death execution. Cancer Res 2004;64:1452-9). **I have been saying all along that H_2O_2 is crucial for pathogen and neoplasia control. It also has to be kept in mind that catalase may inhibit cellular killing of cancer.**

I believe that this shows that apoptosis all begins with EMOD production, especially H_2O_2. H_2O_2 is essential for cancer killing and a shift to an acidic intracellular environment may also aid in its tumoricidal activity.

Fabricating crucial electronically modified oxygen derivatives,
the body's biochemical assembly line hums at
a hellacious nano-second pace,
whilst radicophobes filibuster their essentiality.
It is increasingly apparent
that the acuity of the mind's eye of the oxy-moron
is borderline blind.
R. M. Howes, M.D., Ph.D.
12/26/05

21.0 PEROXIDE, SUPEROXIDE AND CARDIOVASCULAR DISEASE

Some of the following material was abstracted, excerpted or modified from: Role of Oxidative Modifications in Atherosclerosis. Roland Stocker and John F. Keaney, Jr. *Physiol. Rev.* 84: 1381-1478. **I highly recommend this excellent review.**

There is now **a consensus, but not proof, that atherosclerosis represents a state of heightened oxidative stress** characterized by lipid and protein oxidation in the vascular wall.

Despite these abundant data however, **fundamental problems remain with implicating oxidative modification as a (requisite) pathophysiologically important cause for atherosclerosis. These include the poor performance of antioxidant strategies in limiting either atherosclerosis or cardiovascular events from atherosclerosis, and observations in animals that suggest dissociation between atherosclerosis and lipoprotein oxidation (RMH Note: I believe that this indicates the severe lack of predictability of the free radical theory as it relates to atherosclerosis).** Indeed, **it remains to be established that oxidative events are a cause rather than an injurious response to atherogenesis.** In this context, inflammation needs to be considered as a primary process of atherosclerosis, and oxidative stress as a secondary event **(RMH Note: This makes the erroneous assumption that there is a distinct entity called "oxidative stress.")**.

Atherosclerosis claims more lives than all types of cancer combined and the World Health Organization predicts that global economic prosperity could lead to an epidemic of atherosclerosis as developing countries acquire Western habits.

Age is among the most important risk factors for predicting incident cardiovascular disease. **(RMH Note: I believe that it**

is because aging is associated with factors which lead to EMOD deficiency states.).

Numerous observational studies have indicated that males exhibit excess risk for cardiovascular disease compared with age-matched women **(RMH Note: I believe that this is because testosterone decreases EMOD production in the male, thus making males more vulnerable to atherosclerosis.)** (Barrett-Connor E and Bush TL. Estrogen and coronary heart disease in women. *JAMA* 265: 1861–1867, 1991). There has been considerable speculation that **estrogens offer a "protective" effect to women**, as **cardiovascular disease accelerates in women after menopause**. However, this speculation has been **difficult to substantiate**, as the **treatment with estrogen has not reduced the incidence of cardiovascular disease of postmenopausal women** (Hulley S, Grady D, Bush T, Furberg C, Herrington D, Riggs B, and Vittinghoff E. Randomized trial of estrogen plus progestin for secondary prevention of coronary heart disease in postmenopausal women. Heart and Estrogen/progestin Replacement Study (HERS) Research Group. *JAMA* 280: 605–613, 1998). Alternatively, some of this apparent protection could be due to the fact that **women exhibit relatively higher concentrations of high-density lipoprotein (HDL) cholesterol than do age-matched men**. Nevertheless, **incident cardiovascular disease is less common in premenopausal women than their age-matched male** counterparts.

There is now a growing appreciation that obesity, defined as an excess body weight with an abnormal high preponderance of body fat, is a condition that increases the incident risk of cardiovascular disease. **The exact mechanism(s) to explain this phenomenon, however, are controversial.** A number of other risk factors for cardiovascular disease, such as hypertension, low HDL cholesterol, and diabetes mellitus, often **coexist (clustering)** with obesity (Wilson PW, Kannel WB,

Silbershatz H, and D'Agostino RB. Clustering of metabolic factors and coronary heart disease. *Arch Intern Med* 159: 1104–1109, 1999). **I believe that the presence of the double bonded fats, which trap ROS, leads to an EMOD deficiency state and increases the risk of atherosclerosis.**

The Surgeon General's report estimates that smoking increases atherosclerotic disease by 50% and doubles the incidence of coronary artery disease (United States Department of Health and Human Services. Reducing the health consequences of smoking: 25 years of progress. *Report Surgeon General* DHSS CDC 89–8411, 1989). **I believe that this is due to the obvious decrease in available ground state oxygen for tissues, organs and cells and thus, deficiency states of EMODs.** There is now **considerable confidence** that smoking is causally related to coronary artery disease, as smoking **cessation is quite effective in lowering the future risk of the disease.** In fact, the risk of heart attack in ex-smokers approaches that of nonsmokers in only 2 years (Gaziano JM. Epidemiology of risk factor reduction. In: *Vascular Medicine*, edited by Loscalzo J, Creagher M, and Dzau V. Boston, MA: Little Brown, 1996, p. 569–586). **I believe that this is due to "spontaneous regression" of atherosclerosis and is due to resumption of adequate levels of oxygen which can generate adequate levels of EMODs.**

In patients with diabetes, the risk of coronary atherosclerosis is three- to fivefold greater than in nondiabetics despite controlling for other risk factors **("clustering")**(Bierman EL. George Lyman Duff Memorial Lecture. Atherogenesis in diabetes. *Arterioscler Thromb* 12: 647–656, 1992) (Pyorala K, Laakso M, and Uusitupa M. Diabetes and atherosclerosis: an epidemiologic view. *Diabetes Metab Rev* 3: 463–524, 1987). **I believe that this is due to the fact that hyperglycemia results in deficiency levels of EMODs. Also, remember that H_2O_2 has insulin-mimetic activity.**

Familial hypercholesterolemia is an autosomal dominant disorder that **affects 1 in 500 persons. .In heterozygotes, 85% of individuals have experienced a myocardial infarction by the age of 60, and this age is reduced to 15 yr in patients homozygous for the disease** (Gotto AM Jr and Farmer JA. Risk factors for coronary artery disease. In: *Heart Disease: A Textbook of Cardiovascular Medicine,* edited by Braunwald E. Philadelphia, PA: Saunders, 1988, p. 1153–1190).

Early concepts of atherosclerosis involved progressive luminal narrowing until the blood flow was compromised to the point that organ metabolic needs could no longer be met, producing ischemia and infarction of the subtended tissue such as the heart or the brain. **Over the last 15 years, this concept has changed dramatically to include the notion of plaque rupture as both a precipitant of clinical events** but also a component of plaque progression in atherosclerosis. **I believe that this indicates that the old paradigm of cholesterol build-up is wrong.** Clinical events indicate that thrombosis is the consequence **of an abrupt, catastrophic change** in plaque morphology **rather than a gradual narrowing of the lumen** (Davies MJ and Thomas AC. Plaque fissuring—the cause of acute myocardial infarction, sudden ischaemic death, and crescendo angina. *Br Heart J* 53: 363–373, 1985) (Davies MJ. A macro and micro view of coronary vascular insult in ischemic heart disease. *Circulation* 82: 1138–1146, 1990).

I believe that the inflammatory response results in local hypoxia, which ultimately leads to deficiency states of EMODs and this in turn, decreases the ability of the vessel wall to disrupt pre-plaque micro-aggregation. Current theories involve a significant component of inflammation, a known feature of atherosclerosis (Libby P. Inflammation in atherosclerosis. *Nature* 420: 868–874, 2002). **Here, I see a common thread of "hypoxia."**

I believe that the areas of predisposition are areas which have EMOD deficiencies and they subsequently develop

plaque. I believe that the EMODs oxidize the plasma particulates or aggregates thus, making them excretable products.). Such lesion-prone sites tend rather to demonstrate an enhanced retention of atherogenic apolipoprotein B-containing lipoproteins (Schwenke DC and Carew TE. Initiation of atherosclerotic lesison in cholesterol-fed rabbits. II. Selective retention of LDL vs selective increases in LDL permeability in susceptible sites of arteries. *Arteriosclerosis* 9: 908–918, 1989).

In addition to radicals, several nonradical oxidants are important when considering oxidative modifications in the vessel wall. The most abundant of these is hydrogen peroxide (H_2O_2) derived from the action of oxidases such as glucose oxidase on O_2, or from the dismutation of O_2^- :.

Nonradical oxidants like ONOOH and HOCl (Hazell LJ, van den Berg JJM, and Stocker R. Oxidation of low-density lipoprotein by hypochlorite causes aggregation that is mediated by modification of lysine residues rather than lipid oxidation. *Biochem J* 302: 297–304, 1994) appear to react preferentially with proteins rather than lipids (Vissers MC, Stern A, Kuypers F, vandenBerg J, and Winterbourn CC. Membrane changes associated with lysis of red blood cells by hypochlorous acid. *Free Radic Biol Med* 16: 703–712, 1994). This preference for a reaction with proteins differentiates nonradical from radical oxidants, the latter commonly initiating lipid peroxidation.

21.1 Sources of Oxidants in the Vascular Wall

Within the vessel wall, the different oxidants can originate principally from cellular and extracellular sources, and from enzymatic and nonenzymatic paths. The phagocyte NADPH oxidase (Nox) utilizes electrons derived from NADPH to reduce molecular oxygen to O_2^- :. While O_2^- ·is principally a reducing agent, it can give rise to secondary products that include strong oxidants. Once activated appropriately, phagocytic cells produce large amounts of O_2^-· over relatively short periods that are involved in host defense.

NAD(P)H oxidase activity represents a major source of EMODs in the vasculature (Pagano PJ, Ito Y, Tornheim K, Gallop PM, Tauber AI, and Cohen RA. An NADPH oxidase superoxide-generating system in the rabbit aorta. *Am J Physiol Heart Circ Physiol* 268: $H_2$274–$H_2$280, 1995). **NAD(P)H oxidases in vascular cells can also be activated by stimuli such as angiotensin II, thrombin, platelet-derived growth factor, tumor necrosis factor- , interleukin-1, and for endothelial cells, mechanical forces (including shear stress) and vascular endothelial growth factor** (Ushio-Fukai M, Tang Y, Fukai T, Dikalov SI, Ma Y, Fujimoto M, Quinn MT, Pagano PJ, Johnson C, and Alexander RW. Novel role of gp91[phox]-containing NAD(P)H oxidase in vascular endothelial growth factor-induced signaling and angiogenesis. *Circ Res* 91: 1160–1167, 2002).

In vascular smooth muscle cells, O_2^-· and H_2O_2 appear to be produced predominantly inside the cells, and addition of NAD(P)H to the cells augments O_2^-· generation. For endothelial cells, there is evidence for extracellular release of O_2^-· as indicated using cell-impermeable "trapping" agents (Ushio-Fukai M, Tang Y, Fukai T, Dikalov SI, Ma Y, Fujimoto M, Quinn MT, Pagano PJ, Johnson C, and Alexander RW. Novel role of gp91[phox]-containing NAD(P)H oxidase in vascular endothelial growth factor-induced signaling and angiogenesis. *Circ Res* 91: 1160–1167, 2002). **I believe that this is in agreement of my theory that EMODs disrupt microaggregates oxidatively and prevent the formation of plaque.**

However, even under stimulated conditions, **the amounts of O_2^-· produced by vascular cells are only a fraction of those generated by activated phagocytes and are commonly considered to represent second messengers for a number of key regulatory proteins and cellular responses, rather than toxic species that cause oxidative damage.**

If one accepts the notion that **LDL oxidation is an essential feature of atherosclerosis, then inhibiting LDL oxidation should limit atherosclerosis. There is little evidence that strongly oxidizing conditions persist in vivo in atherosclerotic vessels**.

However, **despite their presence, there is no direct evidence in humans that oxysterols contribute to atherosclerosis** (Brown AJ and Jessup W. Oxysterols and atherosclerosis. *Atherosclerosis* 142: 1–28, 1999). **Oxidative damage to proteins may result from electrophilic (2e-) and radical (1e-) reactions, e.g., initiated by electron leakage, metal-ion-dependent reactions, autoxidation of lipids and sugars, and breakdown products of lipid oxidation.**

Myeloperoxidase is the only human enzyme known to generate HOCl. The myeloperoxidase/H_2O_2/Cl⁻ system and HOCl convert -amino acids to their corresponding aldehydes. **Like cyclooxygenase, lipoxygenases require low levels of "seeding peroxides" to oxidize inactive Fe^{2+} to active Fe^{3+} enzyme and are likely affected by the "peroxide tone" of cells.**

Monoamine oxidase in the outer mitochondrial membrane may represent another source of H_2O_2. Within the mitochondria, O_2^- · production occurs primarily at complex I (NADH dehydrogenase) and complex III (ubiquinone-cytochrome bc1).

The activity of EC-SOD, the major SOD isoenzyme in the arterial wall, was reported to be increased in highly cellular rabbit lesions, but **decreased in advanced, connective tissue-rich human lesions** (Luoma JS, Strålin P, Marklund SL, Hiltunen TP, Sarkioja T, and Ylä-Herttuala S. Expression of extracellular SOD and iNOS in macrophages and smooth muscle cells in human and rabbit atherosclerotic lesions: colocalization with epitopes characteristic of oxidized LDL and peroxynitrite-modified proteins. *Arterioscler Thromb Vasc Biol* 18: 157–167, 1998). **I believe that this provides less H_2O_2 to oxidize microaggregates, making them excretable products. Overall, however, the activity of the different SOD isoenzymes does not appear to be altered drastically compared with normal arteries.**

Chronic inhibition of Cu, Zn-SOD in rats has also been reported to result in increased nonenzymatic lipid peroxidation (Lynch SM, Frei B, Morrow JD, Roberts LJ II, Xu A, Jackson T, Reyna R, Klevay LM, Vita JA, and Keaney JF Jr. Vascular superoxide dismutase deficiency impairs endothelial vasodilator function through direct inactivation of nitric oxide and increased lipid peroxidation. *Arterioscler Thromb Vasc Biol* 17: 2975–2981, 1997)**, indicating the potential for a protective role of SODs in atherosclerosis. I believe that the protection afforded by SOD is directly related to the amount of H_2O_2 that it generates.**

These findings indicate that EC-SOD appears to have surprisingly little influence on atherogenesis in mice and that the role of SOD in intimal LDL oxidation and atherogenesis remains unknown.

In lesions of rabbits fed a hyperlipidemic diet, total thiol compounds and selenium-dependent glutathione peroxidase activity has been reported to progressively rise from 10 to 60 days, whereas the activities of catalase, glutathione reductase, and glutathione transferase significantly decrease, and selenium-independent glutathione peroxidase activity is not detectable (Del Boccio G, Lapenna D, Porreca E, Pennelli A, Savini F, Feliciani P, Ricci G, and Cuccurullo F. Aortic antioxidant defence mechanisms: time-related changes in cholesterol-fed rabbits. *Atherosclerosis* 81: 127–135, 1990). **I believe that this again indicates that less H_2O_2 is available to break down plaque precursors.**

21.2 Transition Metals

Transition metals, specifically iron and copper, are essential for the synthesis of a very large range of proteins, including enzymes, like eNOS, that play a central role in the normal function of blood vessels. However, these metals can undergo 1e-transfer reactions that result in autoxidation reactions or the decomposition of peroxides to peroxyl, alkoxyl, and hydroxyl radicals. For example, transition metals can induce oxidative damage to lipoproteins, and copper is commonly used as the in vitro oxidant for LDL (Esterbauer H, Gebicki J, Puhl H, and Jürgens G. The role of lipid peroxidation and antioxidants in oxidative modification of LDL. *Free Radic Biol Med* 13: 341–390, 1992).

Thus, binding of adventitious transition metals to inactive chelates in the vascular wall may represent an antioxidant defense. Several proteins, such as ferritin, transferrin, haptoglobin, hemopexin, and ceruloplasmin, specifically bind biological iron and copper complexes and are considered to be part of the body's antioxidant defense system (Halliwell B and Gutteridge JMC. The antioxidants of human extracellular fluids. *Arch Biochem Biophys* 280: 1–8, 1990).

The concentration of free transition metals in vivo appears to be very low and there is little convincing evidence that they are related to atherosclerosis. Indeed, an autopsy study on patients with hemochromatosis, a genetic disorder that results in elevated plasma and tissue levels of iron, showed that they have less coronary artery disease than age- and sex-matched controls (Miller M and Hutchins GM. Hemochromatosis, multiorgan hemosiderosis, and coronary artery disease. *JAMA* 272: 231–233, 1994). This is exactly what I have been saying. The increase in oxidation, secondary to transition metals, increases EMODs, which decreases atherosclerosis. I believe that this is also the reason that patients with iron and copper deficiencies have greater risk for developing cancer.

Under normal conditions, transferrin is loaded to only 20–30% so that there is substantial iron binding capacity remaining and "free iron" is essentially non-detectable. In addition, human plasma contains haptoglobin and hemopexin that can prevent the pro-oxidant activity of hemoglobin and heme, respectively. For example, hemopexin can inhibit in vitro LDL oxidation induced by heme and hemoglobin. Of course, this means that heme can oxidize LDL.

It has been known for a long time that the oxidative modification of LDL by vascular cells is absolutely dependent on the presence of low concentrations of transition metals, such as copper and iron, in the medium (Garner B and Jessup W. Cell-mediated oxidation of low-density lipoprotein: the elusive mechanism(s). Redox Report 2: 97–104, 1996). For example, it can be completely prevented by the inclusion of metal chelators such as ethylenediamine tetraacetic acid or relatively small amounts of serum (that contains metal-binding proteins).

However, increasing or decreasing plasma and tissue stores of iron does not affect the formation of atherosclerotic lesions in cholesterol-fed rabbits (Dabbagh AJ, Shwaery GT, Keaney JF Jr, and Frei B. Effect of iron overload and iron deficiency on atherosclerosis in the hypercholesterolemic rabbit. Arterioscler Thromb Vasc Biol 17: 2638–2645, 1997). Also, in apolipoprotein E –/– mice, iron overload decreases lesion size despite detectable increases in hepatic concentrations of markers of oxidative events in the liver. Similarly, dietary supplementation with copper decreases atherosclerosis in cholesterol-fed rabbits, while copper deficiency increases atherosclerosis in C57B mice. Stocker and Kearney say that together, these results indicate that iron and copper are not likely important catalysts for oxidation events leading to atherosclerosis and that studies using free transition metals such as Cu(II) to oxidize LDL in vitro may not be meaningful biologically.

Albumin transports dietary copper to the liver where it is incorporated into ceruloplasmin for release into circulation and transport to various tissues. Ceruloplasmin has ferroxidase activity that is required for iron incorporation into ferritin (see above). The protein can also catalyze oxidation of a wide range of phenols and, surprisingly, was reported to induce in vitro and to facilitate cell-mediated, **metal-dependent LDL oxidation.** As a result of this, it has been speculated (**Mukhopadhyay CK, Ehrenwald E, and Fox PL.** Ceruloplasmin enhances smooth muscle cell- and endothelial cell-mediated low density lipoprotein oxidation by a superoxide-dependent mechanism. *J Biol Chem* 271: 14773–14778, 1996) that **ceruloplasmin may participate in LDL oxidation in the arterial wall.**

Cells or intact organs exposed to H_2O_2 exhibit reduced ferritin synthesis and upregulation of transferrin receptor mRNA (Pantopoulos K and Hentze MW. Rapid responses to oxidative stress mediated by iron regulatory protein. *EMBO J* 14: 2917–2924, 1995.). The mechanism for this effect is complex, as H_2O_2 **releases Fe from iron-regulatory protein, but such H_2O_2-treated protein is not able to bind to iron-response elements,** suggesting some other signaling mechanism for changes in iron status mediated by iron-regulatory protein. This contention is supported by observations that H_2O_2 **treatment of cell lysates does not stimulate binding of iron-regulatory protein to response elements.**

21.3 Probucol (antioxidant)

Early studies with probucol demonstrated inhibition of atherosclerosis in rabbits (Tawara K, Ishihara M, Ogawa H, and Tomikawa M. Effect of probucol, pantethine and their combinations on serum lipoprotein metabolism and on the incidence of atheromatous lesions in the rabbit. *Jpn J Pharmacol* 41: 211–222, 1986**) and monkeys. Probucol is a synthetic cholesterol-lowering drug that also possesses antioxidant activity,**

(Parthasarathy S, Young SG, Witztum JL, Pittman RC, and Steinberg D. Probucol inhibits oxidative modification of low density lipoprotein. *J Clin Invest* 77: 641–644, 1986). **The lipophilic drug associates with and effectively protects LDL against in vitro oxidation induced by copper ions.**

The reduction of atherosclerosis was believed to be due to the antioxidant effect of probucol; however, probucol also produced a 17% reduction in serum cholesterol. Subsequent studies in primates, cholesterol-fed rabbits, and hamsters have also demonstrated a reduction in atherosclerosis with probucol. The situation appears more complex in murine models of atherosclerosis, where probucol promotes atherosclerosis in the aortic root (Moghadasian MH, McManus BM, Godin DV, Rodrigues B, and Frohlich JJ. Proatherogenic and antiatherogenic effects of probucol and phytosterols in apolipoprotein E-deficient mice: possible mechanisms of action. *Circulation* 99: 1733–1739, 1999) but inhibits disease formation at more distal sites.

The Probucol Quantitative Regression Study (PQRST) reported probucol to be ineffective in attenuating lumen loss in the femoral arteries in hypercholesterolemic subjects over 3 years, as assessed by quantitative angiography (Walldius G, U E, Olsson AG, Bergstrand L, Hadell K, Johansson J, Kaijser L, Lassvik C, Molgaard J, and Nilsson S. The effect of probucol on femoral atherosclerosis: the Probucol Quantitative Regression Swedish Trial (PQRST). *Am J Cardiol* 74: 875–883, 1994). In contrast, **the Fukoaka Atherosclerosis Trial (FAST) observed probucol to significantly decrease atherosclerosis progression in the carotid artery of hypercholesterolemic patients,** as assessed by the intima-to-media thickness determined by B-mode ultrasound (Sawayama Y, Shimizu C, Maeda N, Tatsukawa M, Kinukawa N, Koyanagi S, Kashiwagi S, and Hayashi J. Effects of probucol and pravastatin on common carotid atherosclerosis in patients with asymptomatic hypercholesterolemia. Fukuoka Atherosclerosis Trial (FAST). *J Am Coll Cardiol* 39: 610–616, 2002).

In studying cardiovascular disease it is important to remember **there is no single animal model in which atherosclerosis truly reflects the human pathogenesis.**

Consistent with its relative chemical reactivity, $O_2^-\cdot$ **is not able to oxidize LDL, in contrast to its protonated form, the hydroperoxyl radical ($HO_2\cdot$)** (Bedwell S, Dean RT, and Jessup W. The action of defined oxygen-centered free radicals on human low-density lipoproteins. *Biochem J* 262: 707–712, 1989). However, **at physiological pH only a fraction of $O_2^-\cdot$ produced is present as $HO_2\cdot$. This suggests that $O_2^-\cdot$-generating systems, including NAD(P)H oxidases, are by themselves not efficient in oxidizing LDL. However, some believe that $O_2^-\cdot$ may act as the precursor for chemically more reactive oxidants, such as $ONOO^-$ and H_2O_2 and oxidants derived from them, and these may participate in LDL oxidation in the vessel wall.**

Stocker and Keaney state that the causative relationship between oxidative events and atherosclerosis in general and the pathophysiological importance of LDL oxidation in particular have been **challenged by the overall poor performance of antioxidant strategies in limiting atherosclerosis and its cardiovascular events, the overall lack of clear disease stage dependency in the vessel wall contents of oxidized molecules and antioxidants, and by the reported dissociation of atherosclerosis and lipoprotein oxidation in the vessel wall of animals** (Role of Oxidative Modifications in Atherosclerosis. Roland Stocker and John F. Keaney, Jr. *Physiol. Rev.* 84: 1381-1478).

I concur.

22.0 CONCLUSIONS

I believe that I have presented strong evidence for the following:

H_2O_2 is normally present in our natural and immediate environment.

Over a billion pounds of H_2O_2 are produced annually in the United States.

H_2O_2 is produced by all aerobic cells.

H_2O_2 is a product of normal metabolism.

H_2O_2 is likely the most prominent oxidant in the body.

H_2O_2 is likely one of the most important secondary cellular messengers.

H_2O_2 helps modulate the redox status of the cell.

Without electronically modified oxygen derivatives (EMODs) we would die.

We have a strong system of prooxidant protection and for oxidative self-healing.

H_2O_2 is an essential component of oxidative killing of pathogens.

H_2O_2 is an essential component of oxidative killing of cancer cells.

EMODs (i.e., H_2O_2, $O_2^{\cdot-}$, $^1O_2$, $HOCl$, etc.) are effective bactericidal, virucidal, fungicidal, parasiticidal and tumoricidal agents.

All antibody reactions involve H_2O_2.

EMOD deficiencies are strongly linked to many illnesses.

H_2O_2 is a very important tumoricidal agent in vitro and likely in vivo.

Cancer cells commit suicide (apoptosis) secondary to EMODs.

Without H_2O_2 our ability to resist infections and neoplasia is seriously compromised, as in CGD and immunosuppressed patients.

Chronic granulomatous disease patients lack EMOD production and suffer repeated infections and growth of tumors called granulomas.

Hypoxia is indicative of inflammation, limits the electron transport chain, reduces EMOD production and serves as a fertile area for infections and neoplasia.

Patients with a complete deficit of myeloperoxidase suffer with repeated infections and are prone to cancer development.

It is reasonable to believe that H_2O_2 can and is being used for therapeutic benefit, based on countless reports worldwide.

H_2O_2 has a record of extremely low toxicity and associated worldwide fatalities for over a quarter of a century number around fourteen.

H_2O_2 is used to purify large municipal water supplies worldwide.

H_2O_2 is a ubiquitous ingredient used safely in and on food products for human and animal consumption.

Free radicals of oxygen are essential to all aerobic metabolism and life.

The free radical theory of oxidative stress and aging is wrong.

All things age whether they use oxygen or not.

All scientists need to be made aware of the biological and biochemical role of H_2O_2.

All oncologists need an in depth knowledge of H_2O_2.

All physicians need a working knowledge of H_2O_2 and its interconnectedness to health and illness.

At this point, here is what I believe we know:
    High levels of **EMODs** can:

- kill and possibly cure cancer
- dissolve and possibly prevent arteriosclerotic plaques
- kill bacteria, fungi, viruses, protozoans and neoplasia

Antioxidants do not prevent or cure:

- **Diabetes**
- **Cancer**
- **Arteriosclerosis**
- **Aging**
- **Cataracts**
- **Arthritis**
- **Post traumatic brain damage or strokes**

Genetics (inheritance, heredity) is a major influence on the following:

- **Diabetes**
- **Cancer**
- **Arteriosclerosis**
- **Aging**
- **Cataracts**
- **Arthritis**
- **Brain function**

The process that transduces the extracellular messages carried by the first messengers such as hormones, growth factors, and neurotransmitters across plasma membranes into the intracellular components is called **"signal transduction or cell signaling."** An important feature of the signal transduction mechanism is that the first messenger does not have to enter the cell and their biological effects are mediated inside the cell by **second messenger molecules such as cAMP, cGMP, inositol 1,4,5-trisphosphate (Ins 1,4,5-P3), nitric oxide and phosphatidylinositol 1,3,4,5-tetrakisphosphate (PtdIns 1,3,4,5-P4).**

H_2O_2 is rapidly becoming recognized as one of the most important cellular signaling molecules.

H_2O_2 is a small, diffusible and ubiquitous molecule that can be synthesized, as well as destroyed rapidly in response to external stimuli and it fulfills the prerequisites for an intracellular messenger. For example, H_2O_2 mimics the stimulatory effects of insulin on glucose transport and lipid synthesis in adipocytes (May, F.M. and De Haen, C. (1979) The insulin-like effect of hydrogen peroxide on pathways of lipid synthesis in rat adipocytes. J. Biol. Chem. 254: 9017-9021).

This refutes the widely held erroneous belief, that is based on the free radi-crap theory, in which **EMODs** serve only as harmful agents in the cell. Even in the absence of extracellular stimulatory effects, superoxide anions are constantly produced by **normal** metabolic reactions in all aerobic organisms. **In addition, cells are extracorporeally subjected to irradiations (x-rays, gamma-rays, ultraviolet light), inflammatory systems, metal-catalyzed oxidation systems, environmental pollutants, which inevitably generate more EMODs** (Stadtman, E.R., and Berlett, B.S. (1998) Reactive oxygen-mediated protein oxidation in aging and disease. Drug Metabolism Reviews 30: 2005-2008).

Thus, I ask, "If the Free Radi-Crap theory is valid (e.g., EMODs are causative of over 200 pathophysiologies, including aging), shouldn't our life spans be getting progressively shorter in a progressively polluted environment and from increased internal oxidative stress?"

Contrary of the teachings of the free radical theory, our lifespans are steadily increasing.

Points of convergence based on my research: Cancer, spontaneous regression, arteriosclerosis, PDT, HIV/ AIDS, malaria, pregnancy, smoking, hydrogen peroxide, sodium hypochlorite, singlet oxygen, respiratory burst, inflammation, oxygen consumption, cellular oxygen levels, ROS levels, exercise, immunosuppression, antioxidants, hypoxia, aging, hypericin, obesity, chronic granulomatous disease, Down's syndrome, diabetes, pregnancy, etc.

UTOPIA CONNECTIONS AND CONVERGENCE

My studies of the biochemical intricacies connecting electronically modified oxygen derivatives (EMODs), which are also referred to as "reactive oxygen radicals and excited states," has led me to the following unifying concepts:

- EMODs have levels or ranges, which I prefer to call zones, which determine certain biological outcomes, relative to the appearance of cancer and infection. Zones of EMODs appear to be multi-phasic and at least triphasic. In general, these zones refer to the whole organism but due to the heterogeneity of tissue, organs or intracellular organelles necessitates that, at times, they be considered on an individual basis.

- **Howes' TRIPHASIC ZONES OF EMODs**

- **Apoptosis Zone** - the **highest zone (hyper-zone)** of EMODs. Based on the results of thousands and thousands of papers, it is well established that very high levels of EMODs which can be produced by PDT, many chemotherapeutic drugs, radiation and the Howes Singlet Oxygen delivery system, **will kill cancer.** Also, a hyper-stimulated immune system, such as is seen in spontaneous regression of cancer, **kills cancer**.

- **Abeyance Zone** - the **middle zone (mid-zone)** of EMODs. Based on the fact that millions and millions of people go through life without the manifestation of cancer is evidence, par excellence, for the existence of this mid zone of EMODs, which **holds cancer cell development in abeyance.** It is an accepted scientific fact that all aerobic cells undergo exponential numbers of potentially mutagenic oxidative damaging events on a continual basis; yet, **millions do not manifest or develop continual infections or tumors in a life time.** This is the zone of **homeostasis**.

- **Allowance Zone** - the **lowest zone (hypo-zone)** of EMODs. This zone is based on the millions of cases of patients with immunosuppression (acquired or innate) and on genetic diseases such as chronic granulomatous disease, obesity and diabetes. We know that low levels of EMODs **allow the development of cancer**.

Hats off to ELECTRONICALLY MODIFIED OXYGEN DERIVATIVES, especially H$_2$O$_2$.

Randolph M. Howes, M.D., Ph.D.

23.0 HYDROGEN PEROXIDE: A REVIEW OF A SCIENTIFICALLY VERIFIABLE OMNIPRESENT UBIQUITOUS ESSENTIALITY OF OBLIGATE, AEROBIC, CARBON-BASED LIFE FORMS

Howes RM. Hydrogen Peroxide: A review of a scientifically verifiable omnipresent ubiquitous essentiality of obligate, aerobic, carbon-based life forms. *The Internet Journal of Plastic Surgery.* 2010;7(1).

Hydrogen Peroxide:
A review of a scientifically verifiable omnipresent ubiquitous essentiality of obligate, aerobic, carbon-based life forms

Prof. Hon. Randolph M. Howes, M.D., Ph.D.

Adjunct Assistant Professor of Plastic Surgery, The Johns Hopkins Hospital, Baltimore, Md., U.S.A., Espaldon Professor of Plastic and Reconstructive Surgery, University of Santo Tomas, Manila, Philippines. Adjunct Professor of Biological Sciences, Southeastern Louisiana University, Hammond, La.

Address for communication: 27439 Highway 441, Kentwood, Louisiana 70444-8152, USA. Email: rhowesmd@hughes.net

Abstract

Electronically modified oxygen derivatives (EMODs), such as superoxide anion and hydrogen peroxide, carry out highly sophisticated intra, inter and extra cellular signaling roles that are essential for normal biochemical functioning. Hydrogen peroxide is freely diffusible through cell membranes, can not be excluded from cells and is required for normal operation of many enzymes that maintain and promote health. Hydrogen peroxide can act as an enzymatic substrate or activate or inhibit redox sensitive enzymes. Large health related organizations, such as the American Cancer Society, continue to disregard and deride the potential beneficial involvement and contribution of EMODs, especially hydrogen peroxide, in the treatment of any disease condition, inclusive of cancer. Their position of disdain is not supported by an exhaustive review of the medical and scientific literature. Although hydrogen peroxide has on occasion been a proposed mutagen, oncogenic transformation primarily leads to an increase of cellular EMODs that renders these same cells selectively vulnerable to additional EMOD production via EMOD induced apoptosis or necrosis. Legitimate medical health agencies are obliged to embrace the widespread scientific supportive findings regarding prooxidant hydrogen peroxide existent in the literature and encourage in depth scientific investigation into prooxidant EMOD disease protection and prevention. Scientific fact must supplant unsupported skepticism or flawed conclusions based on outdated data. While emphasizing hydrogen peroxide, this review is aimed at presenting the scientific facts regarding prooxidant EMOD health applications and cancer therapy. Based on the scientific literature currently available, EMOD use has significant potential benefits in the treatment of a wide range of human pathophysiologies. To deny the crucial role of hydrogen peroxide and prooxidant EMODs in normal metabolic processes and disease protection is to deny scientific truth.

Introduction

It is perhaps amongst the greatest biochemical wonders of evolution that the most crucial and widespread small molecular weight EMODs, which are purportedly the alleged "enemies within," are ever present and essential occupants of the most sensitive biochemical control systems within obligate aerobic cells. They carry on continual cross talk with their chemical kin. The naïve notion (promulgated by the free radical theory), that EMODs are inherently toxic, is counterintuitive to very basis of the evolutionary concept itself. After all, following oxygen's arrival, they evolved with the cell, by the cell and for the cell. Logic and biochemical principles dictate that careful EMOD modulation could serve as a safe means of advancing disease protection or reversal and health promotion.

However, even with hydrogen peroxide, which is an abundant permeating cellular mediator, nonspecific inhibition or augmentation of its activities may lead to homeostatic derangements by exogenous or endogenous over- or under-production.

Refute the Old Unproven Allegation: Free Radicals are Bad, Antioxidants are Good

In discussing the history of oxidants, such as hydrogen peroxide, respected free radical research pioneer, Barry Halliwell, said that, "In the beginning, it was simple: we said free radicals are bad, antioxidants are good." However, much has changed and over half a century later, these unfounded charges remain unproven. Further, the free radial theory, upon which this was based, has failed to be verified by the scientific method because of its lack of predictability. In fact, recent findings from randomized controlled trials (RCTs) have repeatedly failed to support the free radical theory and some trial results have even shown harmful effects and increased risk of mortality from antioxidant use.

Following the 1992 US National Cancer Institute research for testing of beta carotene, Halliwell, from the National University of Singapore, said, "It was a shock. It (beta carotene) not only did no good but had the potential to do harm." Subsequently, an expert panel convened by the National Institutes of Health has concluded that there is no evidence to recommend beta carotene supplements for the general population, and strong evidence to recommend that smokers avoid it.

The story was the same with vitamin E, in which recent studies have been almost universally "disappointing." Further, in 2005, Dr. Edgar Miller of the Johns Hopkins Medical Institutions, published a meta-analysis review of 19 studies in Annals of Internal Medicine showing that vitamin E increased overall mortality. [1] Even though vitamin E appeared to be a good antioxidant in vitro, there is now serious scepticism that it acts in the same manner in vivo. [2]

Following a large RCT on vitamin C, Halliwell said, "Vitamin C is another disappointment. People are still trying to defend it, but you don't get an effect on free radical damage unless you start with people with a vitamin C deficiency. I think it is a lost cause."

Yet, the prevailing prejudice against EMODs is manifestly illustrated in the November 2003 issue of Readers Digest. In quoting Dr. Bruce Ames, a biochemist at the University of California at Berkley, he stated, "free radical oxidation doesn't just rise with aging-- it causes it. The more that mitochondria 'leak' free radicals (i.e., oxygen radicals, EMODs), the more those radicals end up damaging the mitochondria, which in turn leak even more free radicals." In bold print, the article states, "The ultimate irony: The thing we need most to live--oxygen--is what's killing us." Statements such as this, which appear in both the lay press and in scientific publications, point out the currently accepted dogma which states that oxygen and its radicals are highly toxic, even lethal. To the contrary, the overall data shows that these conclusions are, at best, dubious.

History of the Flawed Free Radical Theory

In *Science* in 1954, Rebeca Gerschman and her colleagues first introduced the notion that free radicals are toxic agents. Gerschman published a paper entitled, "Oxygen poisoning and X-irradiation: a mechanism in common." This paper led to the supposed link between oxygen free radicals and cellular damage, which was later used as the basis for the free radical theory of aging and oxidative stress. In 1956, over 53 years ago, Dr. Denham Harman proposed the free radical theory of aging. The free radical theory of aging simply argues that aging results from the accumulated damage generated over time by EMODs (oxygen free radicals). [3]

Harman's theory stated that the aging process resulted from the "stochastic" or random accumulated damage caused by EMODs (reactive oxygen species, ROS), many of which are products of normal cellular metabolism. [4-7]

The mitochondrial electron transport chain (ETC) is an integral player because up to 10% of the reducing equivalents from NADH so-called "leak" to form superoxide anions and H_2O_2, although this is admittedly one of the highest "guestimates" of superoxide production by the ETC. [8] The commonly quoted range for EMOD ETC production is between 1-5%. The negative opinions regarding EMODs have changed from seeing reactive oxygen species (ROS) and redox states as only sources of damage, to viewing them as integral components in signal transduction. [9]

EMODs and the redox state act as messengers in the intricate regulation of gene expression in development, growth, and apoptosis and there is widespread scientific support for the emerging perspective that EMODs are signaling molecules crucial in numerous cellular functions that are under precise control.

EMODs and Cancer Therapy

Cancer treatments using hydrogen peroxide have been around for decades and have been referred to as some of the following: hyperoxygenation, oxymedicine, oxidative therapy, bio-oxidative therapy and oxydology. The older literature based the use of hydrogen peroxide therapy on the work of Otto Warburg, M.D. (two time Nobel Prize in Medicine recipient), who believed that cancer cells grew best and primarily in an environment with hypoxic conditions. A simplistic view of Warburg's advocates was that the administration of hydrogen peroxide, which is an oxygen-rich solution, would restore the proper oxygen balance and selectively attack and kill cancer cells. The website for the University of California, San Diego Medical Center (Moores Cancer Center) states, "According the American Cancer Society (ACS), there is no scientific evidence that hydrogen peroxide is a safe, effective or useful cancer treatment." (Accessed 9-4-09).

A review of the scientific literature is essential to evaluate the accuracy or veracity of the ACS assessment, regarding the use of hydrogen peroxide for therapeutic purposes. Such a review rebuts their assertion.

345

Even though there has been "the poisoning of the oxidative watering hole" by the free radical theory for over a half century, world orthodoxy is now acknowledging that EMODs, inclusive of hydrogen peroxide, are of crucial benefit and play a central role in pathogen and neoplasia protection and cellular signaling. [10]

Hydrogen Peroxide (H_2O_2)

How could the magnanimous wisdom of evolution produce a ubiquitous, omnipresent, allegedly highly damaging, powerful, toxic agent such as the accused hydrogen peroxide molecule, which, by design, is freely mobile and highly permeable through biological membranes, enabling its diffusion out of and within the cell from any intracellular production site? Such a case would defy scientific and evolutionary logic.

Hydrogen peroxide (H_2O_2) is a well-documented and essential component of aerobic living cells. It plays crucial roles in host defense and oxidative biosynthetic reactions. In addition there is growing evidence that at low levels, H_2O_2 also functions as a signaling agent, particularly in higher organisms. All aerobic organisms studied to date, from prokaryotes to humans, appear to tightly regulate their intracellular H_2O_2 concentrations at levels favorable to healthy homeostasis, i.e., 10^{-9} to 10^{-7}M. [11]

Well defined biochemical pathways involved in the response to exogenous H_2O_2 have been described in both prokaryotes and yeast. In animals and plants, many regulated enzymatic systems generate H_2O_2. In addition oxidation-dependent steps in signal transduction pathways are being uncovered, and evidence is accumulating regarding the nature of the EMOD type(s) involved in each of these pathways. Application of physiologic levels of H_2O_2 to mammalian cells has been shown to stimulate biological responses and to activate specific biochemical pathways in these cells. [12]

Oxidation serves as our first line of defense and occurs with the respiratory burst, which should more properly be referred to as a "peroxide spike," secondary to spontaneous or enzymatic dismutation of the superoxide anion. [13] Ergo, our lives are sustained, at least in part, by an innate "prooxidant-cure" and during times of need, to fight invaders or tumors, we rely on this "peroxide-spike" or "Vis medicatrix naturae" (The Healing Power of Nature). Thus, hydrogen peroxide is a formidable and influential orthomolecular agent.

Disruption of the delicate balance between prooxidants and antioxidants has been implicated in the pathophysiology of many chronic diseases, such as atherosclerosis, cancer, diabetes, strokes, arthritis and cataract formation [14] Unfortunately, far too frequently, we have been "radically misled," regarding the overstated toxicity of EMODs. (see "The Howes Selective World Library of Oxygen Metabolism," available at www.thepundit.com). [15, 16]

Prooxidants are fundamental for life and the concentrations of electronically modified oxygen derivatives (EMODs) are important signaling agents, possibly extending to virtually all cellular processes. Oxygen is an important signal in all major aspects of stem cell biology including proliferation and tumorigenesis, cell death and differentiation, self-renewal, and migration. [17] "Redox signaling" is achieved by discrete, localized redox circuitry rather than by so-called "oxidative stress." [18]

This realization represents a significant departure from traditional views that prooxidant EMODs are simply harmful by-products of normal oxidative metabolism or only a tool through which phagocytes accomplish antimicrobial action. With this paradigm shift comes the challenge of understanding how EMOD production is regulated and localized within cells in both normal and pathological circumstances. Current evidence supports a sustaining role for EMODs and a generalized "injury" and protective response in tissues and organs.

Hydrogen Peroxide Overview

The literature illustrates the wide variety of cells and the distribution of EMOD production in the living/breathing cell. This alone demonstrates their low toxicity and the important role of EMODs in aerobic cells and their wide distribution is a counter argument to their supposed pernicious activity. Noted biochemist, Barry Halliwell, said that, "Over a year, a human body makes 1.7 kilograms or 3.74# of EMODs, which is a conservative estimate." This begs the question, "Thus, how toxic are EMODs?"

O_2^- and H_2O_2 are cellular signaling molecules and they change the behavior of proteins as diverse as transcription factors and membrane receptors by virtue of their ability to undergo redox reactions with the proteins with which they interact, converting -SH groups to disulfide bonds and changing the oxidation states of enzyme-associated transition metals.

Prevalent EMOD Presence

EMOD activity has been detected in a wide variety of different cells including mesangial cells, oocytes, Leydig cells, thyroid cells, adipocytes, tumor cells, red blood cells and platelets. O_2^- and H_2O_2 are manufactured by many cell types, encompassing fibroblasts, endothelial and vascular smooth muscle cells, neurons, ova, spermatozoa and cells of the carotid body. Superoxide anions and hydrogen peroxide also participate in the induction of hyperactivated motility and the acrosome reaction. [19]

The carotid body is an organ located at the bifurcation of the common carotid artery that measures the oxygen tension of the blood and it produces hydrogen peroxide on a continual basis. [20]

Halliwell claims that the gastrointestinal tract, especially the stomach, with its highly acidic environment, is constantly generating reactive oxygen species from food. "Every time you drink a cup of coffee it's a dilute bowl of hydrogen peroxide," says Halliwell. The hydrogen peroxide is there because of the presence of the antioxidants — "antioxidants" is really just another way of saying reducing agent, which can react with oxygen in the water to produce hydrogen peroxide. [21]

There is a surprising number of proteins whose operation depends upon the redox state of the cell and includes the general transcription factors NF-kappa B and AP-1 (jun/fos), as well as several transcription factors that induce the synthesis of proteins that protect against so-called oxidative stress (e.g., soxR, soxS, oxyR).

Yet, some have come to view oxygen as a dangerous gift: indispensable for energy production but the alleged cause of damage that accumulates slowly over a lifetime. [22]

Peroxide, the Terrible

Some say that under normal healthy conditions, 90% of H_2O_2 is generated as a toxic by-product of the mitochondrial electron transport chain (ETC) respiratory activity. [23, 24]

In the past, some believed that H_2O_2, which is long lived and highly biomembrane permeable, must be immediately neutralized at the site of production to prevent diffusion throughout the cell or to the extracellular space. [25] Specific enzyme systems exist expressly for this purpose. These H_2O_2 neutralizing anti-oxidant enzymes are catalase (E.C. 1.11.1.6) and glutathione peroxidase (GPx, E.C. 1.11.1.9) with GPx responsible for 91% of H_2O_2 consumption. [26]

Even more alarming, some believe that, if allowed to accumulate, H_2O_2 will diffuse from its site of production and generate hydroxyl radical ($\cdot OH$), which is the most damaging and chemically reactive radical formed by cellular metabolism. They believe that the hydroxyl radical will indiscriminately destroy everything it encounters. [27-29]

The hydroxyl radical is believed to be principally responsible for the cytotoxic effects of oxygen in animals. [29]

Hydrogen Peroxide's Crucial Role in Normal Cellular Function

Oxygen is the ultimate electron acceptor and reacts with all elements in the periodic table except the noble gases, which have no known biological function. The mitochondrial ETC is not perfect and up to 5% of electrons fail to combine with oxygen to produce water. [27] These so-called "leaked" electrons combine directly with molecular oxygen in the immediate vicinity, instead of the next carrier in the chain, to form the superoxide (O_2- ·) radical. [30]

Likely, complex I and III, of the ETC, are the source of so-called electron leakage leading to the eventual intracellular generation of hydrogen peroxide. [31,32] This ETC "leakage" or metabolic reduction of triplet O_2 during cellular respiration produces superoxide anion ($O_2^{·}$), which is spontaneously or enzymatically dismutated to the prooxidant, H_2O_2, within mitochondria by the enzyme superoxide dismutase (SOD). [27]

H_2O_2 has a pervasive presence in cells and is continuously being produced by the plasma membrane, cytosol and different subcellular organelles including mitochondria, peroxisomes, endoplasmic reticulum, nucleus and by almost 100 enzyme systems. [23, 25]

Studies have determined that H_2O_2 is a small, diffusible, and ubiquitous molecule that can be synthesized, modified and/or destroyed rapidly in response to external stimuli, it meets all of the important criteria for an intracellular messenger, and H_2O_2 is now firmly established as a ubiquitous intracellular messenger under subtoxic conditions. [33-36]

As previously mentioned, metabolic reduction of triplet O_2 during cellular respiration produces superoxide anion radical ($O_2^{·}$), which is spontaneously or enzymatically dismutated to the prooxidant, non-radical, H_2O_2. Varying cell types produce low levels of O_2^- and H_2O_2 in response to a variety of extracellular stimuli, including cytokines (TGF-β1, TNF-α, and IL), peptide growth factors (PDGF; EGF, VEGF, bFGF, and insulin), the agonists of heterotrimeric G protein–coupled receptors (GPCR; angiotensin II, thrombin, lysophosphatidic acid, sphingosine 1-phosphate, histamine, and bradykinin), and shear stress. Research continues to uncover additional important sources of hydrogen peroxide in aerobic cells.

Hydrogen peroxide (H_2O_2) is present in exhaled breath and condensate and is produced by airway epithelia. Additionally, H_2O_2 is a vital substrate for the airway lactoperoxidase (LPO) anti-infection system. Duox is the major NADPH oxidase expressed in airway epithelia and therefore a contributor of H_2O_2 production in the airway lumen. [37]

Although specific levels of ubiquitous H_2O_2 have been debatable, animals and humans have between 5.0 and 41 microM for aqueous humor and 115 and 187 microM for urine. [38,39]

Again, this begs the question, "Just how toxic are EMODs?"

It was believed that oxidative stress was the hallmark of asthma and increased levels of oxidants, such as H_2O_2 were considered a marker of the inflammatory process. In contrast to this notion, current studies suggest that hydrogen peroxide serves a role in suppressing both mucus production and airway hyper-responsiveness. [40]

Hydrogen peroxide production has also been found in the nucleus of epithelial cells and it could convey redox signals altering gene expression. [41,42] H_2O_2 is a natural orthomolecular substance and has been detected in serum and in intact liver. [43]

In mouse pancreatic beta cells, H_2O_2 hyperpolarizes the cell membrane coupled with an increase of cell membrane conductance. [44]

Moreover, it has recently been shown that H_2O_2:

> increases intracellular Ca^{2+}
> decreases the ATP/ADP ratio
> and inhibits glucose-stimulated insulin secretion from isolated
> mouse islets. [45]

H_2O_2 as an Insulin Mimetic

Long ago, it was demonstrated that polyamines are able to exert insulin-like effects in fat cells through the production of hydrogen peroxide. [46]

Hydrogen peroxide is now known to cause the reversible inhibition of protein tyrosine phosphatases (PTP) in cells, thereby strengthening insulin signaling. It has also been shown that production of hydrogen peroxide chemically in cells acts as an insulin mimetic. H_2O_2 improves glucose utilization in diabetics. Membrane receptors and transporters, including the insulin receptor and receptors for certain neurotransmitters, are regulated by the redox state of the cell.

Pancreatic β-cells are extremely sensitive to oxidative stress because of the low expression and activity of antioxidant enzymes. The GSH/GSSG (reduced/oxidized glutathione) ratio in islets is low compared with other tissues. [47]

A 10-6-09 article by Tony Tiganis in the journal Cell Metabolism shows that "mice that lacked the antioxidant enzyme Gpx1 were less likely to develop insulin resistance -- an early sign of diabetes -- than normal mice. But when they treated the enzyme-deficient mice with an antioxidant, they lost this advantage and become more diabetic." Tiganis said, "Our work suggests that antioxidants may contribute to early development of insulin resistance, a key pathological hallmark of type 2 diabetes."

Other Roles for Peroxide

Hydrogen peroxide is only one of the many components that help regulate the amount of oxygen getting to cells. Its presence is vital for many other functions as well. It is required for the production of thyroid hormone and sexual hormones. Even the synthesis of thyroxin depends on the requirements of a H_2O_2 substrate for thyroid peroxidase and it stimulates the production of interferon.

A role for EMODs in controlling oxygen-sensitive channel function in excitable cells has been demonstrated previously. Hydrogen peroxide is capable of activating potassium transport pathways in excitable cells and in alveolar epithelial cells. These data suggest that EMODs and the hydroxyl radicals, formed from O_2 in close vicinity to the cell membrane, play an important role in the oxygen-dependent activation of the K^+-Cl^- co-transporter. [48]

H_2O_2 is produced by the autooxidation of ascorbic acid (vitamin C) and catecholamines, such as dopamine, norepinephrine and serotonin. [49]

Amazingly, H_2O_2 is generated at a rate of 1.36 +/- 0.2 microM/h (3.9 +/- 0.6 nmol.h-1.g Hb-1), and a steady-state red blood cell concentration of H_2O_2 which is approximately $2 \times 10(-10)$ M. Kinetic comparisons of H_2O_2 production and oxyhemoglobin autooxidation (which generates O_2^- that dismutases to H_2O_2) suggests that the latter is the main source of H_2O_2 in red blood cells. [50]

Apparently, many articles and agencies are unaware of peroxide's prime importance because studies have shown that the addition of exogenous H_2O_2 or its intracellular production in response to receptor stimulation, affects the function of various proteins, including protein kinases, protein phosphatases, transcription factors, phospholipases, ion channels, and G proteins.

353

EMODs can induce cellular senescence and apoptosis and can therefore function as anti-tumorigenic species. [51]

Another 100+ articles related to hydrogen peroxide's varied roles, including apoptosis, can be found at: http://www.caspases.org/showcitationlist.php?keyword=hydrogen%20peroxide%20h$_2$o$_2$,

H$_2$O$_2$ can Dilate Arteries

H$_2$O$_2$ can dilate blood vessels in the heart and brain. Mechano-sensitive mechanisms that are sensitive to deformation, pressure, stretch, and wall shear stress elicit release of NO and H$_2$O$_2$, resulting in reactive dilation of isolated coronary arterioles. [52]

On June 23, 2009, the Medical College of Wisconsin received a four year, $1.5 million grant from the National Institutes of Health's National Heart, Lung and Blood Institute to study the role of naturally produced hydrogen peroxide in controlling human blood flow. Dr. David Gutterman's lab has observed a unique relationship between dilation in heart blood vessels from patients with coronary artery disease and the endothelial production of hydrogen peroxide and thus far, the association of vessel dilation with mitochondrial hydrogen peroxide has only been reported in human hearts.

EMOD Induced Apoptotic Cancer Cell Death

Cancer accounts for nearly 25% of all human deaths and no definitive cure is available as yet. [53] The most common treatment modalities promising a cure appear to be a combination of radiotherapy and chemotherapy and these methods, in part, utilize the reactivities of prooxidant EMODs, including hydrogen peroxide.

Radiation exposure leads to the hydrolysis of water, thereby generating EMODs, which initiate chemical peroxidative processes that destroy biomolecules. [54]

The postulated mechanism of action for many forms of chemotherapy, radiation therapy, photodynamic therapy, ozone therapy, hyperbaric oxygen therapy, intravenous mega-dose of vitamin C, the Howes singlet oxygen cancer therapy system and hydrogen peroxide therapy is the generation of electronically modified oxygen derivatives (EMODs). The production of EMODs leads to the stimulation of various signaling pathways, and in particular, stress-responsive signal transduction pathways are strictly regulated by the intracellular redox state. [55, 56]

High level acute H_2O_2 treatment of various cells in vitro leads to apoptosis. [57]

However, some investigators believe that hydrogen peroxide can cause apoptosis via a non-apoptotic pathway. Recent studies in a variety of cell types have suggested that cancer chemotherapy drugs induce tumor cell apoptosis in part by inducing formation of reactive oxygen species (EMODs). Investigators demonstrated that, at least in B lymphoma cells, chemotherapy-induced apoptosis occur using a mechanism that does not involve oxidants. Hydrogen peroxide, which reportedly kills cells by a non-apoptotic pathway, caused increases in both protein and lipid oxidation. [58]

Hydrogen Peroxide and Hydroxyl Radical Antineoplastic Cytotoxicity

The cytotoxicity of the antineoplastic quinones doxorubicin, mitomycin C, and diaziridinylbenzoquinone for the Ehrlich ascites carcinoma can be significantly reduced or abolished by the antioxidant enzymes catalase and superoxide dismutase, the hydroxyl radical scavengers dimethyl sulfoxide, diethylurea, and thiourea, and the iron chelators deferoxamine,

2,2-bipyridine, and diethylenetriaminepentaacetic acid. Furthermore, treatment of intact tumor cells with doxorubicin, mitomycin C, and diaziridinylbenzoquinone required hydrogen peroxide, iron, and intact tumor cells. These results suggest that drug-induced hydrogen peroxide and hydroxyl radical production has a role in the antineoplastic action of redox active anticancer quinones. [59]

Photodynamic Therapy (PDT) and Singlet Oxygen

Photodynamic therapy (PDT) is a novel approach for destruction of malignant cells and involves the administration of nontoxic dyes known as photosensitisers (PS) either systemically or topically, followed by illumination of the lesion with visible light (usually red). [60] The PS absorbs the light, and in the presence of oxygen, transfers the energy, thereby producing cytotoxic oxygen species (either singlet oxygen or oxygen radicals, i.e., EMODs). [61, 62]

This reportedly leads to a rapid tumoricidal response mediated by both direct tumor cell toxicity and photodamage to the involved microvasculature and cellular structure. [63]

Investigations have demonstrated that apoptotic and necrotic pathways are both involved in PDT-mediated cell death. [60, 64]

A wide distribution of early response genes, genes associated with signal transduction pathways and cytokine expression, as well as stress response genes, are activated by PDT and primarily singlet oxygen. [65-71]

EMODs can Have Complex Interactions

Interestingly, EMODs can react and interact to produce a family of products. For example, superoxide can react with itself to produce hydrogen peroxide or it can undergo univalent reduction to form hydrogen peroxide. Superoxide can react with the hydroxyl radical to produce singlet oxygen. Superoxide can also react with nitric oxide (NO) (also a radical) to produce peroxynitrate (OONO⁻). Singlet oxygen can react with superoxide to produce hydrogen peroxide. Hydrogen peroxide can react with hypohalous acid to produce singlet oxygen. Hydrogen peroxide, in the presence of metal ions, can react to form a hydroxyl radical (HO) and the hydroxide ion (HO⁻). Ozone can react with water to form hydrogen peroxide. Methylene blue and superoxide dismutase produce H_2O_2. Ascorbate can react with singlet oxygen and produce hydrogen peroxide.

Examples of the cross reactivity of EMODs illustrate the generation of a family of EMODs from the more basic EMOD agents (superoxide, hydrogen peroxide and singlet oxygen).

A Role for Hydrogen Peroxide in the Pro-apoptotic Effects of Photodynamic Therapy

Although the first EMOD formed during irradiation of photosensitized cells is almost invariably singlet molecular oxygen, $^1O_2^*$, other EMODs have been implicated in the phototoxic effects of photodynamic therapy. Among these are superoxide anion radical (O_2^-), hydrogen peroxide (H_2O_2) and hydroxyl radical (OH.). Investigators studied the role of H_2O_2 in the pro-apoptotic response to PDT in murine leukemia P388 cells. A primary route for detoxification of cellular H_2O_2 involves the peroxisomal enzyme catalase. Inhibition of catalase activity by 3-amino-1,2,4-triazole led to an increased apoptotic response. PDT-induced apoptosis was impaired by addition of an exogenous recombinant catalase analog (CAT-skl) that was specifically designed to enter cells and more efficiently localize in peroxisomes. A similar effect was observed upon addition of 2,2'-bipyridine, a reagent that can chelate Fe(+2), a co-factor in the Fenton reaction that results in the conversion of H_2O_2 to the hydroxyl radical (OH). These results provide evidence that formation of H_2O_2 during irradiation of photosensitized cells contributes to PDT efficacy. [72]

H_2O_2, O_2^{-} and OH. are Involved in Phototoxic Tumoricidal Action

Researchers estimated the participation of EMODs, other than singlet oxygen ($^1O_2^*$), in the antitumor effect of PDT with hematoporphyrin derivative (HPD) as well as determined the ability of photoexcited HPD to the formation of protein peroxides that are regarded as a new form of EMOD. Experiments indicated that H_2O_2 and oxygen radicals could mediate the tumoricidal action of HPD-PDT; they found that photosensitization of EAC cells with HPD leads to the formation of significant amounts of H_2O_2, superoxide (O_2^{-}) and hydroxyl (OH.) radicals, which along with $^1O_2^*$ were involved in photoinactivation of the cells in vitro. Their data showed that in EAC cells subjected to HPD-PDT, the generation H_2O_2, O_2^{-} and OH. could be largely mediated by: (i) an increase in the activity of xanthine oxidase (XOD), due most probably to the conversion of xanthine dehydrogenase (XDH) to XOD via a Ca2+-dependent proteolytic process as well as oxidation of SH groups in XDH; and (ii) photooxidation of some cellular constituents (proteins). Another interesting finding of their studies was that in tumor cells subjected to HPD-PDT the Fenton-like reactions could play an important role in the generation of OH., and that cell-bound Cu/Zn-superoxide dismutase as well as catalase can protect tumor cells against the phototoxic action of HPD. They clearly demonstrated the ability of photoexcited HPD to the generation of protein peroxides in tumor cells. Studies suggest that $^1O_2^*$ is the main agent responsible for the generation of protein peroxides in EAC cells treated with HPD-PDT, although other EMODs (H_2O_2, O_2^{-} and OH.) were also implicated in this process. [73]

Photofrin® is a purified form of hematoporphyrin derivative; it is a photosensitizer used in the treatment of cancer. Upon exposure to light it produces singlet oxygen, a highly electrophilic species that initiates oxidations that lead to cell death. [74, 75]

Interestingly, singlet oxygen reacts readily with ascorbate, producing hydrogen peroxide. [76, 77]

Ubiquitous and Omnipresent H_2O_2

The biochemistry of H_2O_2 is also, to a considerable extent, the biochemistry of the superoxide anion. Superoxide anion ($O_2^{\cdot-}$) converts rapidly to H_2O_2 either spontaneously or with the help of one of the superoxide dismutase enzymes (i.e., CuZnSOD, EcSOD, MnSOD, etc.). Since many of the EMODs are rapidly converted and/or transformed into other EMOD types, it also serves as a source of a large family of EMOD agents.

The two primary metabolic EMODs are $O_2^{\cdot-}$ and H_2O_2. $O_2^{\cdot-}$ is the primary stoichiometric precursor of H_2O_2 but considerable H_2O_2 can be produced directly and not via the superoxide anion.

Chance, et al. reviewed the metabolism of H_2O_2 in mammalian systems. [11]

Though controversial, many papers still state that the mitochondria are the major cellular source of hydrogen peroxide. The amount of H_2O_2 produced by brain mitochondria is up to 5% of the amount of O_2 consumed. H_2O_2 may be produced directly as a product of biological oxidations, or it may be produced by the dismutation of superoxide. The relative estimates of subcellular sources of H_2O_2 are as follows:

- Endoplasmic reticulum (mixed function oxidations)   45%
- Peroxisomes (metal-catalyzed oxidations)   35%
- Mitochondria (oxidative phosphorylation)   15%
- Cytosol (xanthine oxidation)   5%

These EMOD agents are formed continuously in all aerobic cells, either via oxygen energy metabolism, through reactions with drugs or toxins or via metabolism of fatty acids.

In 1999, Juan and Buettner calculated the steady state (ss) levels to be as follows:

$[H_2O_2]$ss in red cells is 10^{-10} M
$[H_2O_2]$ss in mitochondrial membrane is 10^{-8} M
$[H_2O_2]$ss in liver cells is 10^{-8} M
$[O_2]$ss is 10^{-5} M, much higher than $[H_2O_2]$
$[O_2^{-}]$ss in cells is 10^{-10} M

An additional source of O_2^{-} and H_2O_2 is the NADPH oxidase families (NOX and DuOX), which are found on various cellular membranes. Once thought to be restricted only to phagocytes, stimulated H_2O_2 production is now known to occur in almost all cells through NOX and/or DuOX activities. Thus, H_2O_2 has been accused of contributing to pathology through its reaction with transition metals that produce hydroxyl radicals via the Fenton reaction. Yet, even though it is not discussed, two hydroxyl radicals can combine to form hydrogen peroxide. This could well represent another salutary pathway for peroxide formation and pathogen and neoplasia defense.

H_2O_2 is involved in the generation of hypohalous acids through catalysis by myeloperoxidases and lactoperoxidase. These oxidizing acids are capable of killing microorganisms and allegedly causing tissue damage during inflammation. Ubiquitous H_2O_2 acts as a secondary messenger in signal transduction through its reaction with key proteins containing critical cysteine residues. [78, 79]

Yet, the antioxidant, cysteine, itself can undergo autoxidation and form H_2O_2. This is somewhat analogous to the prooxidant EMOD activity of ascorbic acid.

The most common prooxidant in vivo is H_2O_2 and under inflammatory conditions, it is abundantly formed by dismutation of O_2^{-} released from activated phagocytes and other enzymatic systems, [80] but physiologically also by intracellular NADPH oxidases. [81]

Although some H_2O_2 appears to be produced constitutively, receptor-mediated H_2O_2 formation appears to be more common. Typical examples are TNFa-induced mitochondrial O_2^- formation, [82] or cytoplasmic increase of H_2O_2 upon growth factor receptor stimulation. [83] Nonetheless, H_2O_2 is argued to be the most common prooxidant in vivo.

In a study on synergism between tumor necrosis factor-alpha and H_2O_2, levels of cellular toxicity were found. With PC12 tumor cells, TNF alpha toxicity was seen at >50 ng/ml, and that of H_2O_2 at > 150 microM. However, when together, sub-lethal levels (25 ng/ml TNF alpha and 30 microM H_2O_2) induced toxicity. [84]

Please remember that the chemistry of superoxide is also the chemistry of hydrogen peroxide. Once activated, phagocytes produce large quantities of superoxide, on the order of 10 nmol· min-1·10^6 neuutrophils^{-1} during the oxidative burst. [80]

The rate of superoxide production in vascular cells is thought to be ~1-10% of that in leukocytes. [85, 86] Basically, all cells continuously form O_2^- and submitochondrial particles generate O_2^- at a rate of 4-7 nmol/min^{-1}/mg protein^{-1}. [11]

Superoxide anion can be viewed as an innate pathway for hydrogen peroxide production. Thus, EMODs are intentionally being generated to serve as salutary cellular products intended to help regulate critical metabolic and reproductive mechanisms. [87] These prooxidant EMODs stimulate numerous transcription factors as well as signaling cascades via activation of kinases and inhibition of tyrosine phosphatases.

Under physiological conditions, the intracellular production of EMODs does not alter the redox state of cells which have large reserves of reducing agents, notably reduced glutathione, as well as extremely effective antioxidant defense mechanisms, such as SOD, catalase, and peroxidases. This allows agonist-induced increases in

EMODs to function as second messengers by limiting their effecting time and space in a manner similar to other well-known intracellular signals, such as cyclic AMP or nitric oxide. [88]

Differing from O_2^- that is charged, hardly permeable, and extremely short-lived, H_2O_2 is uncharged, relatively longer-lived, and freely diffusible. This property makes H_2O_2 an ideal signaling molecule. Clearly, this illustrates the great importance of H_2O_2 in combination with other EMODs, in the regulation of cellular homeostasis and redox status. Under basal conditions, human cells produce about 2 X 10^9 (2 billion) $O_2.-$ and H_2O_2 molecules per cell per day. [89]

EMODs are recognized as controlling key steps in cellular signal transduction cascades. [90, 91] EMODs can reversibly control gene expression and regulation at non-cytotoxic doses. [92] More specifically, there is evidence that hydrogen peroxide, H_2O_2, can modulate cellular functions through altering signal transduction in many cell types, including endothelial cells (ECs), vascular smooth muscle cells (VSMC), and T cells. [93-97]

In fact, H_2O_2 is now widely recognized as a ubiquitous intracellular messenger, under subtoxic conditions. [23, 34, 35, 36, 98-100] As of 2000, at least 127 genes and signal transducing proteins had been reported to be sensitive to reductive and oxidative (redox) states in the cell. [92] That number, as of 2009, now exceeds 200.

EMODs Kill Cancer

Otto Warburg was the primary scientist to implicate oxygen in cancer. [101] Anaerobic metabolism is favorable to many pathogenic organisms and hypoxia is the predominant condition within neoplastic cells. Hypoxia has been closely associated with pathological processes. [102] Requiring adequate oxygen levels, many anticancer drugs and radiation kill cancer cells by inducing prooxidant EMOD apoptosis. [103]

High level acute H_2O_2 treatment of various cells in vitro leads to apoptosis, with the involvement of NADPH oxidase isoforms and Src family kinases. [104]

The chemotherapeutic agents doxorubicin, mitomycin C, etoposide and cisplatin are superoxide generating agents and consequently hydrogen peroxide producers. [105]

Bleomycin and doxorubicin are agents shown to produce prooxidant oxygen agents. [106]

In reactions involving Fe(II) and oxygen, a so-called "activated" bleomycin species is generated that damages DNA through free radical intermediates. [107]

Superoxide and hydrogen peroxide can also react with Fe(II) or Fe(III) bleomycin, respectively, to produce the activated form of the drug. DNA damage from bleomycin and ionizing radiation is similar in both induction and repair. [108] Several other anti-cancer drugs are known to bring about their tumoricidal actions by an EMOD dependent mechanism. A majority of the studies reported that adriamycin, mitocmycin C, etc., augment EMOD production (superoxide anion and hydrogen peroxide) and lipid peroxidation in vitro and in vivo. [109]

The anti-estrogen tamoxifen, increasingly used alongside other breast cancer therapies, has also been shown to induce oxidative stress (EMOD production) within carcinoma cells *in vitro*. [110]

Oxygen levels are important since radiotherapy and photodynamic therapy generate oxygen radicals within the carcinoma cell. Thus, tumor hypoxia is a therapeutic concern since it can reduce the effectiveness of radiotherapy, some O_2-dependent cytotoxic agents, and photodynamic therapy. [111]

H$_2$O$_2$ Increases Doxorubicin Kill of Bladder Tumor Cells

Investigators determined whether the cytotoxicity of doxorubicin hydrochloride would be enhanced by adding hydrogen peroxide as a source of oxygen free radicals. Mouse bladder tumor cells (MBT-2) were grown in RPMI 1640 medium and treated with various concentrations of doxorubicin hydrochloride for 2 hours. They observed a dose dependent inhibition of MBT-2 cell growth after exposure to doxorubicin hydrochloride. Exposure to doxorubicin and hydrogen peroxide resulted in greater cell growth inhibition than exposure to either agent alone. The effects of hydrogen peroxide on cell proliferation were reversed by pre-incubation with alpha-tocopherol. As a source of oxygen free radicals, hydrogen peroxide enhances the antiproliferative effect of doxorubicin hydrochloride on a mouse bladder tumor cell line. [112]

H$_2$O$_2$ Increases Sulindac Kill of Squamous Cell Carcinoma

A skin squamous cell carcinoma (SCC-25) cell line was utilized and treated with sulindac prior to exposure to tert-butyl hydroperoxide (TBHP) or hydrogen peroxide for 2 hours. The combination of sulindac and TBHP enhanced the killing of the skin cancer cells. Sulindac combined with TBHP leads to markedly increased levels of intracellular EMODs in SCC cells.

A small group of patients with actinic keratoses (AKs), were treated with the combination of sulindac and hydrogen peroxide gels. The results revealed that 60% of the treated AKs responded to therapy by exhibiting a decrease in size or becoming not visible to the naked eye. In addition, 50% of the treated AKs showed no residual AK on histopathology specimens after skin biopsy at the end of the study. Researchers concluded that the combination of sulindac and TBHP or H$_2$O$_2$ significantly enhances the killing of SCC cells. [113]

The Baylor Group Peroxide Experience

In the 1960s, a group of investigators at Baylor Medical School (the Baylor group) conducted ground breaking studies with hydrogen peroxide in the treatment of a wide range of disease conditions. Various investigators have studied the value of H_2O_2 and shrinking the size of tumors, [114] and have studied treatment advantages and increased tumor cytotoxicity by the use of regional H_2O_2 infusion. [115]

Earlier work indicated that hydrogen peroxide, a secretory product of mononuclear phagocytes, [116] accounts for a considerable portion of their nonphagocytic lysis of tumor cells in at least three circumstances: when certain secretagogues were added, when antitumor antibody was present, or when the tumor cells were coated with eosinophil peroxidase. [117]

Many clinical and experimental applications of hydrogen peroxide have been demonstrated by the Baylor group. In over 300 patients regional intra-arterial hydrogen peroxide has potentiated the effect of radiation therapy in situations of malignancy involving the head, neck, pelvis and retro-peritoneum. [118]

Increased localization of radioactive isotopes in malignant tumors has been achieved by regional and intra-arterial infusion of hydrogen peroxide. [119, 120]

Granulocytes also secrete H_2O_2, which may participate in their cytotoxic effects in a variety of conditions. Preformed or enzymatically generated H_2O_2, with or without a peroxidase, lyses tumor cells, which was shown by Nathan's group and others. [121-127]

Reports have suggested that hydrogen peroxide released by mononuclear phagocytes and neutrophils may extend the antimicrobial, antitumor, and oxidant-injury activities of these cells to adjacent tissues. [128, 129]

Nathan devised a nontoxic way to deliver hydrogen peroxide to sites of malignancy in vivo and to test its antitumor efficacy. Glucose oxidase was chosen for this purpose because its substrates, glucose and oxygen, are abundant in the body fluids and because its sole products are H_2O_2 and gluconic acid. [130] Glucose oxidase was coupled covalently to polystyrene microspheres (GOL) produced H_2O_2. Injection i.p. prolonged the survival of mice by 27% after injection of 106 P388 lymphoma cells in the same site, consistent with destruction of 97.6% of the tumor cells. Placing mice for several hours in 100% O~, the probable rate-limiting substrate for GOL, afforded a 42% prolongation of survival from P388 lymphoma, consistent with destruction of 99.6% of the tumor cells. A single injection of preformed H_2O_2 readily killed P388 cells in the peritoneal cavity, but only at doses nearly lethal to the mice. In contrast, GOL had very little toxicity. Thus, an H_2O_2-generating system confined to the tumor bed exerted clear-cut antitumor effects with little toxicity to the host.

Studies demonstrated that a combination of sub-lytic concentrations of chemically generated NO and H_2O_2 leads to death of murine lymphoma cells, in part, via induction of apoptosis. [131] In vitro studies have suggested that a reaction of nitric oxide (NO) gas and H_2O_2 produces singlet oxygen (which is the primary cytotoxic agent in PDT) or hydroxyl radicals. [132, 133] Nevertheless, this has not yet been demonstrated in cell cultures.

Others Argue That EMODs May Inhibit Apoptosis

In the past, the main focus of the importance of EMODs in oncology was that these agents were capable of inducing DNA damage, which could theoretically lead to cellular proliferation and a predisposition to cancer.

Even though an overwhelming accumulation of intracellular EMODs can create an oxidatively stressed environment leading to necrosis, a slight increase is a stimulus for cellular proliferation. [134,] [135] Burdon et al interpreted this to mean that sublethal oxidative stress promotes cell proliferation *in vitro*, with both superoxide and hydrogen peroxide stimulating growth. Proliferation in response to hydrogen peroxide may be due to the activation of mitogen-activated protein kinases (MAPKs). HeLa cells treated with hydrogen peroxide undergo a sustained activation of all three MAPK pathways: extracellular signal related protein kinase; c-Jun amino-terminal kinase/stress-activated protein kinase; and p38.

However, Howes believes that a more logical explanation may be that an EMOD insufficiency "allows" for cell proliferation. [15]

Theoretically, the carcinogenic process in animal models involves initiation and promotion. Allegedly, the production of EMODs and hydrogen peroxide occurs with several known tumor promoters, including 12-O-tetradecanoylphorbol-13-acetate (TPA), okadaic acid (OA), thapsigargin, 2,3,7,8-tetrachlorodibenzo-*p*-dioxin (TCDD) and H_2O_2, as well as peroxisome proliferators, steroidal estrogens, phenobarbital, chlordane and aroclor. However, their specific mechanism of action is evasive and speculative. [136]

Severe oxidative stress leads to apoptosis. Conversely, persistent oxidative stress at sublethal levels may cause resistance to apoptosis. The induction of programmed cell death by EMODs is dependent on p53 in both mouse and human cell lines. [137] Current studies indicating a possible mechanism whereby H_2O_2 could promote tumor formation is sparse. [138] Further, many of these studies were carried out using non-physiological levels of H_2O_2, which can have cytotoxic activity.

However, this is in contrast to the work of others, who state that O_2^- and H_2O_2 do not react with DNA bases at all. [139] Yet, the hydroxyl radical (OH·) generates a variety of products from all four DNA bases and this pattern is used as a diagnostic "fingerprint" of OH· attack. [140]

Singlet oxygen selectively attacks guanine to produce the 8-hydroxyguanine (8-OHG), which is also used as an index of oxidative damage to DNA and it can be measured as the nucleoside, 8-hydroxydeoxyguanosine (8-OHdG).

Some investigators believe that H_2O_2 may act as a "genotoxicant" or "epigenetic" agent and act as a promoting agent. However, even if hydrogen peroxide could cause DNA damage, peroxide is at best a very weak mutagen in mammalian cells. [136]

Some endogenous DNA damage arises from intermediates of oxygen reduction that either attack the bases or the deoxyribosyl backbone of DNA. Yet, the study of oxidative DNA damage and its role in carcinogenesis is still controversial. [141]

The International Agency for Research on Cancer (IARC) has determined that hydrogen peroxide is not classifiable as to its carcinogencity to humans. Even though accusations against H_2O_2 have been wide spread, there is no verified data, in man, that H_2O_2 in any way causes or promotes cancer in vivo. The WHO-IARC said, "There is inadequate evidence in humans for the carcinogenicity of hydrogen peroxide."

Hyperoxia

Under conditions of hyperoxia, mitochondrial EMOD generation increases as a linear function of the oxygen tension. [142] Oxygen is critical to aerobic metabolism, but excessive oxygen (hyperoxia) can cause cell injury and death. An oxygen-tolerant strain of HeLa cells, which proliferates even under 80% O_2, termed "HeLa-80," was derived from wild-type HeLa cells ("HeLa-20") by selection for resistance to stepwise increases of oxygen partial pressure. Unpredictably, antioxidant defenses and susceptibility to oxidant-mediated killing do not differ between these two strains of HeLa cells. However, under both 20 and 80% O_2, intracellular reactive oxygen species (EMODs) production is significantly (~2-fold) less in HeLa-80 cells.

In both cell lines the source of EMODs is evidently mitochondrial. Although HeLa-80 cells consume oxygen at the same rate as HeLa-20 cells, they consume less glucose and produce less lactic acid. Most importantly, the oxygen-tolerant HeLa-80 cells have significantly higher cytochrome *c* oxidase activity (~2-fold), which may act to deplete upstream electron-rich intermediates responsible for EMOD generation. Indeed, preferential inhibition of cytochrome *c* oxidase by treatment with *n*-methyl protoporphyrin (which selectively diminishes synthesis of heme a in cytochrome *c* oxidase) enhances EMOD production and abrogates the oxygen tolerance of the HeLa-80 cells. Thus, it appears that the remarkable oxygen tolerance of these cells derives from tighter coupling of the electron transport chain and reduced EMOD production. [143]

Vitamin C

The ultimate agent to treat cancer would be cytotoxic only to tumor cells and non-toxic to normal cells. Vitamin C has been theorized to meet these requirements but has been criticized by conventional medicine in favor of more powerful and toxic chemotherapeutic agents. [144] Riordan found that at a dose of 7.04 mg/dl, vitamin C is completely toxic to cancer cells while being completely non-toxic to normal cells. Only at eight times the dose needed to kill cancer cells does vitamin C become toxic to normal cells. This reveals its considerable clinical potential. [145]

Metabolically, vitamin C produces dehydroascorbate (DHA), an oxidant. Normal cells take in DHA, which is then converted to ascorbate and H_2O_2, by an oxidation/reduction (redox) electron transfer. Benade et al at the National Cancer Institute found that, in Ehrlich ascites carcinoma cell cultures, vitamin C selectively destroyed cancer cells by generating excess intracellular H_2O_2. [146]

It has been observed for a long time that ascorbic acid and ascorbic acid salts are preferentially toxic to tumor cells, which were thought to be related to intracellular generation of hydrogen peroxide. [147-149] It is theorized that cancer cells are less able than normal cells to neutralize H_2O_2 because they are deficient in catalase. Dr. Agus et al reported that cancer cells have extra glucose channels that rapidly bring in glucose and excess DHA. [150]

Cancer cells are defective in that they cannot fully distinguish between glucose and DHA. This may explain why vitamin C is safe in large doses for normal cells but toxic to cancer cells. The good results of Cameron and Hoffer with humans confirm the National Cancer Institute lab tests.

Mark Levine's group published a study on line for PNAS on September 12, 2005, with results showing that, "Pharmacologic ascorbic acid concentrations selectively kill cancer cells: Action as a pro-drug to deliver hydrogen peroxide to tissues." Human lymphoma cells were studied because of their sensitivity to ascorbate (EC50 of 0.5 mM) and suitability for evaluating mechanisms. Extracellular, but not intracellular, ascorbate resulted in cell death, which occurred by apoptosis and pyknosis/necrosis. Cell death was independent of metal chelators and absolutely dependent on H_2O_2 formation. [151]

Investigators stated that it was not known why it killed cancer cells but not normal cells. They felt that it was possible the hydrogen peroxide caused damage that was repaired in normal cells but not in sensitive cancer cells. The main mechanism thought to be responsible for this is the lack or relative deficiency of catalase in tumor cells. [152]

Therefore, it takes a smaller amount of H_2O_2 to reach or "trigger" apoptosis. This is the point of selectivity for toxicity to cancer cells, wherein there is no harm to normal cells. Interestingly, there is a reported 10- to 100-fold greater content of catalase in normal cells than in tumor cells. [146]

Humans lack gulonolactone oxidase, which is necessary to synthesize vitamin C and H_2O_2 is produced as a by-product in the process. It is incredibly ironic, that in the synthesis of one of the most touted of all of the antioxidants, ascorbate, that "dreaded H_2O_2" is generated stochiometrically on a molecule per molecule basis. This illustrates the fact that H_2O_2 is very important in maintaining homeostasis within the cell and as a secondary messenger and that antioxidants and prooxidants may be considered to be flip sides of the same redox coin.

H_2O_2 Induced Apoptosis in Human Gastric Cancer Cells

Investigations were made into the molecular mechanism by which ascorbic acid (AA) induces apoptosis in human gastric cancer cells, AGS cells. High concentration (more than 5mM) of AA increased cellular iron uptake by increasing transferrin receptor (TfR) expression and induced AGS cell apoptosis which was inhibited by catalase. Interestingly, p38 mitogen-activated protein kinase (MAPK) inhibitor inhibited the upregulation of TfR and increased cell survival by AA. TfR-siRNA-transfected cells reduced apoptosis by AA. H_2O_2 increased TfR expression in AGS cells. Taken together, investigators concluded that high concentration of AA, through H_2O_2, induces apoptosis of AGS cells by p38-MAPK-dependent upregulation of TfR. [153]

H_2O_2 Regulation of T Cells

The immune system is vital to protect us against infectious agents (bacteria, viruses, fungi, protozoans and cancer). Patients with T Cell immunodeficiencies are prone to infections and to certain types of cancers, especially leukemias and lymphomas.

There is evidence that T cells themselves produce H_2O_2 upon stimulation of their antigen receptor. [154, 155] A potential source for the unique production of H_2O_2 is the T cell receptor itself. This proposal comes from studies with isolated antibodies, which have the ability to catalyze a light-dependent reaction between molecular oxygen and water that leads to the production of H_2O_2. [156, 157]

These events occur in all antibodies, regardless of source or antigenic specificity. The reaction is initiated by singlet oxygen that reacts with H_2O to ultimately produce H_2O_2 via intermediates such as H_2O_3 and ozone. [158]

H_2O_2 Safety

The Food & Drug Administration (FDA) in Federal Regulation Vol. 46, Number 6, Jan 9, 1981, in effect gave the food industry a green light to use hydrogen peroxide in the "Aseptic" packaging process. The FDA has further ruled that hydrogen peroxide can be used in the processing of cheese and related cheese products (part 133), eggs and egg products (part 160), and as an anti-microbial agent in whey processing. They have also ruled it to be used in cleaning and healing mouth injuries and as a mouthwash (1% to 3% food grade H_2O_2).

As previously stated, "The International Agency for Research on Cancer (IARC) has determined that hydrogen peroxide is not classifiable as to its carcinogencity to humans. Even though accusations against H_2O_2 have been wide spread, there is no verified data, in man, that H_2O_2 in any way causes or promotes cancer in vivo." The WHO-IARC said, "There is inadequate evidence in humans for the carcinogenicity of hydrogen peroxide."

Information from the Hazardous Substances Data Bank (HSDB), a database of the National Library of Medicine's TOXNET system (http://toxnet.nlm.nih.gov) indicates in general, ingestion, ocular or dermal exposure to small amounts of dilute hydrogen peroxide will cause no serious problems.

In 5 persons who accidentally drank 50 mL of a 33% H_2O_2 solution (not the readily available 3%), symptoms included stomach and chest pain, retention of breath, foaming at the mouth and loss of consciousness. Later, motor and sensory disorders, fever, micro-hemorrhages and moderate leukocytosis were noted. Still, *all recovered completely within 2-3 weeks.* [159] Yet, it may rarely be the cause of accidental death. [160]

A review by Howes found a total of 13 deaths due to the accidental or intentional use of H_2O_2 in the entire history of recorded medical literature available on the internet. [16]

Compare the record of safety with hydrogen peroxide with that of pharmaceutical drugs, which kill 12 per hour, every hour of the day, for 365 days a year (106,000/year). A 2000 report published in the Journal of the American Medical Association by Barbara Starfield, M.D., MPH reported that drugs kill over 106,000 annually, as a conservative estimate. [161]

Pravda has discussed the possible role of hydrogen peroxide in the induction of ulcerative colitis secondary to non-physiological concentrations of peroxide used in peroxide enemas. [162]

Caveat: Some references do not provide access to the original article or to an abstract. Most of the references available to Howes on the internet do not go beyond 1979. Thus, there may be cases of which I am unaware. Many of the articles concerning ingestion or infusion of peroxide are non-conclusive. Clinical histories are incomplete and documentation is scanty. One thing for certain is that many cases of over-zealous or accidental ingestion of concentrated hydrogen peroxide (20-40%) have had a surprisingly uneventful recovery. Actually, the ingestion or infusion of 3% H_2O_2 has resulted in very few patients who developed serious complications or severe outcomes.

A retrospective review of all exposures reported to a regional poison center over a 36 month period and found that of 95,052 exposures reported, 325 (.34%) were due to hydrogen peroxide. The pediatric population (< 18 years) accounted for 71% of hydrogen peroxide exposures and ingestion was the most common route of exposure (83%). Nausea and vomiting were the most common symptoms secondary to ingestion. Ocular and dermal exposures to dilute solutions resulted in transient symptoms without permanent sequelae. While most exposures by all routes resulted in a benign outcome (no effect or minor effect), there was a trend toward more severe outcomes in those who ingested a concentration greater than 10% (p = 0.011). [163] (Division of Emergency Medicine, University of Utah School of Medicine, Utah Poison Control Center, Salt Lake City).

Reports have described levels of H_2O_2 over 50 μM as being cytotoxic for a wide range of plants and animal cells in vitro, but is dependent upon many factors such as, pH, media used, cell type used, length of exposure, etc. Paradoxically, acatalasemia in humans appears to produce no significant phenotype, nor does "knockout" of glutathione peroxidase in mice except under conditions of "abnormally high oxidative stress." This is contrary to the teachings of the free radical theory and consistent with Howes' Unified Theory. [164]

Discussion

It is important to reemphasize the fact that antioxidants have repeatedly failed to prevent, control or reverse cancer and a host of so-called oxidative stress diseases. Thus, the free radical theory lacks predictability and consequently, according to the scientific method, it is unfounded. It is inexcusable that researchers continue to incriminate EMODs as only deleterious, noxious or mutagenic agents. In vitro studies may have little resemblance to the events occurring in living/breathing cells, which have considerable EMOD levels omnipresent.

Previously, investigators suggested that anything which served as an antioxidant was good and anything which oxidized something else was bad. That has repeatedly been proven to be untrue. All antioxidants can serve as prooxidants of greater or lesser reactivity. Further, H_2O_2 is now well recognized as an important and widespread second messenger for all aerobic cells. Based on scientific investigations, implying or giving the false impression that the presence of H_2O_2 is categorically bad is another example of unfounded and erroneous reporting.

Rethinking the Free Radical Theory

Any critical evaluation of EMODs must address the misconceptions propagated by the free radical theory of oxidative stress and aging. Hard data has yielded the following: [15]

- high levels of the antioxidant bilirubin cause kernicterus and permanent brain damage
- the antioxidant β-carotene increases the rate of lung cancer development in smokers
- the antioxidant CoQ, ubiquinone, when deleted from the diet of C. elegans, increases its lifespan
- SOD/catalase mimetics decrease the lifespan of house flies
- the antioxidant α-tocopherol, vitamin E, increases the rate and number of heart attacks and strokes
- high levels of the antioxidant, uric acid, cause gout and cardiovascular disease
-acatalasemic patients live basically normal lives

Many molecules are designed to accept and receive electrons as a natural part of their reactivity, especially the transitions metals and the heme proteins. Oxygen's various modified derivatives, electronic configurations and states, are the primary agents that protect us from infections and neoplastic growths throughout our lives, from conception to death. Report after report shows that mitochondria play a crucial role in apoptosis. [165]

A growing body of evidence favors the involvement of intracellular reactive oxygen species (EMODs) at some point during apoptotic execution. [166-170] Apoptosis is carried out by a multistage chain of reactions in which EMODs act as triggers and essential mediators. [171, 172] The level of lipid peroxidation in patients with cancer was significantly reduced compare with that in healthy control subjects. [173] The lower level of lipid peroxidation in the cancer patients may be indicative of low EMOD levels, which would allow for the development of cancer.

Even death signaling by anticancer drugs generally relies on positive input from the mitochondria, as is evidenced by the resistance of tumor cells over-expressing the death-inhibitory protein Bcl-2 that is localized to the membranes of mitochondria, endoplasmic reticulum, and nucleus. [174-176] Repeatedly, the critical role of cellular redox status in the regulation of death signaling has been demonstrated. [177-180]

These findings become more important considering the critical role of the mitochondria during apoptosis and the fact that mitochondria have been implicated directly as a prime source of EMODs during drug-induced apoptosis. [181-183] As the mitochondria are a major source of intracellular EMODs, it is tempting to speculate that EMODs, such as H_2O_2, may function both upstream and downstream of the mitochondria. Tumor cells lacking Bax (Bax–/–) are resistant to the effect of some anti-cancer drugs. [184]

Analysis of subcellular distribution of Bax (in HCT116, HL60, and CEM cells) revealed that Bax redistributed to the mitochondrial fraction from the cytosol on exposure to H_2O_2, which could be significantly blocked by the H_2O_2 scavenger, catalase.

Recruitment of Bax to the mitochondria during apoptotic signaling has been linked to the activation of upstream caspase 8 and caspase 8-mediated cleavage of the proapoptotic protein Bid. This is particularly true on ligation of death receptors, such as CD95 (Apo1/Fas). Additionally, H_2O_2 and anticancer drugs have been shown to up-regulate the expression of the CD95 receptor or its ligand (CD95L) in some systems. [185, 186]

376

Investigators utilized the ability of certain anticancer drugs to increase intracellular production of EMODs, specifically H_2O_2.[187] Indeed, exposure of HCT116 Bax+/– or HL60 cells to a novel anticancer compound C1 resulted in an increase in intracellular H_2O_2 and translocation of Bax to the mitochondria. This translocation of Bax was inhibited by catalase, thus establishing the critical role of intracellular H_2O_2 in mitochondrial recruitment during drug-induced apoptosis of tumor cells. These data indicate that Bax translocation triggered in tumor cells during drug (C1)-induced apoptosis was a direct result of intracellular H_2O_2 production, independent of the upstream caspase 8 or ceramide pathways. [187]

Cytosolic Acidification

Cytosolic acidification is an early event in apoptosis and provides an intracellular milieu permissive for efficient death execution. In this regard, exposure of cells to H_2O_2 or drugs that trigger intracellular increase in H_2O_2 results in a significant drop in cytosolic pH. [187]

Accordingly, signals that inhibit apoptotic acidification impede death signaling as demonstrated in a recent study. [188] Investigators results provided strong evidence that the link between H_2O_2 and Bax translocation could be the drop in cytosolic pH brought about by exposure of cells to exogenous H_2O_2 or endogenous production of H_2O_2 on drug exposure. It is possible that this indicates the pivotal role of H_2O_2 in cancer cell killing or apoptotic execution.

This shows that apoptosis is likely initiated with EMOD production, especially H_2O_2. H_2O_2 is, for the most part, essential for cancer killing and a shift to an acidic intracellular environment may also aid in its tumoricidal activity and the production of other agents within the EMOD family. Studies demonstrated the ability of commonly used chemotherapeutic drugs vincristine and daunorubicin to trigger an early increase in intracellular H_2O_2. [188]

Pro-oxidant intracellular milieu is a hallmark of many tumor cells and is believed to endow tumor cells with a survival advantage over their normal counterparts. [189, 190] It has been shown previously that maintaining a slightly elevated intracellular O_2^- promotes cellular proliferation [135] and inhibits apoptotic signaling. [191] Fortunately, this is one specific feature which provides us with an opportunity to selectively kill cancer cells by increasing EMOD levels even further.

Many investigators have demonstrated the critical role of intracellular H_2O_2 in rendering the cytosolic milieu permissive for efficient apoptotic execution. [169, 170, 192] Further, these data strongly support and underscore the critical role of H_2O_2 in creating a permissive intracellular milieu for efficient drug-induced execution of tumor cells. [193]

Dicumarol Increased EMODs Killing Human Pancreatic Cancer Cells

Dicumarol is a naturally occurring anticoagulant derived from coumarin that induces cytotoxicity and oxidative stress in human pancreatic cancer cells. Dicumarol increased intracellular levels of superoxide (O_2^{-}), as measured by hydroethidine staining, and inhibited cell growth. [194] Mitochondrial production of EMODs mediates the increased susceptibility of cancer cells to dicumarol-induced cytotoxicity. [195]

MnSOD Overexpression and Inhibition of H_2O_2 Removal Increases Cancer Cell Cytotoxicity

Overexpression of manganese superoxide dismutase (MnSOD) and inhibition of H_2O_2 removal, increases cancer cell cytotoxicity. Investigators hypothesized that increasing endogenous O_2^- production in cells that were pretreated with adenoviral MnSOD (AdMnSOD) plus 1,3-bis(2-chloroethyl)-1-nitrosourea (BCNU) would lead to an increased level of intracellular H_2O_2 accumulation and increased cell killing. The cytotoxic effects of Adriamycin or radiation, agents known to produce O_2^-, were determined in MDA-MB-231 breast cancer cells pretreated with AdMnSOD plus BCNU both in vitro and in vivo. In vitro, AdMnSOD plus BCNU sensitized cells to the cytotoxicity of Adriamycin or radiation. In vivo, AdMnSOD, BCNU, and Adriamycin or ionizing radiation inhibited tumor growth and prolonged survival. Thus, agents that produce O_2^- in combination with AdMnSOD plus BCNU may represent a powerful new antitumor regimen against breast cancer.[196]

Myeloperoxidase Involvement in H_2O_2-induced Apoptosis of HL-60 Human Leukemia Cells

Investigators examined the mechanism of H_2O_2-induced cytotoxicity and its relationship to oxidation in human leukemia cells. The HL-60 promyelocytic leukemia cell line was sensitive to H_2O_2, and at concentrations up to about 20-25 uM, the killing was mediated by apoptosis. When HL-60 cells were incubated with methimazole or 4-aminobenzoic acid hydrazide, which are inhibitors of myeloperoxidase, they no longer underwent H_2O_2-induced apoptosis.[197] This strongly supports the primary role of EMOD induced apoptosis in cancer cell cytotoxicity.

Antitumor Therapy via Enzymatic Generation of Hydrogen Peroxide

Investigators studied the antitumor activity of an H_2O_2-generating enzyme, D-amino acid oxidase (DAO), and its conjugate with polyethylene glycol (PEG; PEG-DAO). To generate cytotoxic H_2O_2 at the tumor site, PEG-DAO was first administered i.v. to tumor-bearing mice. After an adequate lag time, the substrate of DAO, D-proline, was injected i.p. This treatment resulted in significant suppression of tumor growth.

PEG-DAO thus delivered together with D-proline produces remarkable antitumor activity via extensive generation of H_2O_2.[198]

Prof Randolph Michael Howes MD,PhD

SOD Over Expression Increases Peroxide Levels and Suppresses Human Prostate Cancer Cells

Investigators studied the role of the antioxidant enzyme manganese superoxide dismutase (MnSOD) in androgen-independent human prostate cancer (PC-3) cells' growth rate in vitro and in vivo. Production of extracellular H_2O_2 was increased in the MnSOD-overexpressing clones. Results are consistent with MnSOD being a tumor suppressor gene in human prostate cancer. [199]

This supports the assertion that prooxidant EMODs, such as H_2O_2, contribute to a continually functional oxidative protective system to curtail cancer growth. The increased SOD resulted in increased peroxide levels, which in turn suppressed tumor growth, via EMOD induced apoptosis.

Increased EMODs Increases Cancer Cell Cytotoxicity

Relative to normal cells, neoplastic cells demonstrate increased sensitivity to glucose-deprivation-induced cytotoxicity. To determine whether oxidative stress mediated by O_2^- and hydroperoxides contributed to the differential susceptibility of human epithelial cancer cells to glucose deprivation, the oxidation of DHE (dihydroethidine; for O_2^-) and CDCFH(2) [5- (and 6-)carboxy-2',7'-dichlorodihydrofluorescein diacetate; for hydroperoxides] was measured in human colon and breast cancer cells (HT29, HCT116, SW480 and MB231) and compared with that in normal human cells [FHC cells, 33Co cells and HMECs (human mammary epithelial cells)]. HCT116 and MB231 cells were more susceptible to glucose-deprivation-induced cytotoxicity and oxidative stress, relative to 33Co cells and HMECs. HT29 cells were also more susceptible to 2DG (2-deoxyglucose)-induced cytotoxicity, relative to FHC cells. Overexpression of manganese SOD (superoxide dismutase) and mitochondrially targeted catalase significantly protected HCT116 and MB231 cells from glucose-deprivation-induced cytotoxicity and oxidative stress and also protected HT29 cells from 2DG-induced

380

cytotoxicity. These results show that cancer cells (relative to normal cells) demonstrate increased steady-state levels of EMODs (reactive oxygen species; i.e. O_2^- and H_2O_2) that contribute to differential susceptibility to glucose-deprivation-induced cytotoxicity and oxidative stress. These studies support the hypotheses that cancer cells increase glucose metabolism to compensate for excess metabolic production of EMODs and that inhibition of glucose and hydroperoxide metabolism may provide a biochemical target for selectively enhancing cytotoxicity and oxidative stress in human cancer cells. [200]

EMODs are Positive Signals in the Fruit Fly Immune System

The September 24, 2009 issue of the journal Nature, carried an article by Dr. Utpal Banerjee et al, UCLA's Jonsson Comprehensive Cancer Center researchers found much to their surprise, that in Drosophila, the common fruit fly, moderately elevated levels of EMODs are a good thing. Banerjee said, "These small molecules act as an internal communicator, signaling certain blood precursor cells, or blood stem cells, to differentiate into immune-bolstering cells in reaction to a threat. After the progenitor cells differentiate, the EMOD levels return to normal, ensuring the safety and survival of the mature blood cells."

Thus, he asks, "could excessive use of antioxidants deplete our immune systems?" Alleged;y, reducing levels of reactive oxygen is usually the goal, and what Banerjee found was surprising, in that when EMODs were taken away from the blood stem cells, they failed to differentiate into the immune-bolstering cells, called macrophages. On the other hand, when levels of EMODs were further increased by genetic means, the blood stem cells "differentiated like gang busters," Banerjee said, making a large number of macrophages.

The EMODs, Banerjee said, acted as a signaling mechanism that kept the blood stem cells in a certain state - when levels rose, it was a message to the cell to differentiate. Keeping their EMOD levels slightly elevated puts the cells on alert, sensitized and ready to respond to any threat quickly.

That work prompted the obvious question: If fruit fly blood stem cells and mammalian blood stem cells operate in the same way, is it a good thing for people to be taking antioxidants? Are antioxidants dulling the immune system and its ability to react to threats? It is interesting, however, that these types of blood progenitors in mammals also give rise to macrophages, Banerjee said.

Banerjee said, "If we find that those blood stem cells aren't primed to respond because the ROS levels are reduced, that would not be a good thing. Our findings raise the possibility that wanton overdose of antioxidant products may in fact inhibit formation of cells participating in innate immune response." Once again, this data emphasizes the crucial role of EMODs in aerobic cells. http://www.medicalnewstoday.com/articles/165268.php Accessed 9-25-09.

Just to Add Further Complications

Pro-senescent Effect of Hydrogen Peroxide on Cancer Cells and Tumor Suppression

Mild oxidative stress is known to induce premature senescence, termed stress-induced premature senescence (SIPS), in normal human diploid cells. Investigators determined whether mild oxidative stress would trigger SIPS in a human tumor cell line, human lung adenocarcinoma A549. The results showed that sublethal concentrations of H_2O_2 induced SIPS in A549 cells and consequently attenuated, but did not completely eliminate, the tumorigenicity of these cells. They next investigated the reasons for this incomplete impairment of tumorigenicity in A549 cells in SIPS. The results suggested that H_2O_2 treated A549 cells are composed of a heterogeneous cell population: one is sensitive to H_2O_2 and the other is resistant or undergoes reversal; the latter reverted to their original tumorigenic form. The molecular mechanisms determining the cellular fate of tumor cells in SIPS should be identified in order to make use of SIPS and oncogene-induced senescence in tumor cells as methods of tumor suppression. [201]

Indirect Evidence for EMOD Induced Apoptosis Via Antioxidant Studies

The US is experiencing epidemics of cancer, diabetes, obesity and fatigue, which may be related to increased ingestion of antioxidant vitamins and dietary supplements, which are now commonly found as supplements or fortifiers of many foods and are aggressively marketed to an ever-growing segment of the population. These agents could be interfering with or modifying our continually operational prooxidant protective system.

Despite two decades of controversy regarding the use of dietary antioxidant supplementation during conventional chemotherapy and radiation therapy, questions remain about their efficacy and safety. However, on the basis of published randomized clinical trials, the use of supplemental antioxidants during chemotherapy and radiation therapy should be discouraged because of the possibility of tumor protection and reduced patient survival. [202]

Several new reports are raising concerns about the safety and efficacy of vitamin and mineral supplements in healthy individuals and cancer patients and survivors. Some experts see a need for further studies; whereas, others say that there are sufficient negative data to stop vitamin trials altogether. [203]

Significant in vitro data exists showing that antioxidants can block EMOD-induced apoptosis for a wide variety of cancerous cell types, such as leukemia, lymphoma, retinoblastoma, myeloma, pheochromocytoma and human cancers of the breast, lung, pancreas, liver, colon, rectum and endometrium. [204] This data can not be ignored.

However, it has recently been shown that EMODs may have an alternative activity, by modulating tumor cell signaling and that tumor cell signaling mediated by EMODs are readily reversible upon treatment with antioxidants. This emerging evidence may serve as bona fide signal transduction modifiers for cancer. A re-examination is warranted. [205]

However, in the words of one investigator, "If you suppress free radicals, you suppress programmed cell death." [206]

One Final Note

Philipp Niethammer, Harvard Medical School postdoctoral researcher and biologist, accidentally discovered while analyzing the severed tail of zebrafish that the hydrogen peroxide in their wounds appeared in bursts at the wound about 17 minutes before the leukocytes that were supposed to be producing them appeared too. On 6-4-09, ScienceNow reported that hydrogen peroxide summons reinforcements from the immune system, and more specifically white blood cells, which in turn aid with the healing process. Please view the video of peroxide migration in the wound of a zebrafish http://www.youtube.com/watch?v=a7PJ8yXyPVU. "Hydrogen peroxide marshals immune system." Accessed 10-9-09. This interesting video illustrates the rapid wound response and permeability of H_2O_2.

However, due to the complex nature of the interactions of EMODs and antioxidants within the body, it is difficult to clearly and definitively interpret the results of many experiments and observations.

CONCLUSION

Unarguably, EMODs are intricately, inextricably and crucially involved in cancer cell killing via their prominent role in apoptosis. Statements of the ineffectiveness in the killing of cancerous cells via hydrogen peroxide or other EMOD types are baseless, inaccurate and irresponsible. The lingering inaccuracies of the free radical theory must be countered by the obvious omnipresent and ubiquitous known salutary effects of the prooxidant EMODs. Their presence in steady state quantities testifies to their essential nature in healthy homeostasis and their low toxicity. EMODs, and especially hydrogen peroxide, are produced throughout the body in steady state levels on an as needed and when needed basis and serve to support the interrelated highly complex redox systems of the body. It is inconceivable that they only exist for pernicious purposes. Because of their relatively short half lives, their localized instantaneous concentrations can remain at low levels. Yet, their synthesis and availability can be called upon at any given moment to combat impending pathogens or neoplasia.

EMODs have bactericidal, fungicidal, virucidal and anti-protozoan and anti-neoplastic roles but also have far reaching cellular signaling control functions. The peroxide spike during the respiratory burst classically serves as a protective role against infectious pathogens, as does EMOD induced apoptosis to combat neoplasia. Hydrogen peroxide is likely the most ubiquitous member of the family of EMOD agents. Its important and prominent biochemical role is ever expanding.

REFERENCES

1. Miller ER III, Pastor-Barriuso R, Dalal D, Riemersma RA, Appel LJ, Guallar E. Meta-analysis: high-dosage vitamin E supplementation may increase all-cause mortality. *Ann Intern Med.* 2005;142:37-46.

2. Howes M.D., PhD., R. (2007). Antioxidant Vitamins A, C & E; Death in Small Doses and Legal Liability? *PHILICA.COM Article number 89.* Published April 5, 2007.

3. Harman D. Aging: a theory based on free radical and radiation chemistry. J Gerontol 11: 298–300, 1956.

4. Harman, D., 1981. The aging process. Proc. Natl Acad. Sci. USA 78, 7124–7128.

5. Beckman, K.B., Ames, B.N., 1998. The free radical theory of aging matures. Physiol. Rev. 78, 547–581.

6. Finkel, T., Holbrook, N.J., 2000. Oxidants, oxidative stress and the biology of ageing. Nature 408, 239–247.

7. Balaban, R.S., Nemoto, S., Finkel, T., 2005. Mitochondria, oxidants, and aging. Cell 120, 483–495.

8. Marnett LJ, Riggins JN, West JD. Endogenous generation of reactive oxidants and electrophiles and their reactions with DNA and protein. J Clin Invest. 2003; 111: 583–593.

9. Darley-Usmar, V., Starke-Reed, P.E., 2000. Antioxidants: strategies for interventions in aging and age-related diseases, a workshop sponsored by the National Institute on aging and by the office of dietary supplements. Antioxid. Redox. Signal. 2, 375–377.

10. Howes R.M. The Free Radical Fantasy: A Panoply of Paradoxes. Ann. N.Y. Acad. Sci. 2006;1067:22-26.

11. Chance B, Sies, H, Boveris A. Hydroperoxide metabolism in mammalian organs. Physiol Rev 1979; 59: 527-605.

12. Hydrogen Peroxide: A Signaling Messenger. James R. Stone, Suping Yang. Antioxidants & Redox Signaling. March/April 2006, 8(3-4): 243-270.

13. Howes, R. M. *U.T.O.P.I.A. - Unified Theory of Oxygen Participation in Aerobiosis.* © 2004. Free Radical Publishing Co. Kentwood, LA, available at www.iwillfindthecure.org.

14. Halliwell B. Oxidants and human disease: some concepts. FASEB J. 1987;1:358–364.

15. Howes, R.M. © 2005. The Medical and Scientific Significance of Oxygen Free Radical Metabolism. Free Radical Publishing Co. Kentwood, LA. available at www.iwillfindthecure.org.

16. Howes, R.M. Hydrogen Peroxide Monograph 1: Scientific, Medical and Biochemical Overview & Monograph 2: Antioxidant Vitamins A, C, & E: Equivocal Scientific Studies, © 2006. Free Radical Publishing Co. Kentwood, LA. available at www.iwillfindthecure. org.

17. Marie Csete. Oxygen in the Cultivation of Stem Cells. Ann. N.Y. Acad. Sci. 1049: 1–8 (2005.

18. Go YM, Gipp JJ, Mulcahy RT, and Jones DP. H_2O_2-dependent activation of GCLC-ARE4 reporter occurs by mitogen-activated protein kinase pathways without oxidation of cellular glutathione or thioredoxin-1. J Biol Chem 279: 5837–5845, 2004.

19. Aitken J, Fisher H. Reactive oxygen species generation and human spermatozoa: the balance of benefit and risk. Bioessays. 1994 Apr;16(4):259-67.

20. Acker H, Bolling B, Delpiano MA, Dufau E, Gorlach A & Holtermann G (1992). The meaning of H_2O_2 generation in carotid body cells for pO_2 chemoreception. Journal of the Autonomic Nervous System, 41: 41-51.

21. Lisa Melton. The antioxidant myth: a medical fairy tale – from New Scientist. http://www.newscientist.com/article/mg19125631.500.html (5 August 2006) New Scientist. Pg. 40-43. volume 191; issue 2563.

22. B.M. Barbior. Superoxide: a two-edged sword. Braz J Med Biol Res, February 1997, Volume 30(2) 141-155.

23. Thannical VJ, Fanburg BL. Reactive oxygen species in cell signaling. Am J Physiol Lung Cell Mol Physiol 2000; 279: L1005-L1028.

24. Eaton JW, Qian M. Molecular basis of cellular iron toxicity. Free Radic Biol Med 2002; 32: 833-840.

25. Harman, D. 1957. Prolongation of the normal life span by radiation protection chemicals. J. Gerontol. 12: 257-263.

26. Boveris A, Cadenas E. Mitochondrial production of hydrogen peroxide regulation by nitric oxide and the role of ubisemiquinone. IUBMB Life 2000; 50: 245-250.

27. Eberhardt MK. Reactive Oxygen Metabolites: Chemistry and Medical Consequences. CRC Press 2001.

28. Chen S, Schopfer P. Hydroxyl radical production in physiological reactions. Eur J Biochem 1999; 260: 726-735.

29. Fridovich I. Oxygen toxicity: A radical explanation. J Exp Biol 1998; 20: 1203-1209.

30. Cadenas E, Davies KJ. Mitochondrial free radical generation, oxidative stress, and aging. Free Radic Biol Med 2000; 29:222-230.

31. Lemasters J, Nieminen A. Mitochondria in Pathogenesis. Kluwer Academic/Plenum Publishers 2001: 281-286) 90.

32. St-Pierre, J., Buckingham, J.A., Roebuck, S.J. and Brand, M.D. Topology of superoxide production from different sites in the mitochondrial electron transport chain. J Biol Chem 2002; 277:44784-44790.

33. Rhee SG, Bae YS, Lee SR, Kwon J: Hydrogen peroxide: A key messenger that modulates protein phosphorylation through cysteine oxidation. Science's stke. Available at: www.stke. sciencemag.org/cgi/content/full/OC_sigtrans; 2000/53/pe1.

34. Rhee SG: Redox signaling: Hydrogen peroxide as intracellular messenger. Exp Mol Med 31: 53–59, 1999.

35. Finkel T: Oxygen radicals and signaling. Curr Opin Cell Biol 10: 248–253, 1998.

36. Suzuki YJ, Ford GD: Redox regulation of signal transduction in cardiac and smooth muscle. J Mol Cell Cardiol 31: 345–353, 1999.

37. Radia Forteza et al. Regulated Hydrogen Peroxide Production by Duox in Human Airway Epithelial Cells. American Journal of Respiratory Cell and Molecular Biology. Vol. 32, pp. 462-469, 2005.

38. Ramachandran S, Morris SM, Devamanoharan P, Henein M, Varma SD. Radio-isotopic determination of hydrogen peroxide in aqueous humor and urine. Exp Eye Res. 1991 Oct;53(4):503-6.

39. García-Castiñeiras S. Hydrogen peroxide in the aqueous humor: 1992-1997. P R Health Sci J. 1998 Dec;17(4):335-43.

40. Niki L. Reynaert et al. Catalase Overexpression Fails to Attenuate Allergic Airways Disease in the Mouse. The Journal of Immunology, 2007, 178: 3814-3821.

41. Li JM and Shah AM. (2002) Intracellular localization and preassembly of the NADPH oxidase complex in cultured endothelial cells. J Biol Chem 277:19952–19960.

42. Grandvaux N, Grizot S, Vignais PV, Dagher MC. (1999) The Ku70 autoantigen interacts with p40phox in B lymphocytes. J Cell Sci 112:Pt 4503–513.

43. IARC, 1985). (IARC. 1985. International Agency for Research on Cancer. Hydrogen Peroxide. In: IARC Monographs on the Evaluation of Carcinogenic Risk if Chemicals to Humans: Allyl compounds, Aldehydes, Epoxides and Peroxides, Vol. 36. IARC, Lyon, pp. 285-314.

44. Krippeit-Drews, P., Lang, F., Haussinger, D. and Drews, G. Pflugers. H_2O_2 induced hyperpolarization of pancreatic β-cells. Pflügers Arch. 426: 552-554, 1994.

45. Krippeit-Drews, P., Kramer, C., Welker, S., Lang, F., Ammon, H.P. and Drews, G. Interference of H_2O_2 with stimulus-secretion coupling in mouse pancreatic β-cells. J Physiol (Lond) 1999; 514(Pt 2): 471-481.

46. Livingston J, Gurny P, Lockwood D: Insulin-like effects of polyamines in fat cells. Mediation by H_2O_2 formation. J Biol Chem 1977, 252:560-562.

47. Lenzen S, Drinkgern J, Tiedge M. Low antioxidant enzyme gene expression in pancreatic islets compared with various other mouse tissues. Free Radical Biology & Medicine. 1996;20:463–466.

48. Anna Yu Bogdanova and Mikko Nikinmaa. Reactive Oxygen Species Regulate Oxygen-sensitive Potassium Flux in Rainbow Trout Erythrocytes. The Journal of General Physiology, Volume 117, Number 2, February 1, 2001 181-190.

49. Halliwell B. Reactive oxygen species and the nervous system. 1992. J. Neurochemistry 59, 1609-1623.

50. C Giulivi, P Hochstein, KJ Davies. Hydrogen peroxide production by red blood cells. Free Radic Biol Med (1994) 16: 123-9.

51. Valko M, Leibfritz D, Moncol J, Cronin MT, Mazur M, Telser J. Free radicals and antioxidants in normal physiological functions and human disease. Int J Biochem Cell Biol. 2007;39(1):44-84.

52. Akos Koller and Zsolt Bagi. Nitric oxide and H_2O_2 contribute to reactive dilation of isolated coronary arterioles. Am J Physiol Heart Circ Physiol 287: H_2461-H_2467, 2004.

53. Balachandran P and Govindarajan R. Cancer—an ayurvedic perspective Pharmacol Res 2005; 51: 19–30.

54. Papa S and Shulachev VP. Reactive oxygen species, mitochondria, apoptosis and aging. Mol Cell Biochem 1997; 174: 305–19.

55. Matsuzawa A, Ichijo H. Stress-responsive protein kinases in redox-regulated apoptosis signaling. Antioxid Redox Signal. 2005;7:472–481.

56. Han H, Wang H, Long H, Nattel S, Wang Z. Oxidative preconditioning and apoptosis in L-cells. Roles of protein kinase B and mitogen-activated protein kinases. J Biol Chem. 2001;276:26357–26364.

57. Reinehr R, Becker S, Eberle A, Grether-Beck S, Haussinger D. Involvement of NADPH oxidase isoforms and Src family kinases in CD95-dependent hepatocyte apoptosis. J Biol Chem. 2005; 280(29):27179-27194.

58. Senturker, S., Tschirret-Guth, R., Morrow, J., Levine, R. and Shacter, E. Induction of apoptosis by chemotherapeutic drugs without generation of reactive oxygen species. Arch of Biochem and Biophy 2002; 397(2): 262-272.

59. J H. Doroshow. Role of Hydrogen Peroxide and Hydroxyl Radical Formation in the Killing of Ehrlich Tumor Cells by Anticancer Quinones. PNAS June 15, 1986, vol. 83, no. 12, 4514-4518.

60. Dougherty TJ, Gomer CJ, Henderson BW, Jori G, Kessel D, Korbelik M, Moan J, Peng Q (1998) Photodynamic therapy. J Natl Cancer Inst 90: 889–905.

61. Ochsner M (1997) Photophysical and photobiological processes in the photodynamic therapy of tumours. J Photochem Photobiol B 39: 1–18.

62. Fisher A. M. R., Murphree A. L., Gomer C. J. Clinical, and preclinical photodynamic therapy. Lasers Surg. Med., 17: 2-31, 1995.

63. Henderson B. W., Dougherty T. J. How does photodynamic therapy work? Photochem. Photobiol., 55: 145-157, 1992.

64. Oleinick N. L., Evans H. E. The photobiology of photodynamic therapy: cellular targets and mechanisms. Radiat. Res., 150: S146-S156, 1998.

65. Luna M. C., Wong S., Gomer C. J. Photodynamic therapy mediated induction of early response genes. Cancer Res., 53: 1374-1380, 1994.

66. Gollnick S. O., Liu X., Owczarczak B., Musser D., Henderson B. W. Altered expression of interleukin 6 and interleukin 10 as a result of photodynamic therapy in vivo. Cancer Res., 57: 3904-3909, 1997.

67. Tao J-S., Sanghera J. S., Pelech S. L., Wong G., Levy J. G. Stimulation of stress-activated protein kinase and p38 HOG1 kinase in murine keratinocytes following photodynamic therapy with benzoporphyrin derivative. J. Biol. Chem., 271: 27107-27115, 1996.

68. Gomer C. J., Luna M., Ferrario A., Rucker N. Increased transcription and translation of heme oxygenase in Chinese hamster fibroblasts following photodynamic stress or Photofrin II incubation. Photochem. Photobiol., 53: 275-279, 1991.

69. Gomer C. J., Ferrario A., Rucker N., Wong S., Lee A. Glucose regulated protein induction and cellular resistance to oxidative stress mediated by porphyrin photosensitization. Cancer Res., 51: 6574-6579, 1991.

70. Gomer C., Ryter S., Ferrario A., Rucker N., Wong S., Fisher A. Photodynamic therapy mediated oxidative stress can induce heat shock proteins. Cancer Res., 56: 2355-2360, 1996.

71. Curry P. M., Levy J. Stress protein expression in murine tumor cells following photodynamic therapy with benzoporphyrin derivative. Photochem. Photobiol., 58: 374-379, 1993.

72. Price M, Terlecky SR, Kessel D. A Role for Hydrogen Peroxide in the Pro-apoptotic Effects of Photodynamic Therapy. Photochem Photobiol. 2009 Jul 21.

73. Chekulayeva LV, Shevchuk IN, Chekulayev VA, Ilmarinen K. Hydrogen peroxide, superoxide, and hydroxyl radicals are involved in the phototoxic action of hematoporphyrin derivative against tumor cells. J Environ Pathol Toxicol Oncol. 2006;25(1-2):51-77.

74. Redmond RW, Gamlin JN. A compilation of singlet oxygen yields from biologically relevant molecules. Photochem. Photobiol. 1999;70:391–475.

75. Dysart JS, Patterson MS. Characterization of Photofrin photobleaching for singlet oxygen dose estimation during photodynamic therapy of MLL cells in vitro. *Phys. Med. Biol.* 2005;50:2597–2616.

76. Buettner GR, Need MJ. Hydrogen peroxide and hydroxyl free radical production by hematoporphyrin derivative, ascorbate and light. Cancer Lett. 1985;25:297–304.

77. Galina G. Kramarenko, Stephen G. Hummel, Sean M. Martin, and Garry R. Buettner. Ascorbate Reacts with Singlet Oxygen to Produce Hydrogen Peroxide. Photochem Photobiol. 2006; 82(6): 1634–1637.

78. Henry Jay Forman. Hydrogen Peroxide: The Good, The Bad, and The Ugly. Contained in: *Oxidants in Biology*. Springer Netherlands. ISBN 978-1-4020-8398-3. 2008.

79. James R. Stone, Suping Yang. Hydrogen Peroxide: A Signaling Messenger. Antioxidants & Redox Signaling. March/April 2006, 8(3-4): 243-270.

80. Babior, B.M. NADPH oxidase: An update. Blood 1999; 93: 1464-1476.

81. Bayraktutan, U., Blayney, L. and Shah, A.M. Molecular characterization and localization of the NADPH oxidase components gp91-phox and p22-phox in endothelia cells. Arterioscler Thromb Vasc Biol 2000; 20: 1903-1911.

82. Goossens, V., Grooten, J., DeVos, K. and Fiers. W. Direct evidence for tumor necrosis factor-induced mitochondrial reactive oxygen intermediates and their involvement in cytotoxicity. Proc Natl Acad Sci USA 1995; 92: 8115-8119.

83. Finkel, T. Redox-dependent signal transduction. FEBS Lett 2000; 476: 52-54.

84. Trembovler, V., Abu-Raya, S. and Shohami, E. Synergism between tumor necrosis factor-alpha and H_2O_2 enhances cell damage in rat PC12 cells. Neurosci Lett. 2003 Dec 19; 353(2):115-118.

85. Hohler, B.; Holzapfel, B., and Kummer W. NADPH oxidase submits and superoxide production in porcine pulmonary artery endothelial cells. Histochem Cell Biol 2000; 114: 29-37.

86. Rueckschloss, U. Galle, J., Zerkowski H. R. and Morawietz, H. Induction of NAD(P)H oxidase by oxidized low-density lipoprotein in human endothelial cells: antioxidative potential of hydroxymethylglutaryl coenzyme A reductase inhibitor therapy. Circulation 2001; 104: 1767-1772.

87. Signal Transduction by reactive Oxygen and Nitrogen Species: Pathways and Chemical Principles. Edited by H.J. Forman, J. Fukuto and M. Torres, Kluwer Academic Publishers, 2003.

88. Schafer, F. Q. and Buettner, G. R. Redox environment of the cell as viewed through the redox state of the glutathione disulfide/glutathione couple. Free Radic Biol Med 2001; 30: 1191-1212.

89. Hoidal, J.R. Reactive oxygen species and cell signaling. Am J Respir Cell Mol Biol 2001; 25: 661-663.

90. Schreck, R., Rieber, P. and Baeuerle, P.A. Reactive oxygen intermediates as apparently widely needed messengers in the activation of the NK-k B transcription factor and HIV-1. Embo J 1991; 10: 2247-2258.

91. Sen, C.K. and Packer, L. Antioxidant and redox regulation of gene transcription. Faseb J 1996; 10: 709-720.

92. Allen, R.G. and Tresini, M. Oxidative stress and gene regulation. Free Rad Biol Med 2000; 28: 463-499.

93. Los, M., W. Droege, K. Stricker, P.A. Baeuerle, K. Schulze-Osthoff. 1995. Hydrogen peroxide as a potent activator of T lymphocyte functions. Eur. J. Immunol. 25:159.

94. Harlan, J. M., K. S. Callahan. 1984. Role of hydrogen peroxide in the neutrophil-mediated release of prostacyclin from cultured endothelial cells. J. Clin. Invest. 74:442.

95. Lewis, M. S., R. E. Whatley, P. Cain, T. M. McIntyre, S. M. Prescott, G. A. Zimmerman. 1988. Hydrogen peroxide stimulates the synthesis of platelet-activating factor by endothelium and induces endothelial cell-dependent neutrophil adhesion. J. Clin. Invest. 82:2045.

96. Sundaresan, M., Z-X. Yu, V. J. Ferrans, K. Irony, T. Finkel. 1995. Requirement for generation of H_2O_2 for platelet-derived growth factor signal transduction. Science 270:296.

97. Rao, G. N., B. C. Berk. 1992. Active oxygen species stimulate vascular smooth muscle cell growth and proto-oncogene expression. Circ. Res. 70:593.

98. Griendling, K.K. and Ushio-Fukai, M. Reactive oxygen species as mediators of angiotensin II signaling. Regul Pept 2000; 91: 21-27.

99. Patel, R.P., Moellering, D., Murphy-Uhrich, J., Jo., H., Beckman, S. and Darley-Usmar, V.M. Cell signaling by reactive nitrogen and oxygen species in atherosclerosis. Free Radic Biol Med 2000; 28: 1780-1794.

100. Forman, H.J. and Torres, M. Signaling by the respiratory burst in macrophages. IUBMB Life 2001; 51: 365-371.

101. Warburg, O. On the origin of cancer cells. Science 1956; 123: 309-314.

102. Einar K. Rofstad, Heidi Rasmussen, Kanthi Galappathi, Berit Mathiesen, Kristin Nilsen and Bjørn A. Graff. Hypoxia Promotes Lymph Node Metastasis in Human Melanoma Xenografts by Up-Regulating the Urokinase-Type Plasminogen Activator Receptor. Cancer Research 62, 1847-1853, March 15, 2002.

103. Hickman, J.A. Apoptosis induced by anticancer drugs. Cancer Metast Rev 1992; 11: 121-139.

104. Reinehr R, Becker S, Eberle A, Grether-Beck S, Haussinger D. Involvement of NADPH oxidase isoforms and Src family kinases in CD95-dependent hepatocyte apoptosis. J Biol Chem. 2005; 280(29):27179-27194.

105. Yokomizo A, Ono M, Nanri H, Makino Y, Ohga T, Wada M, Okamoto T, Yodoi J, Kuwano M, Kohno K. Cellular levels of thioredoxin associated with drug sensitivity to cisplatin, mitomycin C, doxorubicin, and etoposide. Cancer Res 1995;55:4293–4296.

106. Hasinoff B. B., Davey J. P. Adriamycin and its iron(III) and copper(III) complexes, glutathione-induced dissociation, cytochrome c oxidase inactivation and protection: binding to cardiolipin. Biochem. Pharmacol., *37:* 3663-3669, 1988.

107. Burger R. M. Cleavage of nucleic acids by bleomycin. Chem. Rev., *98:* 1153-1169, 1998.

108. Byfield J. E., Lee Y. C., Tu L., Kullhanian F. Molecular interactions of the combined effects of bleomycin and X-rays on mammalian cell survival. Cancer Res., *36:* 1138-1143, 1976.

109. Sangeetha, P., Das, U.N., Koratkar, R. and Suryaprabha, P. Increase in free radical generation and lipid peroxidation following chemotherapy in patients with cancer. Free Radic Biol Med 1990; 8(1): 15-19.

110. Ferlini C, Scambia G, Marone M, Distefano M, Gaggini C, Ferrandina G, Fattorossi A, Isola G, Benedetti Panici P, Mancuso S. Tamoxifen induces oxidative stress and apoptosis in estrogen receptor-negative human cancer cell lines. Br J Cancer 1999;79:257–263.

111. P. Vaupel and L. Harrison. Tumor Hypoxia: Causative Factors, Compensatory Mechanisms, and Cellular Response. Oncologist, November 1, 2004; 9(suppl_5): 4 – 9.

112. Loughlin KR; Manson K; Cragnale D; Wilson L; Ball RA; Bridges KR. The use of hydrogen peroxide to enhance the efficacy of doxorubicin hydrochloride in a murine bladder tumor cell line J Urol. 2001; 165(4):1300-4.

113. Lionel Resnick, Harold Rabinovitz, David Binninger, Maria Marchetti, Herbert Weissbach. Topical sulindac combined with hydrogen peroxide in the treatment of actinic keratoses.

Journal of Drugs in Dermatology. January 1, 2009. Volume: 8 Issue: 1 Page: 29(4).

114. Aronoff, B.L. Regional oxygenation in neoplasms. Cancer 1965; 18: 1250.

115. Mallams, J.T., Balla, G.A. and Finney, J.W. Regional oxygenation and irradiation in the treatment of malignant tumors. Prog in Clin Cancer 1965; 1: 137.

116. Nathan, C. F., and R. K. Root. 1977. Hydrogen peroxide release from mouse peritoneal macrophages. Dependence on sequential activation and triggering.]. *Exp. Med.* 146:1648.

117. Nathan CF, Cohn ZA. Antitumor effects of hydrogen peroxide in vivo. J Exp Med. 1981 Nov 1;154(5):1539–1553.

118. Mallams, J.T., Balla, G.A. and Finney, J.W. Regional oxygenation and irradiation in the treatment of malignant tumors. Prog Clin Cancer 1965; 1: 137.

119. Finney, J.W., Collier, R.E., Balla, G.A., Tomme, J.W., Wakley, J., Race, G.J., Urschel, H.C., D'Errico, A.D. and Mallams, J.T. The preferential localization of radioisotopes in malignant tissue by regional oxygenation. Nature 1961; 202: 1172.

120. Finney, J.W., Balla, G.A., Collier, R.E., Wakely, J., Urschel, H.C. and Mallams, J.T. Differential localization of isotopes in tumors through the use of intra-arterial hydrogen peroxide: Part I: Basic science. Amer J Roentgen 1965; 94: 783.

121. Nathan, C. F., L, H. Brukner, S. C. Silverstein, and Z. A. Cohn. 1979. Extracellular cytolysis by activated macrophages and granulocytes. I. Pharmacologic triggering of effector cells and the release of hydrogen peroxide. J. Exp. Med. 149:84.

122. Philpott, G. W., W. T. Shearer, R. J. Bower, and C. W. Parker. 1973. Selective cytotoxicity of hapten-substituted cells with an antibody-enzyme conjugate. J. Immunol. 111:921.

123. Edelson, P. J., and Z. A. Cohn. 1973. Peroxidase-mediated mammalian cell cytotoxicity. J. Exp. Med. 138:318.

124. Clark, R. A., S. J. Klebanoff, A. B. Einstein, and A. Fefer. 1975. Peroxidase-H$_2$0-halide system: cytotoxic effect on mammalian tumor cells. Blood. 45:161.

125. Nathan, C. F. 1979. The role of oxidative metabolism in the cytotoxicity of activated macrophages after pharmacologic triggering. In Immunobiology and Immunotherapy of Cancer. W. D. Terry and Y. Yamamura, editors. Elsevier North-Holland, Inc., New York. 59.

126. Philpott, G. W., A. Kulczycki, Jr., E. H. Grass, and C. W. Parker. 1980. Selective binding and cytotoxicity of rat basophilic leukemia cells (RBL-1) with immunoglobulin E-biotin and avidin-glucose oxidase conjugates. J. Immunol. 125:1201.

127. Nathan, C. F., B. A. Arrick, H. W. Murray, N. M. DeSantis, and Z. A. Cohn. 1981. Tumor cell antioxidant defenses: inhibition of the glutathione redox cycle enhances macrophage mediated cytolysis. J. Exp. Med. 153:766.

128. Nathan CF, Brukner LH, Silverstein SC, Cohn ZA. Extracellular cytolysis by activated macrophages and granulocytes. I. Pharmacologic triggering of effector cells and the release of hydrogen peroxide. J Exp Med. 1979 Jan 1;149(1):84–99.

129. Nathan CF, Silverstein SC, Brukner LH, Cohn ZA. Extracellular cytolysis by activated macrophages and granulocytes. II. Hydrogen peroxide as a mediator of cytotoxicity. J Exp Med. 1979 Jan 1;149(1):100–113.

130. Keilin, D., and E. F. Hartree. 1948. Properties of glucose oxidase (notatin). Biochem. J. 42:221.

131. Filep, J.G., Lapierre, C., Lachance, S. and Chan, J.S.D. Nitric oxide cooperates with hydrogen peroxide in inducing DNA fragmentation and cell lysis in murine lymphoma cells. Biochem J 1997; 321: 887-901.

132. Kanner, J., Harel, S. and Granit, R. Arch Biochem Biophys 1991; 289: 130-136.

133. Noronha-Dutra, A.A., Epperlein, M.M. and Woolf, N. FEBS Lett 1993; 321: 59-62.

134. Burdon R. H., Gill V., Rice-Evans C. Cell proliferation and oxidative stress. Free Radic. Res. Commun., 7: 149-159, 1989.

135. Burdon R. H. Superoxide and hydrogen peroxide in relation to mammalian cell proliferation. Free Radic. Biol. Med., 18: 775-794, 1995.

136. Takeuchi, T., Matsugo, S. and Morimoto, K. (1997) Mutagenicity of oxidative DNA damage in Chinese hamster V79 cells. Carcinogenesis, 18, 2051–2055.

137. Yin Y, Solomon G, Deng C, Barrett JC. Differential regulation of p21 by p53 and Rb in cellular response to oxidative stress. Mol Carcinog 1999;24:15–24.

138. Huang, et al, Tumor promotion by hydrogen peroxide in rat liver epithelial cells. Carcinogenesis, Vol. 20, No. 3, pp. 485-492, 1999.

139. Dizdaroglu, M. (1993) In DNA and Free Radicals (Halliwell, B., and Aruoma, O.I. eds.), pp. 19-39, Ellis Horwood, Chichester.

140. Halliwell, B. and Aruoma, O.I. DNA damage by oxygen-derived species. (1991) FEBS Lett. 281, 9-19.

141. L.J. Marnett. Oxyradicals and DNA damage. Carcinogenesis 2000 Mar;21(3):361-70.

142. Turrens, J.F. Mitochondrial formation of reactive oxygen species. (2003) Journal of Physiology-LONDON 552(2):335-344.

143. Campian, J.L., Qian, M., Gao, X., and Eaton, J.W. Oxygen tolerance and coupling of mitochondrial electron transport. 279(45): 46580-46587, 2004.

144. Riordan N, Riordan H and Casiari J. Clinical and experimental experiences with intravenous vitamin C. Journal of Orthomolecular Medicine, Special Issue: Proceedings from Vitamin C as Cancer Therapy Workshop, Montreal. 15(4): 201-13. 1999.

145. Riordan N et al. Intravenous ascorbate as a tumour cytotoxic chemotherapeutic agent. Medical Hypothesis. 9(2): 207-13. 1994.

146. Benade L, Howard T and Burke D. Synergistic killings of Ehrlich ascites carcinoma cells by ascorbate and 3 amino-1, 2, 4-triazole. Oncology. 1969;23:33-43.

147. Tsao C, Dungham B and Ping Y. In vivo antineoplastic activity of ascorbic acid for human mammary tumour. In vivo. 2: 147-50. 1988.

148. Bram S et al. Vitamin C preferential toxicity for malignant melanoma cells. Nature. 284: 629-31. 1980.

149. Matsuda, T., Kuroyanagi, M., Sugiyama, S., Umehara, K., Ueno, A. and Nishi, K. Role of hydrogen peroxide for cell death

induction by sodium 5,6-Benzylidene-L-ascorbate. Chem Pharm Bull 1994; 6: 1216-1225.

150. Agus DB, Vera JC and Golde DW. Stromal cell oxidation: a mechanism by which tumors obtain vitamin C. Cancer Research. 1999;59:4555-4558.

151. Chen Q, Espey MG, Krishna MC, Mitchell JB, Corpe CP, Buettner GR, Shacter E, and Levine L. Pharmacologic ascorbic acid concentrations selectively kill cancer cells: Action as a pro-drug to deliver hydrogen peroxide to tissues. PNAS. September 20, 2005. Vol. 102. No. 38. pp. 13604-13609.

152. Maramag C et al. Effect of vitamin C on prostate cancer cells in vitro: effect on cell number, viability, and DNA synthesis. Prostate. 32: 188-95. 1997.

153. Ha YM, Park MK, Kim HJ, Seo HG, Lee JH, Chang KC. High concentrations of ascorbic acid induces apoptosis of human gastric cancer cell by p38-MAP kinase-dependent up-regulation of transferrin receptor. Cancer Lett. 2009 May 8;277(1):48-54.

154. Devadas S, Zaritskaya L, Rhee SG, Oberley L, Williams MS. Discrete generation of superoxide and hydrogen peroxide by T cell receptor stimulation: selective regulation of mitogen-activated protein kinase activation and Fas ligand expression. J Exp Med 195(1):59-70, 2002.

155. Williams MS, Kwon J. T cell receptor stimulation, reactive oxygen species and cell signaling. Free Rad Biol Med 37(8):1144-1151, 2004.

156. Wentworth et al., 2000) (Wentworth AD, Jones LH, Wentworth P Jr, Janda KD, Lerner RA. Antibodies have the intrinsic capacity to destroy antigens. PNAS 97(20):10930-10935, 2000).

157. Wentworth P Jr, Jones LH, Wentworth AD, Zhu X, Larsen NA, Wilson IA, Xu X, Goddard WA III, Janda KD, Eschenmoser A, Lerner RA. Antibody catalysis of the oxidation of water. Science 293 (5536):1806-1811, 2001.

158. Wentworth P Jr, Wentworth AD, Zhu X, Wislon IA, Janda KD, Eschenmoser A, Lerner RA. Evidence for the production of trioxygen species during antibody-catalyzed chemical modification of antigens. PNAS 100(4):1490-1493, 2003.

159. IARC. 1985. International Agency for Research on Cancer. Hydrogen Peroxide. In: IARC Monographs on the Evaluation of Carcinogenic Risk if Chemicals to Humans: Allyl compounds, Aldehydes, Epoxides and Peroxides, Vol. 36. IARC, Lyon, pp. 285-314.

160. Cina SJ, Downs JC, Conradi SE. Hydrogen peroxide: a source of lethal oxygen embolism. Case report and review of the literature. Am J Forensic Med Pathol. 1994 Mar;15(1):44-50.

161. Starfield, B. Is US Health Really the Best in the World? JAMA 2000 Jul 26;284[4]:483-5.

162. Jay Pravda. Radical induction theory of ulcerative colitis. J Gastroenterol April 28, 2005 April;11(16):2371-2384.

163. Dickson KF, Caravati EM. Abstract: Hydrogen peroxide exposure--325 exposures reported to a regional poison control center. J Toxicol Clin Toxicol. 1994;32(6):705-14.

164. Howes, R. M. *U.T.O.P.I.A. - Unified Theory of Oxygen Participation in Aerobiosis.* © 2004. Free Radical Publishing Co. Kentwood, LA Available at www.iwillfindthecure.org.

165. Kroemer, G., Zamzami, N. and Susin, S.A. Mitochondrial control of apoptosis. Immunol Today 1997; 18: 44-51.

166. Fleury C, Mignotte B, Vayssiere JL Mitochondrial reactive oxygen species in cell death signaling. Biochimie 2002;84:131-41.

167. Mansat-de Mas V, Bezombes C, Quillet-Mary A, et al Implication of radical oxygen species in ceramide generation, c-Jun N-terminal kinase activation and apoptosis induced by daunorubicin. Mol Pharmacol 1999;56:867-74.

168. Simizu S, Umezawa K, Takada M, Arber N, Imoto M Induction of hydrogen peroxide production and Bax expression by caspase-3(-like) proteases in tyrosine kinase inhibitor-induced apoptosis in human small cell lung carcinoma cells. Exp Cell Res 1998;238:197-203.

169. Hirpara JL, Clement MV, Pervaiz S Intracellular acidification triggered by mitochondrial-derived hydrogen peroxide is an effector mechanism for drug-induced apoptosis in tumor cells. J Biol Chem 2001;276:514-21.

170. Clement MV, Ponton A, Pervaiz S Apoptosis induced by hydrogen peroxide is mediated by decreased superoxide anion concentration and reduction of intracellular milieu. FEBS Lett 1998;440:13-18.

171. Kerr, J.F.R., Winterfold, C.M. and Harmon, B.V. Apoptosis, its significance in cancer and cancer therapy. Cancer 1994; 73: 2013-2026.

172. Blackstone, N.W. and Green, D.R. The evolution of a mechanism of cell suicide. Bio Essays 1999; 21: 84-88.

173. Khyshiktyev BS, Khyshiktueva NA, Ivanov VN, Darenskaia SD, Novikov SV. Diagnostic value of investigating exhaled air condensate in lung cancer. Vopr Onkol 1994; 40: 161-164.

174. Tsujimoto Y., Shimizu S. VDAC regulation by the Bcl-2 family of proteins. Cell Death Differ., 7: 1174-1181, 2000.

175. Korsmeyer S. J. *BCL-2* gene family and the regulation of programmed cell death. Cancer Res., *59:* 1693-1700S, 1999.

176. Harris M. H., Thompson C. B. The role of the Bcl-2 family in the regulation of outer mitochondrial membrane permeability. Cell Death Differ, 7: 1182-1191, 2000.

177. Clement M.V., Pervaiz S. Reactive oxygen intermediates regulate cellular response to apoptotic stimuli: an hypothesis. Free Radic. Res., *30:* 247-252, 1999.

178. Clement M.V., Pervaiz S. Intracellular superoxide and hydrogen peroxide concentrations: a critical balance that determines survival or death. Redox. Rep., *6:* 211-214, 2001.

179. Pervaiz S., Clement M.V. Hydrogen peroxide-induced apoptosis: oxidative or reductive stress?. Methods Enzymol., *352:* 150-159, 2002.

180. Pervaiz S., Clement M.V. A permissive apoptotic environment: function of a decrease in intracellular superoxide anion and cytosolic acidification. Biochem. Biophys. Res. Commun., *290:* 1145-1150, 2002.

181. Fleury C, Mignotte B, Vayssiere JL Mitochondrial reactive oxygen species in cell death signaling. Biochimie 2002;84:131-41.

182. Childs AC, Phaneuf SL, Dirks AJ, Phillips T, Leeuwenburgh C Doxorubicin treatment in vivo causes cytochrome C release and cardiomyocyte apoptosis, as well as increased mitochondrial efficiency, superoxide dismutase activity, and Bcl-2:Bax ratio. Cancer Res 2002;62:4592-8.

183. Quillet-Mary A, Jaffrezou JP, Mansat V, Bordier C, Naval J, Laurent G Implication of mitochondrial hydrogen peroxide generation in ceramide-induced apoptosis. J Biol Chem 1997;272:21388-95.

184. Zhang L, Yu J, Park BH, Kinzler KW, Vogelstein B Role of BAX in the apoptotic response to anticancer agents. Science 2000;290:989-92.

185. Hug H, Strand S, Grambihler A, et al Reactive oxygen intermediates are involved in the induction of CD95 ligand mRNA expression by cytostatic drugs in hepatoma cells. J Biol Chem 1997;272:28191-3.

186. Suhara T, Fukuo K, Sugimoto T, et al Hydrogen peroxide induces up-regulation of Fas in human endothelial cells. J Immunol 1998;160:4042-7.

187. Hirpara JL, Clement MV, Pervaiz S. Intracellular acidification triggered by mitochondrial-derived hydrogen peroxide is an effector mechanism for drug-induced apoptosis in tumor cells. J Biol Chem 2001;276:514-21.

188. Ahmad KA, Clement MV, Hanif IM, Pervaiz S. Resveratrol inhibits drug-induced apoptosis in human leukemia cells by creating an intracellular milieu nonpermissive for death execution. Cancer Res 2004;64:1452-9.

189. Cerutti P.A. Prooxidant states and tumor promotion. Science (Wash. DC), 227: 375-381, 1985.

190. Burdon R. H., Gill V., Rice-Evans C. Oxidative stress and tumour cell proliferation. Free Radic. Res. Commun., 11: 65-76, 1990.

191. Fadeel B., Ahlin A., Henter J. I., Orrenius S., Hampton M. B. Involvement of caspases in neutrophil apoptosis: regulation by reactive oxygen species. Blood, 92: 4808-4818, 1998.

192. Hampton M. B., Orrenius S. Dual regulation of caspase activity by hydrogen peroxide: implications for apoptosis. FEBS Lett., 414: 552-556, 1997.

193. Tze Wei Poh and Shazib Pervaiz. LY294002 and LY303511 Sensitize Tumor Cells to Drug-Induced Apoptosis via Intracellular Hydrogen Peroxide Production Independent of the Phosphoinositide 3-Kinase-Akt Pathway. Cancer Research 65, 6264-6274, July 15, 2005.

194. Cullen, J. J., Hinkhouse, M. M., Grady, M., Gaut, A. W., Liu, J., Zhang, Y., Weydert, C. J. D., Domann, F. E., and Oberley, L. W. (2003) Cancer Res. 63, 5513–5520.

195. Juan Du, David H. Daniels, Carla Asbury, Sujatha Venkataraman, Jingru Liu, Douglas R. Spitz, Larry W. Oberley, and Joseph J. Cullen. Mitochondrial Production of Reactive Oxygen Species Mediate Dicumarol-induced Cytotoxicity in Cancer Cells. The Journal of Biological Chemistry Vol. 281, No. 49, pp. 37416–37426, December 8, 2006.

196. Sun Wenqing; Kalen Amanda L; Smith Brian J; Cullen Joseph J; Oberley Larry W. Enhancing the antitumor activity of adriamycin and ionizing radiation. Cancer research 2009;69(10):4294-300.

197. Wagner B A; Buettner G R; Oberley L W; Darby C J; Burns C P. Myeloperoxidase is involved in H_2O_2-induced apoptosis of HL-60 human leukemia cells. The Journal of biological chemistry 2000;275(29):22461-9.

198. Jun Fang, Tomohiro Sawa, Takaaki Akaike and Hiroshi Maeda. Tumor-targeted Delivery of Polyethylene Glycol-conjugated D-Amino Acid Oxidase for Antitumor Therapy via Enzymatic Generation of Hydrogen Peroxide. Cancer Research 62, 3138-3143, June 1, 2002.

199. Venkataraman Sujatha; Jiang Xiaohong; Weydert Christine; Zhang Yuping; Zhang Hannah J; Goswami Prabhat C; Ritchie Justine M; Oberley Larry W; Buettner Garry R. Manganese superoxide dismutase overexpression inhibits the growth of androgen-independent prostate cancer cells.

200. Oncogene 2005;24(1):77-89.

201. Aykin-Burns Nùkhet; Ahmad Iman M; Zhu Yueming; Oberley Larry W; Spitz Douglas R. Increased levels of superoxide and H_2O_2 mediate the differential susceptibility of cancer cells versus normal cells to glucose deprivation. The Biochemical Journal 2009;418(1):29-37.

202. Yoshizaki K, et al. Pro-senescent effect of hydrogen peroxide on cancer cells and its possible application to tumor suppression. Biosci Biotechnol Biochem. 2009 Feb;73(2):311-5.

203. Brian D. Lawenda, Kara M. Kelly, Elena J. Ladas, Stephen M. Sagar, Andrew Vickers, Jeffrey B. Blumberg. Should Supplemental Antioxidant Administration Be Avoided During Chemotherapy and Radiation Therapy? JNCI Journal of the National Cancer Institute 2008 100(11):773-783.

204. Vicki Brower. An Apple a Day May Be Safer Than Vitamins. JNCI Journal of the National Cancer Institute 2008 100(11):770-772.

205. Howes M.D., PhD., R. (2009). Dangers of Antioxidants in Cancer Patients: A Review. PHILICA.COM Article number 153. Published 7th February, 2009.

206. Nima Sharifi. Commentary: Antioxidants for Cancer: New Tricks for an Old Dog? The Oncologist, Vol. 14, No. 3, 213-215, March 2009.

207. Salganik, R. I., Albright, C. D., Rodgers, J., Kim, J., Zeisel, S. H., Sivashinskiy, M. S. & Van Dyke, T. A. (2000) Dietary antioxidant depletion: enhancement of tumor apoptosis and inhibition of brain tumor growth in transgenic mice. Carcinogenesis 21: 909–914.

24.0 DR. HOWES' RESPONSE TO A MURDER CHARGE INVOLVING THE USE OF H_2O_2 BY AN ALTERNATIVE PRACTITIONER

Dr. Smith Case:

The Randolph M. Howes, M.D., Ph.D. response to the Dr. Steven Bratman Report/Notes

The primary issue at hand, in the Dr. Smith case, is the safety or the lethality of hydrogen peroxide (H_2O_2), administered to a patient intravenously in a 0.03% saline solution over a period of 1-3 hours and the use of multiple infusions of the same. The issue of safety is directly related to the known safety or toxicity of H_2O_2 during normal cellular metabolism and to the known breakdown products of H_2O_2, when it is mixed with components in the human blood stream.

The answers to these issues could be in the form of the following questions: A) Is intravenous 0.03% H_2O_2 safe or lethal, when used in humans? and B) Are the breakdown products of H_2O_2 safe or lethal when H_2O_2 is combined with human blood?

Secondary issues related to this case include: 1) can H_2O_2 be of benefit to patients, 2) can H_2O_2 be harmful to patients, 3) can H_2O_2 administered intravenously in a 0.03% solution increase or raise vascular O_2 levels, 4) whether or not increasing vascular oxygen (O_2) could be of benefit or harm to patients, 5) what is the probable significance and the biochemical role of H_2O_2 in establishing a condition of homeostasis and health in humans. The data, which I present in my monograph, will also shed some light on these points.

As regards Dr. Steven Bratman Report/Notes, on page 2, paragraph 3, Dr. Bratman states verbatim that, "However, a tiny uncontrolled non-randomized study conducted eight-five years ago cannot be regarded as meaningful evidence. Curiously, Dr. Bratman then proceeds to support his woefully inadequate arguments by quoting "tiny uncontrolled non-randomized studies, which cannot be regarded as meaningful evidence." In fact, he quoted unsubstantiated singular events, usually with unknown quantities of H_2O_2 or unknown concentrations, as being meaningful evidence implicating the toxicity of H_2O_2. There is no information provided as to presence of other potential harmful disease conditions in these patients or whether or not H_2O_2 was also used in combination with harmful or lethal pharmaceuticals, both of which must be considered as variables in these cases. To single out H_2O_2 as the only potential source of lethality in this handful of cases is grossly misleading and it is scientifically unsubstantiated. Associations are not proof of causality.

Thus, utilizing his criteria for meaningfulness, his "Adverse Effects Table" is a short series of anecdotes of meaningless "unknowns." It has no scientific medical significance or value. Since there are many more appropriate examples in the world literature than those quoted by Dr. Bratman, it is obvious that he has either not reviewed the current literature on H_2O_2 or he has chosen not to present timely relevant H_2O_2 data.

In referring to the work of Dr. Farr, on Page 2, paragraph 4, line 1, he states that Dr. Farr's study "fails to meet modern standards of evidence." Certainly, one can find points which require clarification in Dr. Farr's work but it is obvious that Dr. Bratman went on with his discussion and failed to present any "blinded, randomized, meaningful evidence," per his definition of meaningful evidence. By his own criteria, his discussion and "irrelevant" offerings are meaningless.

There is overwhelming scientific evidence that H_2O_2 has bactericidal, fungicidal, virucidal and tumoricidal activity. This represents an incredible range of salutary properties for prooxidant protection of the human condition. H_2O_2 has inherent oxidant properties and it can be transformed into other EMODs (electronically modified oxygen derivatives) by EMOD-EMOD interactions (i.e., reactions with superoxide anion, hydroxyl radical, singlet oxygen, hypochlorous acid, peroxynitrite, nitric oxide, etc.) or via myeloperoxidase.

I have worked in the area of oxygen metabolism for over 40 years and I have concluded that H_2O_2 is one of the most important redox molecules to favorably influence human health and homeostasis. It is present in steady state levels in all aerobic cells and its absence results in increased infections and neoplasia. There was a time when all EMODs, including H_2O_2, were considered to be damaging or harmful to aerobic cells. However, that time has passed and scientists are increasingly recognizing and acknowledging the multitude of reactions in which H_2O_2 and EMODs are essential for normal cellular functioning.

Recently, I condensed the available world data on H_2O_2 into a single monograph and in order for the reader to get an accurate picture of the importance and safety of H_2O_2, I will refer you to that volume: **HYDROGEN PEROXIDE: MONOGRAPH 1: SCIENTIFIC, MEDICAL AND BIOCHEMICAL OVERVIEW. Randolph M. Howes, M.D., Ph.D. Free Radical Publishing Co. 2006. Pages 1-203.** Since information from clinical studies on H_2O_2 is either scanty or lacking, animal and laboratory data may provide insights as to the safety and toxicity of H_2O_2 in humans.

I will now provide a very brief profile of the scientific and medical information discussed in **HYDROGEN PEROXIDE: MONOGRAPH 1: SCIENTIFIC, MEDICAL AND BIOCHEMICAL OVERVIEW. Randolph M. Howes, M.D., Ph.D. Free Radical Publishing Co. 2006.**

NORMAL METABOLISM UTILIZES OXYGEN AND PRODUCES HYDROGEN PEROXIDE. All aerobic organisms, including humans, derive most of their metabolic energy from the reduction of oxygen and, consequently, produce significant amounts of O_2- and H_2O_2 that are generated during the metabolism of oxygen. **(Genetic Contributions to Plasma Total Antioxidant Activity. Xing Li Wang; David L. Rainwater; Jane F. VandeBerg; Braxton D. Mitchell; Michael C. Mahaney. Arteriosclerosis, Thrombosis, and Vascular Biology. 2001;21:1190). This is a key factor when considering the safety of** H_2O_2.

The consumption of oxygen during cellular respiration is the fundamental pathway that sustains aerobic life, which always and continually produces electronically modified oxygen derivatives (EMODs), especially superoxide anion and hydrogen peroxide. In other words, we can not live without them.

Healthy tissue maintains a steady state of H_2O_2 **of 10-9 to 10-7 M** (Chance, B., Sies, H. and Boveris, A. Hydrogen peroxide metabolism in mammalian organs. Physiol Rev 1979; 59: 527). **The synthesis of thyroxine depends on the actions of** H_2O_2 **and thyroid peroxidase. Hydrogen peroxide** is only one of the many components that help regulate the amount of oxygen getting to your cells. Its presence is vital for many other functions as well. **It is required for the production of thyroid hormone and sexual hormones** (Mol Cell Endocrinol 86;46(2): 149-154) (Steroids 82;40(5):5690579). **It stimulates the production of interferon** (J Immunol 85;134(4):24492455). **It dilates blood vessels in the heart and brain** (Am J Physiol 86;250 (5 pt 2): H815-821 and (2 pt 2):H157-162). **It improves glucose utilization in diabetics** (Proceedings of the IBOM Conference 1989, 1990, 1991). These are just a few examples of the crucial areas in which H_2O_2 functions continuously.

H_2O_2 **has been detected in the human breath at levels ranging from 1.0 µg/L to 0.34 µg/L (IARC, 1985), and even in the breath of babies.** H_2O_2 **is a naturally occurring substance.** H_2O_2 **has been detected in serum and in intact liver** (IARC, 1985). (IARC. 1985. International Agency for Research on Cancer. Hydrogen Peroxide. In: IARC Monographs on the Evaluation of Carcinogenic Risk if Chemicals to Humans: Allyl compounds, Aldehydes, Epoxides and Peroxides, Vol. 36. IARC, Lyon, pp. 285-314).

In 1999, Juan and Buettner calculated the steady state levels to be as follows:

$[H_2O_2]$ss in red cells is 10-10 M
$[H_2O_2]$ss in mitochondrial membrane is 10-8 M
$[H_2O_2]$ss in liver cells is 10-8 M
$[O_2]$ss is 10-5 M, much higher than $[H_2O_2]$
$[O_2.-]$ss in cells is 10-10 M

Non-destructive and reversible oxidative modifications may be achieved by H_2O_2 and other hydroperoxides with or without the aid of redox mediators such as GSH or thioredoxin. **The most common oxidant in vivo is H_2O_2 that, in inflammatory conditions, is amply formed by dismutation of $O_2.-$ released from activated phagocytes** (Babior, B.M. NADPH oxidase: An update. Blood 1999; 93: 1464-1476), but physiologically also by intracelular NADPH oxidases (Bayraktutan, U., Blayney, L. and Shah, A.M. Molecular characterization and localization of the NADPH oxidase components gp91-phox and p22-phox in endothelia cells. Arterioscler Thromb Vasc Biol 2000; 20: 1903-1911), and other enzymatic systems. Although some H_2O_2 appears to be produced constitutively, receptor-mediated H_2O_2 formation appears to be more common. Typical examples **are TNF-α-induced mitochondrial $O_2.-$ formation** (Goossens, V., Grooten, J., DeVos, K. and Fiers. W. Direct evidence for tumor necrosis factor-induced mitochondrial reactive oxygen intermediates and their involvement in cytotoxicity. Proc Natl Acad Sci USA 1995; 92: 8115-8119), or **cytoplasmic increase of H_2O_2 upon growth factor receptor stimulation** (Finkel, T. Redox-dependent signal transduction. FEBS Lett 2000; 476: 52-54).

Mitochondrial respiration is an important proximal component of the signaling response to H_2O_2. These data implicate the **mitochondrion as a proximal component of redox-sensitive events in cell signaling** (K Chen, SR Thomas, A Albano, MP Murphy, and JF Keaney, Jr. Mitochondrial Function Is Required for Hydrogen Peroxide-induced Growth Factor Receptor Transactivation and Downstream Signaling. J. Biol. Chem., Vol. 279, Issue 33, 35079-35086, August 13, 2004).

Cellular concentrations of H_2O_2 are important and **low levels of H_2O_2** regulate physiological processes such as:

- receptor-mediated cell signaling pathways
- normal cell proliferation and
- transcription activation (Simon, H.U. et al Role of reactive oxygen species (ROS) in apoptosis function. Apoptosis, 5: 415-418, 2000, Huang, R.P. et al, UV activates growth factor receptors via reactive oxygen species. J Cell Biol., 133: 211-220, 1996).

Confidently, **I predict that H_2O_2 will be proven to be one of the most important cellular secondary messengers and this will lead to new therapeutic applications and interventions. H_2O_2 will conform to the pattern of initial discovery, to be later followed by clinical and therapeutic application.** (Howes, R. M. 2004. U.T.O.P.I.A. - Unified Theory of Oxygen Participation in Aerobiosis. (767 page text) Free Radical Publishing Co. Kentwood, LA) (Howes, R.M. 2005. The Medical and Scientific Significance of Oxygen Free Radical Metabolism. (931 page text) Free Radical Publishing Co. Kentwood, LA).

Peroxide is becoming a recognized second messenger just like cAMP, Ca2+, Ins 1,4,5-P3, and NO (Rhee, S.G. Redox signaling: hydrogen peroxide as intracellular messenger. Exp. and Mol. Med., Vol. 31, No. 2, 53-59, June 1999).

H_2O_2 is a normal product of metabolism and is continually produced in the human body. **I believe that one of the most compelling arguments for the harmless nature of H_2O_2 in the human body is the fact that individuals, who lack one of the primary enzymes to break down H_2O_2 (acatalasemia), their peroxide levels essentially do not cause them harm. Patients lacking catalase (the primary enzyme for breaking down hydrogen peroxide) appear to live relatively normal lives and the Swiss type acatalasaemic patients show no signs of oxidative damage** (Goth, L and Pay, A. Genetic heterogeneity in acatalasemia. (1992) Electrophoresis 17: 1302-1303).

Catalase does not appear to be nearly so important as SOD, judging from the weak phenotypes of cells that lack it (Imlay, J. A., and Linn, S. (1988) *Science* 240, 1302-1309**) and persons with acatalasemia** (Eaton, J. W., and Ma, M. (1995) in *The Metabolic and Molecular Bases of Inherited Disease* (Scriver, C. R., Beaudet, A. L., Sly, W. S., and Valle, D., eds), 7th Ed., pp. 2371-2383, McGraw-Hill, Inc., New York).

H_2O_2 **is involved in any metabolic pathway which utilizes oxidases, peroxidases, cyclo-oxygenases, lipoxygenases, myeloperoxidase, catalase, etc. In some it is generated and in others, it is altered or removed. The most important sources of EMOD generation, including H_2O_2, are:**

-endoplasmic reticulum (cytochrome P450)
-peroxisomes (fatty acid oxidation)
-mitochondrial electron transport system (univalent reduction of molecular oxygen NADH dehydrogenase complex)
-endothelial cells (xanthine oxidase reaction)
-inflammatory cells (myeloperoxidase, NADPH oxidase)
-catecholamine oxidation
—and arachidonic acid metabolism

Hydrogen Peroxide Production:

Also, Copper Containing Oxidases Produce H_2O_2
Cytochrome oxidase
Laccase
Ferroxidase I
2) **cytochrome P-450, cytochrome B5 and Xanthine oxidase** which produce superoxides;
3) **oxidases** for fatty acids, urate, L-pipecolic acid, D-amino acids, alcohols, polyamines, a-hydroxy acids and cholestanoic acid which produce H_2O_2;

Activated phagocytes can produce as much as 47 nmol of H_2O_2/106 cells within 30 minutes corresponding to a concentration of 47 uM H_2O_2 in a diluted volume of 1 ml. The rapid dismutation of O_2.- to H_2O_2 is (spontaneous, 105 [mol/L]-1 ·s-1, SOD-catalyzed, 109 [mol/L]-1. s-1).

Usually, (O_2.-) is the stoichiometric precursor of H_2O_2. The amount of H_2O_2 produced by brain mitochondria is up to 5% of the amount of O_2 consumed. However, some H_2O_2 is produced directly and not via the superoxide anion.

Enzyme Tissue Location	Tissue	Location
Monoamine oxidase	liver	mitochondrial
outer membrane		
D-amino acid oxidase	kidney	peroxisome
Glycolate oxidase	liver	peroxisome
Fatty acyl-CoA oxidase	liver	peroxisome
L-Gulonolactone oxidase	liver	microsomal
Pyridoxamine-5'-phosphate	liver	cytosol
Diamine oxidase	placenta	
Thiol oxidase	kidney	plasma
Urate oxidase	liver	peroxisome
Xanthine oxidase	milk	

Sulfite oxidase	liver	mitochondria
Xanthine oxidase	neutrophil	specific granules
Aldehyde oxidase		

Superoxide and H_2O_2 are Produced Enzymatically By

- NADPH oxidases (phagocytosis)
- Mitochondrial cytochrome c oxidase (cell respiration)
- Liver Cytochrome P 450 (oxidation of xenobiotics)
- Xanthine oxidase (ischemic reperfusion)
- Prostaglandin synthetase
- Lipoxygenase
- Aldehyde oxidase
- Amino acid oxidase
- Myeloperoxidase (uses H_2O_2 to oxidize chloride ions to form HOCl)

H_2O_2 is also generated by:

Arachidonic acid-metabolizing enzymes
Xanthine oxidase
Nitric oxide synthase
Cytochrome P450
as well as in the cellular response to ultraviolet radiation.

Any mitochondrial substrate incorporated in the respiratory chain through NADH or ubiquinone, will generate H_2O_2. Thus, H_2O_2 generation is a physiologic event under aerobic conditions.

The main sites for H_2O_2 and $O_2.-$ production are the:
1) NADH-ubiquinone-reductase (complex I)
2) ubiquinol-cytochrome c-reductase (complex III)
Both have ubiquinone as a common component, and act **as prooxidants**.

(Signal Transduction by reactive Oxygen and Nitrogen Species: Pathways and Chemical Principles. Edited by H.J. Forman, J. Fukuto and M. Torres, Kluwer Academic Publishers, 2003. **H$_2$O$_2$ as Intracellular Messenger.** C. Giulivi and M.J. Oursler. Page 313).

Virtually all types of vascular cells produce O$_2$-. and H$_2$O$_2$ (Griendling, K. K., Sorescu, D. and Ushio-Fukai, M. NAD(P)H oxidase: role in cardiovascular biology and disease. Cir Res 2000: 86; 494–501). **The smooth muscle cell response to growth factors is now known to be dependent on the intracellular generation of H$_2$O$_2$** (Bae YS, Kang SW, Seo MS, Baines IC, Tekle E, Chock PB, and Rhee SG. Epidermal growth factor (EGF)-induced generation of hydrogen peroxide. Role in EGF receptor-mediated tyrosine phosphorylation. *J Biol Chem* 272: 217–221, 1997) (Sundaresan M, Yu ZX, Ferrans VJ, Irani K, and Finkel T. Requirement for generation of H$_2$O$_2$ for platelet-derived growth factor signal transduction. *Science* 270: 296–299, 1995).

A number of smooth muscle cell mitogens actually require H$_2$O$_2$ production for a proliferative response (Sundaresan M, Yu ZX, Ferrans VJ, Irani K, and Finkel T. Requirement for generation of H$_2$O$_2$ for platelet-derived growth factor signal transduction. *Science* 270: 296–299, 1995).

The amount of H$_2$O$_2$ produced by brain mitochondria is up to 5% of the amount of O$_2$ consumed. Even though the brain is only 2% of the body by weight, it consumes 20% of the body's oxygen.

Hydrogen peroxide (H$_2$O$_2$) is produced by the cornea and neighboring tissues. Aqueous humor itself generates H$_2$O$_2$ with reportedmaximum levels of approximately **0.09 mM H$_2$O$_2$ in bovine aqueous** (Spector A, Ma W, Wang RR. The aqueous humor is capable of generating and degrading H$_2$O$_2$. Invest Ophthalmol Vis Sci 1998;39:1188–97).

Peroxisomes produce H₂O₂, but not O₂.- under physiological conditions **(Chance et al. 1979). Peroxisomes are now found to be present in virtually all eukaryotic cells (except mature red blood cells). Peroxisomes account for a large fraction of total cellular H₂O₂ production** (Boveris, A., Oshino, N. and Chance, B. The cellular production of hydrogen peroxide. Biochem J 1972; 128: 617-630).

Peroxisomes contain **H₂O₂-generating enzymes including:**

> **glycollate oxidase**
> **D-amino acid oxidase**
> **urate oxidase**
> **L-*a*-hydroxylases oxidase**
> **and fatty acyl-CoA oxidase.**

The section, **ACUTE H₂O₂ TOXICITY,** demonstrates the incredibly low toxicity of H₂O₂. Ideally, we should discuss the effects of IV H₂O₂ in humans but there is very little in the literature to quote, which involved IV H₂O₂ infusions in humans utilizing 0.03% H₂O₂. Thus, perhaps the best source of such information is from the evaluations of physicians, who routinely use IV H₂O₂ in their practices. It is common knowledge amongst tens of thousands of physicians who practice oxidative therapy using IV H₂O₂ that it is effective in treating a wide range of illnesses and carries an extremely low risk of adverse reactions, especially for the 0.03% H₂O₂.

Hydrogen peroxide is used to cleanse and irrigate wounds. **As it decomposes immediately into water and oxygen on contact with organic tissue, it is usually regarded as a safe agent. (**Oxygen embolism due to hydrogen peroxide irrigation during cervical spinal surgery. Morikawa H, Mima H, Fujita H, Mishima S. Can J Anaesth. 1995 Mar;42(3):231-3). **When applied to tissue, solutions of H₂O₂ have poor penetrability** (HSDB. 1995. Hazardous Substances Data Bank. Medlars Online Information Retrieval System, National Library of Medicine).

Hydrogen peroxide has a half-life of 0.75 to 2.0 seconds in human blood. Catalase breaks down peroxide into water and ground state oxygen, both of which are harmless and are needed by the body. Thus, H_2O_2 given by a peripheral vein is decomposed before it can be carried out of the upper extremity.

The Baylor University School of Medicine H_2O_2 studies of Harold Urschel and Thomas Mallams et al indicate the following:

Hydrogen peroxide is broken down very rapidly when introduced into the blood stream in both rabbits and humans; **in dilute solutions, intravascular hydrogen peroxide has no unacceptable deleterious effect on formed blood elements** (with the exception of dogs, where, due to an apparent deficient in RBC and plasma catalase, methemoglobin is produced); (Mallams, J.T., Balla, G.A. and Finney, J.W. Regional oxygenation and irradiation in the treatment of malignant tumors. Progress in Clinc Cancer 1965; 1: 137), and **the breakdown of hydrogen peroxide by biological fluids results in the supersaturation of these fluids with oxygen** (Jay, B.E., Finney, J.W., Balla, G.A. and Mallams, J.T. The supersaturation of biologic fluids with oxygen by decomposition of hydrogen peroxide. Texas Rep Biol & Med 1964; 22: 106). **The magnitude of the supersaturation is equivalent to several atmospheres of oxygen.**

The Baylor authors have noted a reduction in the subintimal lipid deposits and atheromatous plaques in the arteries of individuals being infused intra-arterially with hydrogen peroxide.

Several patients who have been infused intra-arterially with hydrogen peroxide as an adjunct to irradiation therapy in the management of their malignant disease have undergone postmortem examination. During the autopsy, the catheter was left in place, the aorta was split longitudinally, and the tip of the catheter marked. Sections were prepared from the aorta immediately above and below tip for comparative histologic evaluation by oil red-O and H and E stains.

All patients were being **infused into the abdominal aorta with 0.48 percent hydrogen peroxide in Ionosol T**. Venous samples were taken before and during the last minute of infusion and the results of the two samples compared. During the entire infusion period (20 minutes), the patient was reclined and relaxed.

In all cases studied to date, the patients have received hydrogen peroxide infusion alone as an adjunct to other modes of therapy for a variety of conditions over extended periods of time ranging from 4 to 16 weeks. During this time, the individuals received daily infusions of 250 ml of hydrogen peroxide in Ionosol T with **a peroxide concentration ranging from 0.36 to 0.48 percent.**

Upon gross examination, the segment of the aorta being infused was found to be different from the area not being infused. **This difference was marked by a decrease in the number and severity of atheromatous plaques, and an increase in flexibility and elasticity of the vessel.** Histologic evaluation by oil red-O stained sections **showed a decrease in total subliminal lipid deposits.** When weighed samples of the vessels were extracted and total lipids determined, **it was found that approximately a 50 percent reduction in total lipids had occurred in the area being infused with hydrogen peroxide.** In my opinion, this work is some of the most exciting work in the last 50 years!

In vitro studies on human aortas incubated with hydrogen peroxide, the results indicate a bi- or multiphase reaction which starts immediately with the elution of relatively large quantities of cholesterol, cholesterol esters, phospholipid, triglyceride and free fatty acids: the total concentration of these components in the supernatant fluid decreases over a period of the next few hours. This decrease if followed by a subsequent increase in total concentration at 12 to 24 hours. **The same general results have been obtained with human aorta in saline exposed to oxygen at five atmospheres absolute pressure.** (Finney, J.W., Jay, B.E., Race, G.J., Urschel, H.C., Mallams, J.T. and Balla, G.A. Removal of cholesterol and other lipids from experimental animal and human atheromatous arteries by dilute hydrogen peroxide. Angiology 1966; 17: 223-228.). **I believe that this data indicates, in part, the signaling capability of H_2O_2 because, even though it is present for a very short time, it can activate processes which occur sometime later. This effect is being reported with increasing frequency for many of the EMODs.**

During the early studies in the treatment of patients with intra-arterial hydrogen peroxide and irradiation therapy, two observations were made. In some of the patients, **not only did the tumor respond more rapidly to irradiation, but also it was found that the wounds would heal at a much faster rate and with less scar formation.**

Following the failure of conventional resuscitation methods, hydrogen peroxide was employed in one human case with temporary reversal of ventricular fibrillation to regular sinus rhythm and elevation of the blood pressure to normal (Urschel, H.C., Jr., Finney, J.W., Morales, A.R., Balla, G.A. and Mallams, J.T. Cardiac resuscitation with hydrogen peroxide. Abstract of the 38th Scientific Sessions. 1965; Suppl II, Vol. 31 & 32).

Regional H_2O_2 for Clostridia Myositis

The intra-arterial infusion of hydrogen peroxide has been used as a method for producing a hyperoxic environment in experimental animals for the treatment of experimentally induced clostridia myositis. Eighty-five rabbits were employed in this study; 43 were controls and 42 were experimental animals. In the experimental study, 21 animals were treated with hydrogen peroxide by each route of administration. In this group, **52.4% of the animals receiving the intra-arterial H$_2$O$_2$ infusion and 66.6% receiving intramuscular clysis with H$_2$O$_2$ survived. There were no survivors past 72 hours in the control group.** (Finney, J.W., Haberman, S., Race, G.J., Bala, G.A. and Mallams, J.T. Local and regional application of hydrogen peroxide in the control of clostridia myositis in rabbits. J Bacterio 1967; 93: 1430-1437).

Hydrogen peroxide is broken down very rapidly when introduced into the blood stream in both rabbits and humans; **in dilute solutions, intravascular hydrogen peroxide has no unacceptable deleterious effect on formed blood elements** (with the exception of dogs, where, due to an apparent deficient in RBC and plasma catalase, methemoglobin is produced); (Mallams, J.T., Balla, G.A. and Finney, J.W. Regional oxygenation and irradiation in the treatment of malignant tumors. Progress in Clinc Cancer 1965; 1: 137), and **the breakdown of hydrogen peroxide by biological fluids results in the supersaturation of these fluids with oxygen** (Jay, B.E., Finney, J.W., Balla, G.A. and Mallams, J.T. The supersaturation of biologic fluids with oxygen by decomposition of hydrogen peroxide. Texas Rep Biol & Med 1964; 22: 106). **The magnitude of the supersaturation is equivalent to several atmospheres of oxygen.**

The time required to remove all hydrogen peroxide from the blood system when one-sixth of the total volume is 0.5% hydrogen peroxide is less than 0.1 second in human blood and 0.2 second in rabbit blood. This total peroxide volume would not be encountered under in vivo conditions; therefore, the life of the peroxide molecule in the vascular system would be considerably shorter than this. **I believe that this data shows that H$_2$O$_2$ is present for extremely short times intervals in the vascular system and that it is rapidly broken down into ground state oxygen and water. This serves to negate many of the criticisms directed towards intravenous infusion of 0.03% H$_2$O$_2$ in humans.**

427

It has also been shown that **the time of maximum oxygen concentration in a dilute blood system was at a point immediately following the complete disappearance of hydrogen peroxide from the solution.**

Elevated oxygen tensions have been observed during the intra-arterial infusion of hydrogen peroxide under a variety of experimental conditions in both animals and humans. In animals being infused into the thoracic aorta, samples collected from the femoral artery revealed **a total oxygen content equivalent to 4 to 6 atmospheres of pressure. In humans who were being infused into the thoracic aorta, blood samples were collected from the femoral artery and showed an oxygen content equivalent from 2 to 4 atmospheres of pure oxygen.**

It has been repeatedly observed that high concentrations of oxygen are present on both the arterial and venous side of a regional system being infused with dilute hydrogen peroxide solutions. The rate of the diffusion and final concentration in a given tissue will ultimately govern the degree to which the peroxide will exert its beneficial effect.

I find the H_2O_2 resuscitation data so important that it is unbelievable that it has not received intense scientific investigation. I believe that the Baylor H_2O_2 study results are extremely important observations and that they have potential application in all cases involving cardiac resuscitation. The Baylor data was taken from: Howes, R. M.

2004. U.T.O.P.I.A. - Unified Theory of Oxygen Participation in Aerobiosis. (767 page text) Free Radical Publishing Co. Kentwood, LA

Again, I emphasize the great importance of the Baylor group. Their work emphasizes the safety of intravenous

and intra-arterial H_2O_2 infusion and intramuscular H_2O_2 injection. High concentrations of H_2O_2, up to 0.7% were well tolerated and did not produce hemolysis. H_2O_2 dissolved plaques, produced successful cardiac resuscitations and increased wound healing rates. All physicians need to be made aware of this landmark work with H_2O_2 in humans.

Data from poison control centers offers insight into the extremely low toxicity of H_2O_2 ingestion. The following 2 studies are representative of the overall data and demonstrates the fact that patients usually have an uneventful and full recovery from H_2O_2 ingestion:

1) Isolated case reports have documented that **hydrogen peroxide exposure** can be associated with serious toxicity by various routes of exposure. The purpose of the following study was to better delineate the epidemiology, medical outcome, and potential health hazards of hydrogen peroxide exposures to the general public. They performed **a retrospective review of all exposures reported to a regional poison center over a 36 month period and found that of 95,052 exposures reported, 325 (.34%) were due to hydrogen peroxide.** The pediatric population (< 18 years) accounted for 71% of hydrogen peroxide exposures and ingestion was the most common route of exposure (83%). Nausea and vomiting were the most common symptoms secondary to ingestion. **Ocular and dermal exposures to dilute solutions resulted in transient symptoms without permanent sequelae. While most exposures by all routes resulted in a benign outcome (no effect or minor effect),** there was **a trend toward more severe outcomes in those who ingested a concentration greater than 10%** ($p = 0.011$). (Abstract: Hydrogen peroxide exposure--325 exposures reported to a regional poison control center. Dickson KF, Caravati EM. J Toxicol Clin Toxicol. 1994;32(6):705-14).Division of Emergency Medicine, University of Utah School of Medicine, Utah Poison Control Center, Salt Lake City.

2) The following was a retrospective chart review of exposures to **hydrogen peroxide 3%** reported to the Long Island Regional Poison Control Center from **January 1992 to April 1995 (39 months)**. Data extracted included age, route of exposure, amount of agent, symptoms, therapy, and medical outcome. RESULTS: **There were 670 exposures to hydrogen peroxide 3% of 81,126 total exposures reported during the 40 months. Most exposures were by oral route (77%), occurred in children < 17 years old (67%), and were asymptomatic (85.6%). All but one exposure resulted in a benign outcome.** One child, who presented with bloody emesis, developed multiple gastric ulcers and duodenal erosions after ingestion of hydrogen peroxide 2-4 oz. CONCLUSIONS: **Exposure to hydrogen peroxide 3% is usually benign;** however, severe gastric injury may occur following small ingestions in children. Patients who report persistent vomiting or bloody emesis require medical evaluation and consideration of endoscopy to evaluate gastrointestinal injury. (Abstract: Hydrogen peroxide 3%, exposures. Henry MC, Wheeler J, Mofenson HC, Caraccio TR, Marsh M, Comer GMSinger AJ. J Toxicol Clin Toxicol. 1996;34(3):323-7).

Hydrogen peroxide is a readily available clear, odorless liquid that is commonly used as an irrigant for superficial wounds. It is not widely thought of as a poison; however, **it may rarely be the cause of accidental death.** (Hydrogen peroxide: a source of lethal oxygen embolism. Case report and review of the literature. Cina SJ, Downs JC, Conradi SE. Am J Forensic Med Pathol. 1994 Mar;15(1):44-50).

In 5 persons who accidentally drank 50 mL of a 33% H_2O_2 solution, symptoms included stomach and chest pain, retention of breath, foaming at the mouth and loss of consciousness. Later, motor and sensory disorders, fever, micro-hemorrhages and moderate leukocytosis were noted. **All recovered completely within 2-3 weeks** (IARC. 1985. International Agency for Research on Cancer. Hydrogen Peroxide. In: IARC Monographs on the Evaluation of Carcinogenic Risk if Chemicals to Humans: Allyl compounds, Aldehydes, Epoxides and Peroxides, Vol. 36. IARC, Lyon, pp. 285-314).

In my opinion, this represents the low toxicity of H_2O_2 and demonstrates the body's ability to handle excess amounts of H_2O_2. **Alternative medicine clinics around the world have given thousands upon thousands of I.V. doses of H_2O_2 without untoward effects. Additionally, their patients readily testify as to the benefits of these H_2O_2 infusions. I fully realize that testimonials do not meet scientific standards but that fact does not negate the relief of pain and suffering in thousands of patients.**

Information from the Hazardous Substances Data Bank (HSDB), a database of the National Library of Medicine's TOXNET system (http://toxnet.nlm.nih.gov) **indicates in general, ingestion, ocular or dermal exposure to small amounts of dilute hydrogen peroxide will cause no serious problems.**

Homozygous CAT knockout mice, which are completely deficient in catalase expression, develop normally and show no gross abnormalities. This fact should allay any misgivings regarding the harmful nature of H_2O_2. (Y-S Ho, Y Xiong, W Ma, A Spector, and D S Ho. Mice Lacking Catalase Develop Normally but Show Differential Sensitivity to Oxidant Tissue Injury. J. Biol. Chem., Vol. 279, Issue 31, 32804-32812, July 30, 2004).

Mouse L cells and rat aortic smooth muscle cells **overexpressing catalase display heightened oxidant sensitivity and retarded growth with increased cell death. I believe that this indicates that too much H_2O_2 is being destroyed and this increases the incidence of death.**

Cell H_2O_2 Reaction is Concentration Dependent

The following abstract by K.J. Davies contains very important information relative to a cell's response to varying concentrations of H_2O_2 and information of a time course over which these responses occur. Although I

disagree with the use of the concept of "oxidative stress," I applaud his assemblage of data for this paper.

Proliferating mammalian cells exhibit a broad spectrum of responses to oxidative stress, depending on the stress level encountered.

Very low levels of hydrogen peroxide, e.g., 3 to 15 microM, or 0.1 to 0.5 micromol/107 cells, **cause a significant mitogenic response**, 25% to 45 % growth stimulation.

Greater concentrations of H_2O_2, 120 to 150 microM, or 2 to 5 micromol/107 cells, **cause a temporary growth arrest** that appears to protect cells from excess energy use and DNA damage. **After 4-6 h** of temporary growth arrest, many **cells will exhibit up to a 40-fold transient adaptive response in which genes for oxidant protection and damage repair are preferentially expressed. After 18 h of H_2O_2 adaptation** (including the 4-6 h of temporary growth arrest) **cells exhibit maximal protection against oxidative stress.**

The **H_2O_2** originally added **is metabolized within 30-40 min,** and if no more is added the **cells will gradually de-adapt, so that by 36 h after the initial H_2O_2 stimulus they have returned to their original level of H_2O_2 sensitivity.** (Davies KJ. The broad spectrum of responses to oxidants in proliferating cells: a new paradigm for oxidative stress. IUBMB Life. 1999 Jul;48(1):41-7). This provides a time line for the secondary cellular effects of **H_2O_2.**

5 uM H_2O_2 is non-toxic (The Oxygen Paradox," Eds. K.J.A. Davies and F. Ursini. Cleup University Press, 1995. O_2 Paradox, page 574).

In 1976, the highly respected Dr. Klebanoff stated that H_2O_2 is one of the most important antimicrobial and antitumor weapons of polymorphonuclear leukocytes (Klebanoff SJ. Phagocytic cells: products of oxygen metabolism. In: Gallin JI,

Goldstein IM, Snyderman R, eds. Inflammation: basic principles and clinical correlates, 1 ed. New York: Raven Press Ltd, 1988).

Phagocytes are a key feature of defense against microorganisms (The Jeremiah Metzger Lecture. Microbial defenses against killing by phagocytes. Mandell GL, Frank MO. Trans Am Clin Climatol Assoc. 1992;103:199-209).

Hydrogen peroxide generated in mononuclear phagocytes and polymorphonuclear cells is of pivotal importance in the intracellular killing of several pathogens (Babior BM. Oxygen-dependent microbial killing by phagocytes (second of two parts). N Engl J Med. 1978 Mar 30;**298**(13):721–725).

Phagocytic cells attack and destroy invading organisms and cancer cells by consuming large amounts of oxygen in a process called **the "respiratory burst." Of the oxygen consumed, 70-90% is converted into the superoxide anion, which readily forms H_2O_2.** This action literally produces a peroxide spike.

Intracellular H_2O_2 molecules may also mediate, in part, the antineoplastic activity of macrophages (Nathan C, Cohn Z. Role of oxygen-dependent mechanisms in antibody-induced lysis of tumor cells by activated macrophages. J Exp Med. 1980 Jul; 152(1):198–208) (Nathan CF, Cohn ZA. Antitumor effects of hydrogen peroxide in vivo. J Exp Med. 1981 Nov 1;154(5):1539–1553). (see section 20.0)

Both nonlethal *Plasmodium yoelii* and lethal *Plasmodium berghei* **(malaria) were killed in vitro by hydrogen peroxide at concentrations as low as 10^{-5} M. Higher concentrations** were required in the presence of added normal erythrocytes. Injection of hydrogen peroxide in vivo significantly reduced *P. yoelii* parasitemia but had less effect on *P. berghei* (Dockrell, Hazel M.; Playfair, John H L. Killing of Blood-Stage Murine Malaria Parasites by Hydrogen Peroxide. Infect Immun. 1983 Jan;**39**(1):456–459).

Prof Randolph Michael Howes MD,PhD

Providing additional support for a potential therapeutic role for parenterally administered hydrogen peroxide, (Dockrell, HJ. M., and J. H. L. Playfair. 1983. Killing of blood-stage murine malaria parasites by hydrogen peroxide. Infect. Immun. 16:75-80) reported that **murine Plasmodium yoelii parasitemia was reduced after the intravenous administration of hydrogen peroxide**.

These observations, together with reports of successful infusions of hydrogen peroxide into patients (Mallams JT, Finney JW, Balla GA. The use of hydrogen peroxide as a source of oxygen in a regional intra-arterial infusion system. South Med J. 1962 Mar;**55**:230–232) (Oliver, T.H., and D.V. Murphy. 1920. Influenzal pneumonia: the intravenous injection of hydrogen peroxide. Lancet 1:432-433) (Balla GA, Finney JW, Aronoff BL, et al: Use of Intra-arterial Hydrogen Peroxide to Promote Wound Healing. Am J Surg 1964; 108: 621-629), **suggest that exogenous hydrogen peroxide might be effective in the therapy of selected infectious and neoplastic diseases.**

Researchers have long known that certain **bacteria are associated with a lower incidence of bacterial and yeast infection of the vagina.** It has been found that **the overall microbicidal activity of lactobacilli is primarily due to the presence in many women of species that produce hydrogen peroxide as well as lactic acid.** Studies comparing the incidence of STDs such as chlamydial infection, candidiasis, gonorrhea, and syphilis in women with and without peroxide-producing strains of vaginal lactobacilli show that **infection is much lower when peroxide-producing strains are present.** Even more intriguing, a number of studies now indicate that **the risk of acquiring HIV through heterosexual contact is also substantially lower in women with peroxide-producing lactobacilli (**Hillier SL. The vaginal microbial ecosystem and resistance to HIV. 1998;14(suppl 1):S17-S21**).**

Klebanoff et al. proposed that hydrogen peroxide-producing lactobacilli and peroxidase in the vagina of healthy women

might be responsible for the prevention of vaginosis and also might exert an antitumor effect (1). Based on recent evidence on superoxide anion generation by transformed cells (2,3) and on the potential of myeloperoxidase for selective apoptosis induction in transformed cells (4), a model for specific reactive oxygen species interaction during lactobacilli-mediated tumor control in the vagina is presented here. He proposed that **peroxidase, which converts hydrogen peroxide into hypochlorous acid, is responsible for creating a microbicidal vaginal milieu by maintaining a balanced, non-toxic, steady state level of the microbicides H_2O_2 and HOCl** (Lactobacilli-mediated control of vaginal cancer through specific reactive oxygen species interaction. Bauer G. Med Hypotheses 2001 Aug;57(2):252-7**).

Hydrogen Peroxide and Hydroxyl Radical Antineoplastic Cytotoxicity

The **cytotoxicity** of the clinically important antineoplastic quinones doxorubicin, mitomycin C, and diaziridinylbenzoquinone for the Ehrlich ascites carcinoma was **significantly reduced or abolished by the antioxidant enzymes catalase and superoxide dismutase, the hydroxyl radical scavengers dimethyl sulfoxide, diethylurea, and thiourea, and the iron chelators deferoxamine, 2,2-bipyridine, and diethylenetriaminepentaacetic acid. These results suggest that drug-induced hydrogen peroxide and hydroxyl radical production may play a role in the antineoplastic action of redox active anticancer quinones** (J H. Doroshow. Role of Hydrogen Peroxide and Hydroxyl Radical Formation in the Killing of Ehrlich Tumor Cells by Anticancer Quinones. PNAS June 15, 1986, vol. 83, no. 12, 4514-4518).

Ascorbic acid and ascorbic acid salts are preferentially toxic to tumour cells, which is thought to be related to intracellular generation of hydrogen peroxide (Tsao C, Dungham B and Ping Y. In vivo antineoplastic activity of ascorbic acid for human mammary

Prof Randolph Michael Howes MD,PhD

tumour. In vivo. 2: 147-50. 1988; Bram S et al.Vitamin C preferential toxicity for malignant melanoma cells. Nature. 284: 629-31. 1980).

Mark Levine's group published on line for PNAS on September 12, 2005 results showing that, "**Pharmacologic ascorbic acid concentrations selectively kill cancer cells: Action as a pro-drug to deliver hydrogen peroxide to tissues.**" Cell death was independent of metal chelators and absolutely dependent on H_2O_2 formation.

Oxidants such as H_2O_2, have been found to mimic the intracellular signals initiated by TCR (T cell receptors) aggregation and have also been used to study this signaling pathway. **In short, H_2O_2 can trigger T cell proliferation and activation.** (Wange, R. L., and Samelson, L. E. (1996) Immunity 5, 197-205).T cells are one of the most important components of the human immune system, which protects us from pathogens. **Patients with T Cell immunodeficiencies are prone to infections and to certain types of cancers, especially leukemias and lymphomas.** The immune system is vital to protect us against infectious agents (bacteria, viruses, fungi, protozoa and cancer) and there is strong evidence that our immune system uses H_2O_2 to fight infectious diseases and cancer.

One final note concerning the integrity of Dr. Mallams, insinuated by Dr. Bratman. Dr. Mallams has always been a man of unquestioned integrity.After his stent as head of radiology at Yale, he now resides in Florida and is restricted by age and health problems.

I consider the work of the Baylor University Medical School investigators to be of unequaled scientific importance and their medical studies serve as a model to demonstrate the safety of H_2O_2 in humans.

Please see section 8.1,Adverse Drug Reactions: Fatalities and Hemorrhage in my H_2O_2 monograph.

Perhaps we should look at factors more likely to cause adverse drug reactions other than H$_2$O$_2$ and which are considered to be causative of serious reactions and/or death (Hospitalizations caused by adverse drug reactions (ADR): a meta-analysis of observational studies. H.J Beijer and C.J. de Blaey. Pharmacy World & Science 2002 24:46-54.). A 2000 report published in JAMA by Barbara Starfield, M.D., MPH, showed that in the U.S. there are:

106,000 deaths/year from adverse effects of medications

80,000 deaths/year from nosocomial infections in hospitals

20,000 deaths/year from other errors in hospitals

12,000 deaths/year from unnecessary surgery

7,000 deaths/year from medication errors in hospitals

In the **2000 JAMA article, Dr. Barbara Starfield** presents well-documented facts that **the U.S. ranks 12th of 13 industrialized countries when judged by 16 health status indicators**. Starfield notes that many deaths attributable to medical error today are likely to be coded to indicate some other cause of death (JAMA 2000;284:483-485).

A five-country survey published in the *Journal of Health Affairs* found that 18-28% of people who were recently ill had suffered from a medical or drug error in the previous two years. The study surveyed 750 recently ill adults. The breakdown by country showed the percentages of those suffering a medical or drug error were 18% in Britain, 23% in Australia and in New Zealand, 25% in Canada, and **28% in the US**.

The Lazarou study analyzed records for prescribed medications for **33 million US hospital admissions from** four electronic databases which were searched from 1966 to 1996. **It discovered 2.2 million serious injuries due to prescribed drugs;** 2.1% of inpatients experienced a serious adverse drug reaction, 4.7% of all hospital admissions were due to a serious adverse drug reaction, and **fatal adverse drug reactions occurred in 0.19%** of inpatients and 0.13% of admissions. Starfield **estimated that 106,000 deaths occur annually due to adverse drug reactions.** Using a cost analysis from a 2000 study in which the increase in hospitalization costs per patient suffering an adverse drug reaction was $5,483, costs for the Lazarou study's 2.2 million patients with serious drug reactions amounted to $12 billion (Incidence of Adverse Drug Reactions in Hospitalized Patients: A Meta-analysis of Prospective Studies. Jason Lazarou, MSc; Bruce H. Pomeranz, MD, PhD; Paul N. Corey, PhD. *JAMA.* 1998;279:1200-1205).

According to Dr. Joseph Mercola, if you go into the hospital, there is a one in 15 chance that you will have an adverse reaction to a drug. Those are quite high numbers. Even more startling, is that **there is a one in 312 chance that the adverse reaction will result in death.** This is such a high number that it is the FIFTH leading cause of death in this country. It is important to remember that this analysis was only done for hospitalized patients. The number is clearly higher as many more prescriptions are written for patients outside of the hospital. (J Clin Pharm Ther. October, 2000;25(5):355-61).

In a survey of over 28,000 patients, ADRs (adverse drug reactions) were considered to be the cause of 3.4 percent of hospital admissions. Of these, 187 ADRs were coded as severe. Gastrointestinal complaints (19 percent) represented the most common events, followed by metabolic and **hemorrhagic complications (nine percent).** The drugs most frequently responsible for these ADRs were diuretics, calcium channel blockers, nonsteroidal antiinflammatory drugs and digoxin (Adverse drug reactions as cause of hospital admissions: results from the Italian Group of Pharmacoepidemiology in the Elderly (GIFA). Onder G,

Pedone C, Landi F, Cesari M, Della Vedova C, Bernabei R, Gambassi G. J Am Geriatr Soc. 2002 Dec;50(12):1962-8).

As was concluded in the article by Weingart et al, "For these reasons the precise prevalence and magnitude of medical error is unknown, but it is probably enormous. We are aware of no study showing that medical care can be provided without error. In fact, the more closely we examine patient care, the more error we find. No setting is free from hazards and no specialty is immune, and patients are at risk no matter what their age, sex, or health status." (Epidemiology of medical error. Saul N Weingart, Ross McL Wilson, Robert W Gibberd, Bernadette Harrison. *BMJ* 2000;320:774-777 (18 March).

Clearly, H_2O_2 does not cause anywhere near the adverse drug reactions or fatalities that are caused by common pharmaceuticals. Even common drugs such as aspirin and Tylenol (acetaminophen) cause far more deaths in a single year, than H_2O_2 has caused in its entire recorded history. H_2O_2 has one of the safest records in clinical use that I can find, including topical, oral and intravenous routes of administration. This is not to say that it can not cause a fatality but this outcome has only occurred when it was used in inappropriate concentrations, was inappropriately administered (i.e., accidentally) or was administered without medical supervision.

CONCLUSION

In general, I believe that most physicians have very little, if any, scientific knowledge concerning the crucial role that H_2O_2 occupies in the maintenance of our cellular redox status and in the modulation of homeostasis. Additionally, I believe that they have the erroneous impression that there can be minimal benefit, or perhaps harm, from oxidative therapeutic interventions in the treatment of human diseases, since the old school's flawed teachings associated reactive oxygen species with widespread disease causation. Fortunately, that has changed.

Prof Randolph Michael Howes MD,PhD

In my opinion, which I based on available worldwide scientific medical information, the following are the answers to the key questions: A) Is intravenous 0.03% H_2O_2 safe or lethal, when used in humans? and B) Are the breakdown products of H_2O_2 safe or lethal when H_2O_2 is combined with human blood?

Intravenous 0.03% H_2O_2, when given as an infusion over a 1-3 hour period is safe in humans. At this concentration and rate of infusion, I see no significant risk of air embolism or of hemolysis of erythrocytes.

The breakdown products of H_2O_2 by human catalase are ground state oxygen and water. Both of these molecules are absolute and necessary requirements to sustain human life and to maintain a redox condition of health and homeostasis.

Prof. Randolph M. Howes, M.D., Ph.D.
Adjunct Assistant Professor of Plastic Surgery,
The Johns Hopkins Hospital
Baltimore, Maryland, USA

http://www.pbraunmd.org/pbraunmd/howes_response_to_bratman_on_h₂o₂.pdf

CANCER THERAPY: A REVIEW WITH SCIENTIFIC VALIDATION FOR THE ROLE OF ELECTRONICALLY MODIFIED OXYGEN DERIVATIVES IN ONCOLOGIC TREATMENT MODALITIES

Prof. Hon. Randolph M. Howes, M.D., Ph.D.

Adjunct Assistant Professor of Plastic Surgery, The Johns Hopkins Hospital, Baltimore, Md., U.S.A., Espaldon Professor of Plastic and Reconstructive Surgery, University of Santo Tomas, Manila, Philippines. Adjunct Professor of Biological Sciences, Southeastern Louisiana University, Hammond, La.

Address for communication: 27439 Highway 441, Kentwood, Louisiana 70444-8152, USA. Email: rhowesmd@hughes.net

Abstract

The American Cancer Society and the British Columbia Cancer Agency state that electronically modified oxygen derivatives, such as hydrogen peroxide and other "oxidative therapies," are basically ineffective, harmful or even lethal in the treatment of cancer. A compelling body of evidence over the past few decades demands that the therapeutic role of oxygen derivatives be reevaluated. The free radical theory defined oxygen free radicals or reactive oxygen species as being destructive and as the cause of the majority of common human diseases. Yet, decades of experimentation have shown that the free radical theory lacks predictability, fails to meet the requirements of the scientific method and is therefore invalidated. This nullification requires reexamination of oxidative oncologic complementary, alternative and integrative treatment modalities.

Prooxidants, some of which are oxygen free radicals or reactive oxygen species, have been blamed for cancer causation and unscrupulous marketers have brought discredit to oxygen based therapies and disregard to oxidative centered treatments. In contrast, a review of currently effective tumoricidal methods reveals a "commonality of oxygen based, anti-neoplastic action," in that many successful cytotoxic agents, procedures or methods have been shown to proceed primarily via prooxidants. Discussions will compare chemotherapy, radiation therapy, megadose intravenous vitamin C therapy, photodynamic therapy, sonodynamic therapy, the Howes' singlet oxygen tumoricidal system, ozone therapy, hyperbaric oxygen therapy and hydrogen peroxide therapy. Various prooxidant delivery systems currently offer beneficial, unique tumoricidal properties and approach the "Holy Grail" for cancer treatments, allowing for selective killing of cancer cells while sparing normal cells. This review describes these prooxidant EMOD agents and areas of possible complementarity of oxidative therapies (prooxidant stacking) based on the available scientific literature. Decades of scientific study have shown that prooxidant antineoplastic therapeutic agents provide significant clinical advantage and offer safe, effective and economical promise in the future treatment of cancer.

Introduction

The widely held flawed notions promulgated by the free radical theory have so biased world orthodoxy, regarding the true role of oxygen in disease causation and prevention that it is best to start over with a new, well configured, open minded scientific paradigm. To this end, prior "oxidative" prejudicial terminology will be eschewed.

Unproven therapies and misrepresented products, offered over the internet and at various clinics, local and abroad, have created a generalized negative attitude towards so-called "oxygen therapies" and "oxidative medicine," because it has been used to refer to any number of worthless products or ineffective treatments, which were not based on scientific facts regarding oxygen metabolism. The therapeutic potential of prooxidant electronically modified oxygen derivatives (EMODs) have been demonstrated for decades by their use in academic oncology treatment programs. Many so-called oxidative therapies prompted the British Columbia Cancer Agency (a part of the Canadian Provincial Health Services Authority) and the American Cancer Society (ACS) to recommend against their use. These therapies go by many names including "Oxygen Therapies, Hyperoxygenation Therapy, Oxymedicine, Bio-Oxidative Therapy, Oxidative Therapy, Oxidology, Ozone therapy, Autohemotherapy, Hydrogen peroxide therapy and Germanium sesquioxide therapy." To be sure, some of these approaches are subject to fraudulent practices and lack credibility but others are based on a solid scientific principles and investigations. (ACS website accessed 12-7-09).

The BC Cancer Agency website presents the following summary: "Patients with cancer should not consider oxygen therapies as either alternative (first-line) or adjunct (complementary) therapies. Researchers now understand that cancer cells "lower-than-normal respiration" is due to the fact that tissue surrounding cancer cells receives less oxygen because it has fewer blood vessels feeding it. Oxygen therapies have not been found useful against cancer and are not used as mainstream cancer treatments." They also state that, "Oxygen therapy can destroy cells, including those of the blood-forming organs. Very high doses can seriously damage health or even cause death." (BC Cancer Agency website accessed 8-31-09).

The American Cancer Society website gives the following overview: "Available scientific evidence does not support claims that putting oxygen-releasing chemicals into a person's body is effective in treating cancer. It may even be dangerous. There have been reports of patient deaths from this method."

Contrary to disputed statements of major cancer agencies, this review clearly demonstrates that prooxidant EMODs have been scientifically confirmed as essential, effective and safe clinical agents in the battle against cancer. Undeniably, for decades, prooxidant EMOD cancer therapeutic modalities have been a mainstay for our most effective oncologic treatment programs, which utilize chemotherapy, radiation therapy and photodynamic therapy.

Simultaneously, a persuasive assemblage of scientific data shows that EMODs are crucial agents for gene regulation, maintenance of cellular oxidation/reduction (redox) homeostasis and pathogen and neoplasia protection.

At first glance, oxygen has obvious medical benefits in emergency or critical care situations but upon closer review of the available scientific literature, it becomes readily apparent that EMODs have already made significant contributions in fighting disease, maintaining healthy homeostasis and in combatting cancer. As it relates to cancer therapy, prooxidant EMOD-induced apoptosis and necrosis is currently used in a wide spectrum of modalities to successfully treat neoplasia. There appears to be "a prooxidant point of convergence" in these EMOD applications, which includes a role in chemotherapy, radiation therapy, intravenous vitamin C mega-dose therapy, photodynamic therapy, sonodynamic therapy, the Howes singlet oxygen tumoricidal system, ozone therapy, hyperbaric oxygen therapy and intravenous hydrogen peroxide therapy.

Conversely, hypoxia and so-called antioxidants can effectively modify or block cancer cell kill by interfering with electronically modified oxygen derivative (EMOD)-induced apoptosis. EMODs possess the levels of reactivity to serve as tumoricidal agents.

Ground state triplet oxygen (O_2) does not have the same level of reactivity as the prooxidants referred to in this article, such as: the superoxide anion ($O_2 \cdot -$), hydrogen peroxide (H_2O_2), metastable excited singlet oxygen ($^1O_2^*$), the hydroxyl radical

(OH.), hypochlorous acid (HOCl), nitric oxide (NO), peroxynitrite (OONO-), ozone (O_3), etc. However, ground state triplet oxygen serves as the source for the production of the entire family of EMOD agents. EMODs are formed by basic alterations of the electron structure of ground state triplet oxygen, such as addition or removal of electrons, altered electron spin configurations, altered pi electron orbital positions, combinations with nitrogen, exposure to ultraviolet light or wave specific white light, altered pressure other than atmospheric, etc.

Gathering EMOD agents into inaccurate and misleading categorizations is no longer suitable with the use of terms such as oxygen free radials or reactive oxygen species. The usage of incorrect biochemical terminology is no longer acceptable and its taint must be abandoned. Ignorance of the literature does not allow health care agencies the latitude of making scientifically unsupported statements. As Carl Nathan said in a 2003 *Journal of Clinical Investigation* article, "terms of discourse" need to be addressed.

Because of the common use of varying terms, such as reactive oxygen species (ROS), reactive oxygen intermediates (ROI), reactive oxygen metabolites (ROM), active oxygen species (AOS), oxygen species (OS), etc., confusion abounds as to precise nature of the oxygen entities being discussed in various articles. Thus, in 2005, in *The Medical and Scientific Significance of Oxygen Free Radical Metabolism*. pg. 39, I stated, "It is also time to discard ROS, RONS, OS, ROI, ROM, AOS, etc. and utilize a more meaningful and accurate term. I propose the term "electronically modified oxygen derivative(s)" (EMODs). This term does not imply charge, radicality, or reactivity. It merely indicates that an electron(s) of oxygen has (have) been altered or changed from its ground state orbit. This avoids all of the inaccuracies of terms such as reactive oxygen species, reactive oxygen metabolites, or oxygen intermediates, all of which should be discarded from usage. Thus, EMODs include superoxide anion, singlet oxygen, hydrogen peroxide, hypochlorous acid, peroxynitrite, hydroxyl radical, nitric oxide, alkyl radicals, alkoxyl radicals, etc. The term does not limit itself to oxygen covalent bonding or hydrogen abstraction and addition. Thus, oxygen-containing sulfates, nitrates, phosphates, etc. would also qualify as EMODs. Further, it includes all of the nitrative and oxidative forms of oxygen."

Further, according to Barry Halliwell, EMODs such as superoxide anion are barely "reactive" at all and are redox ambivalent at a physiological pH. EMODS, such as hydrogen peroxide, singlet oxygen, ozone and hypochlorous acid are not free radicals but are frequently erroneously placed in this chemical category.

In 1971, President Nixon launched the "War Against Cancer," which was designed to fight the escalating incidence of cancer that had assumed epidemic proportions. According to Samuel S. Epstein's book, *Cancer-GATE: How to Win the Losing Cancer War*, only incremental progress has been made in this overall crusade. The development of agents that improve or enhance the efficacy of cancer therapy is one of the most important areas of research in current medical oncology. Biological oxidation/reduction (redox) reactions are central to metabolism, cellular energy production and cancer therapy.

Many *in vitro* studies have shown support of prooxidant cancer therapies and even though it should not be assumed that they will be identically effective *in vivo* in the cure of cancer, clinical studies cited in this review are increasingly showing support for this thesis.

Discussion

Harman's free radical theory

Harman's free radical theory hypothesized that diseases, such as cancer and aging, resulted from the random or "stochastic" accumulation of oxidative damage purportedly caused by EMODs, from environmental sources and from by-products of normal cellular metabolism. [1-5] When investigators found that their results were not as predicted by the free radical theory, they either discounted their results or referred to them as a paradox. Countless examples of this are in the literature but can be best illustrated by the 1995 tome edited by Kelvin J.A. Davies and Fulvio Ursini entitled, *THE OXYGEN PARADOX.*

The alleged damaging derivatives of oxygen were defined as being inherently deleterious and harmful. However, this notion has been rebuffed by Howes.[6] Apoptosis, necrosis, and growth arrest have been shown to be regulated to a significant degree by prooxidant EMOD species.[7-10] Apoptosis, in part, controls the neoplastic process as genetically damaged or mutated cells can be eliminated by inducement of the apoptotic process.[11] Apoptosis involves caspases (cysteine proteases cleaving after particular aspartate residues), mitochondrial pathways and/or EMODs, which are usually, but not always, key components.[12] Many apoptosis-inducing agents function as prooxidants *in vitro.*[13]

Prooxidant EMOD generating agents have repeatedly been shown to kill cancer cells selectively, while sparing normal cells and this tumoricidal action can be modified or blocked by antioxidants, which may accelerate cancer growth both *in vitro* and *in vivo.*[14-17] Since therapeutic agents (radiation therapy, chemotherapy or photodynamic therapy, PDT) work, to a considerable extent, by releasing prooxidant free radicals (EMODs), it is logical that antioxidants likely interfere with their action. EMOD levels and cellular redox tone appear to be uniquely exploitable targets in cancer chemoprevention via the stimulation or induction of cytoprotection in normal cells and/or the induction of apoptosis in transformed malignant cells.

Antioxidants and apoptosis

Yet, some believe that antioxidants may play a central role in apoptosis and cancer therapy. Some investigators have made claims that antioxidants can actually kill cancer cells and argue

that antioxidants are beneficial during chemotherapy. A review
on the use of antioxidants during chemotherapy, published
in Cancer Treatment Reviews, was a collaborative effort
led by Dr. Keith Block and researchers from the University
of Illinois at Chicago and M.D. Anderson Cancer Center in
Houston. After reviewing articles, only 33 of 965 articles
considered, including 2,446 subjects, met the inclusion criteria.
Antioxidants evaluated were: glutathione, melatonin, vitamin A,
an antioxidant mixture, N-acetylcysteine, vitamin E, selenium,
L-carnitine, Co-Q10 and ellagic acid. Nine studies reported
no difference in toxicities between the 2 groups. Only 1 study
(vitamin A) reported a significant increase in toxicity in the
antioxidant group. This review provides some evidence that
antioxidant supplementation during chemotherapy might
reduce dose-limiting toxicities but it must be kept in mind
that many of these so-called antioxidants have considerable
prooxidant activity to which their salutary effects could also
be attributed. Larger, well-designed studies of antioxidants
impact on PDT, chemotherapy and tumoricidal radiation
therapy are warranted. [18]

However, until such data is available, considerations for
utmost patient safety must prevail. The mechanisms of action
of chemotherapeutic drugs and antioxidants are sufficiently
understood to predict their resultant interactions and to suggest
that considerable care should be exercised with respect to
both clinical decisions and study interpretations. [19] Additionally,
antioxidants have a wide variety of biochemical actions and are
capable of interfering selectively with EMOD initiation, propagation
and termination. EMODs have been studied for their positive effects
in the prevention or cure of many cancers, cardiovascular disease,
age-related diseases, and other disorders. [20-23]

Nonetheless, there seems to be agreement that the antioxidant
N-acetylcysteine (NAC), a derivative of the naturally occurring
amino acid cysteine, should be avoided by cancer patients because of

studies showing interference with chemotherapeutic agents, such as cisplatin and doxorubicin. [24, 25] A 2005 report concluded that cancer patients should avoid antioxidant supplements while receiving chemotherapy or radiation treatment. [26] Directed towards informing the public, a *Wall Street Journal* article argued that antioxidants could block the beneficial effects of standard cancer therapy. [27]

Those who recommend the use of antioxidants in cancer patients claim that antioxidants such as vitamin C, vitamin E, coenzyme Q10, glutathione, and selenium can reduce the toxicity of free radicals. [28-31] Thus, EMOD-induced prooxidant apoptosis and the cancer conundrum leave us with unanswered questions regarding their interactions, auto-oxidation of antioxidants and the prooxidant character of many antioxidants. [32]

A 2007 article not only defends the use of antioxidants in cancer patients, it states that, "In 15 human studies, 3,738 patients who took non-prescription antioxidants and other nutrients actually had increased survival." [33] In contrast, a 2008 article in the *Journal of the National Cancer Institute* reviewed randomized trial data, which suggested that cancer patients should avoid the routine use of antioxidant supplements because they may potentially decrease the efficacy of cancer therapy by protecting the tumor and reducing survival. They looked at clinical trials investigating the impact of antioxidants on radiation therapy and found evidence suggesting that antioxidant supplementation reduced overall survival. [34]

Hypoxia (low oxygen levels)

Threshold levels of oxygen (O_2)

Hypoxia (defined as the fraction of measured O_2 partial pressures of <5 mmHg) is a statistically significant adverse prognostic factor of disease-free survival. Considerable data indicates that low O_2 in tumor cells is an adverse prognostic sign. In general, low tumor O_2 is associated with: increased aggressiveness of primary cancerous lesions, their ability to metastasize, and an increased resistance to treatments with irradiation, chemotherapeutics and surgery.

In general, median O_2 partial pressures of less than 10 mmHg result in intracellular acidosis, ATP depletion, a drop in the energy supply and increasing levels of inorganic phosphate. Mitochondrial oxidative phosphorylation is limited at O_2 partial pressures of less than approximately 0.5 mmHg but there are exceptions to this generality.

Overall, a number of key findings have been described as follows: 1) most tumors have lower median O_2 partial pressures than their tissue of origin; 2) many solid tumors contain areas of low O_2 partial pressure than cannot be predicted by clinical size, stage, grade, histology and site; 3) tumor-to-tumor variability in oxygenation is usually greater than intra-tumoral variability in oxygenation; and 4) recurring tumors have a poorer oxygenation status than the corresponding primary tumors.

Cancer cell apoptosis or cellular suicide (apoptotic execution) is considered to be a needed means for controlling the growth or proliferation of neoplastic cells, which is highly desirable and the goal of cancer therapy.

Tumor hypoxia and oxygen deficiency is strongly implicated in the growth of tumors and is a known adverse factor in the effectiveness of conventional radiation and chemotherapy. [35, 36] Hypoxia can induce programmed (apoptotic) cell death in normal and neoplastic cells. The level of p53 in cells increases under hypoxic conditions, and the increased level of p53 induces apoptosis by a pathway involving Apaf-1 and caspase-9 as downstream effectors. [37] However, hypoxia also initiates p53-dependent apoptosis pathways involving hypoxia-inducible factor-1 (HIF-1), genes of the BCL-2 family, and other unidentified genes. [38]

Hypoxia stimulates the transcription of glycolytic enzymes, glucose transporters (GLUT1 and GLUT3), angiogenic molecules, survival and growth factors (e.g. vascular endothelial growth factor [VEGF], angiogenin, platelet-derived growth factor-B, transforming growth factor-B, and insulin-like growth factor-II), enzymes, proteins involved in tumor invasiveness (e.g., urokinases-type plasminogen activator), chaperones, nuclear factor kB (NFkB) and other resistance-related proteins.

Anoxia/hypoxia-induced proteome changes in neoplastic and stroma cells may lead to the arrest or impairment of neoplastic growth through molecular mechanisms, resulting in cellular quiescence, differentiation, apoptosis and necrosis. Cells exposed to hypoxia are generally arrested at the G1/S-phase boundary.[39] Under anoxia, most cells are arrested immediately, regardless of their position in the cell cycle.

Studies on tumors of the uterine cervix have demonstrated that tumor hypoxia is independent of patient and tumor characteristics such as, patient age, menopausal status, and parity, International Federation of Gynecology and Obstetrics (FIGO) stage, clinical tumor size, histopathological and grade of malignancy. In fact, tumor oxygenation was the strongest independent prognostic factor.[40]

Adequate levels of oxygen are essential to effectively generate adequate tumoricidal prooxidant EMOD levels and to kill a wide range of cancer cell types and tumor hypoxia can be a serious limiting factor in reducing the effectiveness of radiotherapy, some O_2-dependent cytotoxic agents and photodynamic therapy.[41]

Prooxidant Chemotherapeutic Agents

Cancer therapy can be aimed at the cell cycle, which consists of four phases, i.e., the G_1, S, G_2, and M phases. Based on their specificity, chemotherapy drugs can be classified as cell-specific agents (effective during certain cell cycle phases) and cell-cycle non-specific (effective during all phases of the cell cycle). Based on their specific characteristics and nature of treatment, chemotherapeutic agents can be classified as alkylating agents, anti-metabolites, anthracyclines,

451

antitumor antibiotics, monoclonal antibodies, platinums, or plant alkaloids.

Prooxidant EMOD production by chemotherapeutic agents

Many chemotherapeutic drugs have well-defined mechanisms of actions, including traditional alkylating agents and anthracycline antitumor antibiotics, which generate EMODs. Depending upon specifics of oxidation/reduction potentials, these EMODs are uniformly subject to transformation to altered compounds by antioxidants through the simple process of electron transfer.

Doxorubicin, arsenic-induced apoptosis and 2-Methoxyestradiol induced apoptosis

Antineoplastic therapy can be based on the cell cycle and/or it can be based on the involvement of electronically modified oxygen derivatives (EMODs), formerly called oxygen free radicals or reactive oxygen species. These prooxidant EMOD reactants induce apoptosis and appear to be essential as activators for removing or killing cells that have accumulated mutations. 2-Methoxyestradiol induces apoptosis in Ewing sarcoma cells through mitochondrial hydrogen peroxide production. [42-44] Daunorubicin and doxorubicin can undergo redox cycling and produce EMODs, which can have a variety of effects, including damage to cell membranes and DNA-damage. [45]

Bleomycin and doxorubicin

Bleomycin and doxorubicin are two agents known to generate prooxidant oxygen species. [46] In reactions involving Fe(II) and oxygen, an "activated" bleomycin species is formed that damages DNA through free radical intermediates. [47] Superoxide and hydrogen peroxide can also react with Fe(II) or Fe(III) bleomycin, respectively, to produce the activated form of the drug. DNA damage from bleomycin and ionizing radiation is similar in both induction and repair. [48]

Tamoxifen, doxorubicin, mitomycin C, etoposide and cisplatin

Many chemotherapeutic drugs, such as tamoxifen, doxorubicin, mitomycin C, etoposide and cisplatin are superoxide (EMOD) generating agents and induce oxidative stress and apoptosis. [49, 50]

Anthracyclines

Reduction in EMOD levels generated by chemotherapeutic agents has the same effect as a reduction in dose. [51] NADPH-flavin reductase, cytochrome p450 reductase and mitochondrial NADH reductase can all reduce anthracyclines to a semiquinone radical. [52] This semiquinone radical can donate its free electron to molecular oxygen to generate the superoxide radical ($O_2^{\cdot-}$). [52] Like hydrogen peroxide (H_2O_2), $O_2^{\cdot-}$ can generate hydroxyl radicals ($^{\cdot}OH$) upon interaction with metal ions. [52] This results in lipid peroxidation of plasma membranes, leading to a loss of mitochondrial inner membrane potential and consequent cytochrome c release and apoptosis. EMODs can also directly damage DNA through generation of strand breaks and oxidized nucleic bases such as guanine to 8-hydroxyguanine, giving rise to G-T transversions. [52]

However, as a caution, free radical generation by anthracyclines is thought to be responsible for the cardiotoxicity that puts some limits on their therapeutic use. [53, 54]

Additional prooxidant EMOD apoptosis inducing agents

Ideal treatment should aim to selectively kill the cancer cells, without harming normal cells. Elegant regulation of prooxidant EMOD levels may be a means to this exalted goal.

Cancer therapy seeks to utilize the sensitivity of transformed cells towards apoptotic signals, which allows the execution of apoptotic cell death. [55, 56] Contrary to Harman's free radical theory in which

EMODs are only deleterious, EMODs have been found to play a crucial beneficial role in intracellular apoptotic execution (cellular suicide). [57-61]

Glioma pathogenesis-related protein 1 (GLIPR1), a p53 target gene

Glioma pathogenesis-related protein 1 (GLIPR1), a novel p53 target gene, is down-regulated by methylation in prostate cancer and has p53-dependent and -independent proapoptotic properties in tumorous cells. Investigators reported that the expression of GLIPR1 is significantly reduced in human prostate tumor tissues compared with adjacent normal prostate tissues and in multiple human cancer cell lines and that overexpression of GLIPR1 in cancer cells leads to suppression of colony growth and induction of apoptosis. Mechanistic analysis indicated that GLIPR1 up-regulation increases EMOD production leading to apoptosis through activation of the c-Jun–NH$_2$ kinase (JNK) signaling cascade. These results identify GLIPR1 as a proapoptotic tumor suppressor acting through EMODs and the ROS-JNK pathway and support the therapeutic potential for this protein. [62]

Elesclomol (formerly STA-4783)

Elesclomol (formerly STA-4783) is a novel small molecule undergoing clinical evaluation in a pivotal phase III melanoma trial (SYMMETRY). In a phase II randomized, double-blinded, controlled, multi-center trial in 81 patients with stage IV metastatic melanoma, treatment with elesclomol plus paclitaxel showed a statistically significant doubling of progression-free survival time compared with treatment with paclitaxel alone. Elesclomol induces apoptosis in cancer cells through the induction of oxidative stress (EMOD generation). Treatment of cancer cells *in vitro* with elesclomol resulted in the rapid generation of EMODs and the induction of a transcriptional gene profile characteristic of an oxidative stress response. Inhibition of oxidative stress by the antioxidant N-acetylcysteine (NAC) blocked the induction of gene transcription by elesclomol. In addition, N-acetylcysteine blocked drug-induced apoptosis, indicating that EMOD generation is the primary mechanism responsible for the proapoptotic activity of elesclomol. Excessive EMOD production and elevated levels of oxidative stress is believed by some to cause critical biochemical alterations that contribute to cancer cell growth. Thus, the induction of oxidative stress by elesclomol exploits this unique characteristic of cancer cells by increasing EMOD levels beyond a threshold that triggers cell death. [63]

Imexon

The antitumor agent imexon activates oxidative stress and antioxidant gene expression, which is evidence for EMOD production. Results show that a predominant biological effect of imexon is a change in redox state that can be detected in surrogate normal tissues as increased redox-sensitive transcription factor binding, EMOD generation and increased antioxidant gene expression. [64]

Chaetocin

Investigators found that Chaetocin, a thiodioxopiperazine natural product previously unreported to have anticancer effects, was found to have potent antimyeloma activity in IL-6–dependent and –independent myeloma cell lines in freshly collected sorted and unsorted patient CD138+ myeloma cells and in vivo. Chaetocin displays superior ex vivo antimyeloma activity and selectivity than does doxorubicin and dexamethasone, and dexamethasone- or doxorubicin-resistant myeloma cell lines are largely non–cross-resistant to chaetocin. Mechanistically, chaetocin is dramatically accumulated in cancer cells via a process inhibited by glutathione and requiring intact/unreduced disulfides for uptake. Its anticancer (antimyeloma) in vitro and in vivo activity appears to be mediated primarily via the imposition of oxidative stress (prooxidant EMODs) and consequent apoptosis induction. [65]

PCI-24781 (histone deacetylase [HDAC] inhib)

Investigators examined the cytotoxicity and mechanisms of cell death of the broad-spectrum histone deacetylase (HDAC) inhibitor PCI-24781, alone and combined with bortezomib in Hodgkin lymphoma and non-Hodgkin lymphoma cell lines and primary lymphoproliferative (CLL/SLL) cells. PCI-24781 resulted in increased EMODs, oxidative stress and NF-κB inhibition, leading to caspase-dependent apoptosis. They showed that bortezomib is synergistic with PCI-24781. This combination or PCI-24781 alone has potential therapeutic value in lymphoma. [66]

Zinc

Zinc is becoming increasingly important in regulating cancer cell growth and proliferation. Investigators showed that the anticancer agent motexafin gadolinium (MGd) disrupted zinc metabolism in A549 lung cancer cells, leading, in the presence of exogenous zinc, to cell death. They reported the effect of MGd and exogenous zinc on intracellular levels of free zinc, oxidative stress, proliferation, and cell death in exponential phase human B-cell lymphoma and other hematologic cell lines. They found that increased levels of oxidative stress, EMOD production and intracellular free zinc precede and correlate with cell cycle arrest and apoptosis. [67]

Quinones

Many naturally occurring quinones can be isolated from biological tissues. [68] Also, chemotherapeutic drugs (adriamycin, daunorubicin, and mitomycin), acetaminophen (Tylenol), and air pollutants (cigarette smoke and automobile exhaust) are common source of quinones. Some quinones have potential to markedly induce the generation of prooxidant EMODs and may serve as the molecular mechanism of quinone cytotoxicity. [68]

Radiation Therapy

Hypoxic cancer cells are radio-resistant, which contributes dramatically to the inability of radiotherapy to control neoplastic growth and metastasis. Methods or therapies that provide increased prooxidant oxygen to cancer cells help radiation work more effectively by enabling more EMOD or free-radical formation. Radiation kills cancer cells by concentrating massive amounts of prooxidant free radicals directly into tumors.

Ionized radiation releases reactive oxygen species, i.e., EMODs, from the water molecule. [69] Thus cancer patients who undergo radiation therapy may be exposed to significant quantities of reactive prooxidant species. This may produce overkill or generate dangerously high prooxidant levels in areas outside of the treatment target site. Radiotherapy aims to alter cellular homeostasis, modify signal transduction pathways, alter redox states and induce cellular apoptosis. Exposure to ionizing radiation produces prooxidant oxygen-derived free radicals including hydroxyl radicals (the most damaging), superoxide anion radicals, hydrogen peroxide and other oxidants. [70]

And finally, as reported on 2-04-09 in the journal Nature, Stanford researcher, Robert Cho, found that breast cancer stem cells make much higher levels of protective antioxidants than other cancer cells. Use of a drug to block the antioxidant, glutathione, caused the cancer stem cells to become far more vulnerable to radiation. Using cells from mice and human breast cancer, the antioxidant glutathione protected the cancer cells from being killed by radiation EMOD-induced apoptosis.

However, even though EMODs are effective in killing tumor cells, they may threaten the integrity and survival of surrounding normal cells, which is dependent upon inherent tissue sensitivity and repair. Yet, the bottom line is that oxygen and its prooxidant EMOD agents are usually essential for effective radiation therapy and the induction of either apoptosis and/or necrosis.

Hydrogen Peroxide Therapy

Hydrogen peroxide appears to have medical attributes but has received little support in modern medicine. Hydrogen peroxide (H_2O_2) is a moderate oxidant that induces apoptosis of tumor cells *in vitro*. [71]

Even though the Baylor group's research on cancer, heart disease, wound healing and infections in the 1960s on hydrogen peroxide was ground breaking, it has remained in obscurity. Still, it teaches the therapeutic potential of hydrogen peroxide in the treatment of cancer, wound healing, atherosclerosis, shock management and infectious diseases. Peroxide has been used widely in Europe and has had an impressive record of safety and effectiveness.

Many clinical and experimental applications of hydrogen peroxide have been demonstrated. In over 300 patients regional intra-arterial hydrogen peroxide potentiated the effect of radiation therapy for malignancy involving the head, neck, pelvis and retro-peritoneum. [72] Increased localization of radioactive isotopes in malignant tumors was achieved by regional and intra-arterial infusion of hydrogen peroxide. [73, 74] Oxygen enhanced environments were shown to be bactericidal for most clostridia species and inhibited alpha toxin release. Hyperbaric oxygen was shown to be a beneficial adjunct to therapy in Bacteroides fragilis, Fusobacterium infections and nonclostridial anaerobic soft tissue infections. [75]

Results with hyperbaric oxygen are similar to that obtained by the Baylor investigators using intra-arterial and intra-venous H_2O_2.

Hydrogen peroxide appears to have two distinct effects. It initially inhibits the caspases_ and delays apoptosis. Then, depending on the degree of the initial oxidative stress, the_caspases are activated and the cells die by apoptosis, or they remain inactive and necrosis occurs. [76, 77] Some investigators believe that AIDS and cancer can be helped with hydrogen peroxide because of its induction of interferon-gamma production and its interactions which can produce a wide variety of oxygen derivatives. [78]

In a simple but rather elegant experiment, Davies showed that cellular division or cell death is EMOD concentration dependent, when utilizing the EMOD, H_2O_2. Cellular responses go from proliferation, to arrest, to apoptosis. [77] Those opposing hydrogen peroxide use have accused it of acting as a "genotoxicant or epigenetic" agent but although H_2O_2 can cause DNA damage, it is, at best, a very weak mutagen in mammalian cells. [79]

Intravenous Vitamin C Megadoses and Hydrogen Peroxide

Vitamin C (ascorbate, ascorbic acid) has had a controversial history in the prevention of cancer. Based on the pioneering work of Dr. Hugh Riordan, there have been some significant subsequent developments. One clinical case report by Drisko et al showed that vitamin C together with other oxidants, when added adjunctively to first-line chemotherapy, prevented recurrence in two ovarian cancer patients. [80] This high dose, intravenous vitamin C therapy was believed to operate through the generation of hydrogen peroxide. Ascorbate-mediated cell death was due to protein-dependent extracellular H_2O_2 generation (i.e., prooxidant EMOD generation). Ascorbate, an electron-donor in such reactions, ironically initiates prooxidant chemistry and H_2O_2 formation. It was concluded that ascorbate at pharmacologic concentrations in blood is a pro-drug for H_2O_2 delivery to tissues. [81, 82]

Vitamin C acts as a cosubstrate for hydroxylase and oxygenase enzymes for the biosynthesis of procollagen, carnitine, and neurotransmitters. [83] These enzymes produce EMODs and ascorbate acts as a cosubstrate for them and thus, acts as a prooxidant. [84] Chen et al showed that at pharmacologic concentrations, ascorbate acts as a prooxidant, hydrogen peroxide generating agent, which exhibits selective cytotoxicity towards a wide variety of cancer cells *in vitro* and *in vivo*. [85, 86] Even though there is much to be discovered in the ascorbate and hydrogen peroxide system, this appears to be an area of great potential. [87]

Yet, in contrast, several vitamin C and iron co-supplementation studies, both in animals and humans, indicate that vitamin C inhibits rather than promotes iron-dependent oxidative damage. [88]

Photodynamic Therapy

Photodynamic therapy (PDT) holds considerable promise in treating cancer but current terminology leads to confusion.

First, we need a definition of terms:

> Phototherapy - light, UV, etc., is shown on to the skin, such as treating hyperbilirubinemia in babies.
> Photochemotherapy - uses a photosensitizer like, psoralin
> Photodynamic therapy - uses a photosensitizer given to the patient to produce $^1O_2$* (excited singlet oxygen).
> Photo-oxidative therapy - also referred to as photo irradiative therapy, uses UV light shown on blood which is returned to the body.
> Bio-oxidative therapy - aerobic exercise.
> Autohemotherapy - ozone.
> Photodynamic effect - a photon is absorbed by a photosensitizer and raises it to its lowest triplet excited state, it diffuses until it collides with O_2 and raises it to its lowest singlet state.

Photodynamic therapy requires a photosensitive compound and a light source (usually a laser) capable of energizing electrons to higher orbitals (excited states). These excited molecules in turn excite triplet oxygen to one of its singlet excited states in accordance with the amount of energy transferred to oxygen's outer orbital electrons.

The unique property of photosensitizers to selectively accumulate in malignant and dysplastic tissues is exploited in the treatment of malignancies. PDT can selectively destroy tumors with this simple concept. Compared to surgery and conventional thermal Yag and argon laser treatment, there is much less damage and disruption of the underlying and adjacent normal tissue structures with photodynamic therapy, since there is essentially no thermal damage to the tissues. Superficial treatments do not require sterile theater conditions and can be delivered in an outpatient setting. There is little post-treatment discomfort and the only significant side effect is residual photosensitivity.

Availability of ground state oxygen within the tumor can dramatically influence and limit direct tumor cell kill.[89] Photodynamic therapy (PDT) is a novel therapeutic method for the treatment of malignant tumors, which utilizes prooxidant EMOD generation and in particular metastable singlet oxygen ($^1O_2^*$). By combining PDT with hyperoxygenation, any underlying hypoxic condition is improved and the cell killing rate at various time points after PDT is dramatically enhanced.[90,91]

In 1991, investigators described an apoptotic response to PDT.[92] Prooxidant species, especially singlet oxygen, produced by photosensitization or derived from cytotoxic agents, can activate apoptotic pathways.[93] However, malignant cell types can exhibit an impaired ability to undergo apoptosis. PDT-mediated oxidative stress induces a transient increase in the downstream early response genes c-fos, c-jun, c-myc, and egr-1.[94]

The in vivo tumoricidal reaction after PDT is accompanied by a complex immune response. PDT is a highly effective means of generating tumor-sensitized immune cells that can be recovered from lymphoid sites distant to the treated tumor at protracted time intervals after PDT, which asserts their immune memory character.[95,96] Vascular shutdown is clearly an important aspect of PDT.[97]

Clearly, when generated under carefully controlled conditions using exogenous sensitizers and light in the visible range (400 -700 nm), $^1O_2^*$ can be exploited for therapeutic purposes, as in antineoplastic photodynamic therapy (PDT). In biological systems, singlet oxygen has a short lifetime of <0.04 ms and has also been shown to have a short radius of action of <0.02 mm. [98]

However, in a cell with quenchers or scavengers abounding, $^1O_2^*$ lifetime can be <50 nsec with a diffusion distance <10 nm from its point of origin, which is less than 0.1% of the radius of an average eukaryotic cell. This short distance of reactivity can have clinical and therapeutic benefits and limit the target area or "zone of reactivity."

Although controversial, it is important to remember that all antibodies apparently go through a singlet oxygen and ozone step. Antibodies can generate hydrogen peroxide (H_2O_2) from singlet molecular oxygen ($^1O_2^*$). This process is catalytic, and investigators identified the electron source for a quasi-unlimited generation of H_2O_2. Antibodies produce up to 500 mole equivalents of H_2O_2 from $^1O_2^*$, without a reduction in rate. This work shows the enormous potential for H_2O_2 production by antibodies and their prooxidant mechanism of action. [99, 100]

The Howes Singlet Oxygen ($^1O_2^*$) Cancer Therapy System

Howes proposed a singlet oxygen generating system composed of physiological agents for the eradication of cancer, which did not have the limitations of conventional photodynamic therapy, radiation therapy or chemotherapeutic systems. In a pilot study at Tuft's Medical School, athymic mice, which had received human squamous cell carcinoma, experienced a 22.7% tumor disappearance rate in the "high dose group" following injection with the Howes singlet oxygen producing system. [101]

Even more encouraging results were seen, with an initial 80% disappearance rate, when basal cell skin cancers were similarly injected with this singlet oxygen delivery system. [102]

PDT generates similar products, in particular $^1O_2^*$, with similar chemical reactivity as the Howes Singlet Oxygen Delivery system.

Commonality Between PDT and the Howes Singlet Oxygen Therapy System

Pioneering work in the 1970s by Howes and Steele on microsomal lipid peroxidation [103] and aryl-hydroxylations [104] demonstrated evidence for the generation and participation of electronic excitation states, namely singlet oxygen. This was the first demonstration of a functional generation of an electronic excitation state, exclusive of vision, in mammalian systems. Their proposal, that singlet oxygen is the identity of the long sought out "active oxygen" acting on the cytochrome P 450 microsomal mixed function oxidases, has more recently been supported by the work of Yasui et al in 2002. [105]

While studying widely divergent biological electronic excitation generating systems, such as the microsomal mixed function oxidases, the neutrophil respiratory burst [106] and proline hydroxylation for collagen biosynthesis, one of the investigators (Howes) believed that these oxidative systems shared a point of convergence, expressed in the Howes Excytomer Pathway, involving superoxide anion and electronically excited singlet oxygen. [107]

Furthermore, Howes saw an additional commonality with generation of singlet oxygen produced by the steady-state physiological oxidative reagents containing an organic peroxide and the salt of hypohalous acid [108]

Subsequently, Howes reasoned that the peroxide/hypochlorite oxidative system may represent an ideal method of singlet oxygen delivery for effectively treating premalignant and malignant lesions, while simultaneously eliminating many of the drawbacks associated, not only with PDT, but with all other conventional methods of cancer therapy, including chemotherapy and irradiation. The peroxide/hypochlorite oxidative system has been shown to generate primarily singlet oxygen exclusively, as opposed to hydroperoxide/hypochlorite systems which have been shown to produce peroxyl and alkoxyl radicals. [109]

Ozone Therapy

Ozone therapy is practiced in most mainland European countries and the recently passed Alternative Therapy Legislation has made ozone therapy an option for patients in the USA in Alaska, Arizona, Colorado, Georgia, Minnesota, New York, New Jersey, North Carolina, Ohio, Oklahoma, Oregon, South Carolina, and Washington. Ozone therapy is not prohibited in Bulgaria, Cuba, Czech Republic, France, Germany, Greece, Israel, Italy, Japan, Malaysia, Mexico, Poland, Romania, Russia, Switzerland, Turkey, United Arab Emirates and Ukraine. Still, it remains on the fringe of mainstream medicine in America and the American Cancer Foundation has always strongly advised cancer patients against ozone therapy, as it does for other "Questionable methods of cancer management: hydorgen peroxide and other 'hyperoxygenation' therapies." [110]

However, scientific studies have found support for ozone therapy and investigators at Washington University discovered ozone inhibited growth of lung, breast and uterine cancer cells in a dose dependent manner while healthy tissues were not damaged by ozone. [111]

French studies have shown that ozone enhanced the treatment of chemo-resistant tumors and acted adjunctively with 5-fluorouracil chemotherapy in tumors derived from the colon and breast. [112]

Research has shown that ozone therapy can improve oxygenation in hypoxic tumors. [113-115] A 2004 study at Oxford University, using a human trial of ozone therapy, involving 19 patients with incurable head and neck tumors receiving radiotherapy and tegafur, plus either chemotherapy or ozone therapy, concluded that results warrant further research of ozone as a treatment for cancer. [116]

Cuban studies in rats [117, 118] and Russian human trials report benefits of complimentary ozone treatment and as regards drug complications. [119-121]

A 2008 study by Schulz et al, published in the International Journal of Cancer, found that survival of New Zealand White rabbits with head and neck squamous cell carcinoma could be enhanced by peritoneal insufflation of a medical ozone/oxygen gas mixture.

Hyperbaric Oxygen Therapy

It has been reported that hyperbaric oxygen therapy, using pressures at or less than 2.5 ATA, do not significantly increase EMODs in the presence of normal antioxidant defenses. Hyperbaric oxygen increases the oxygen in tumor tissue, as well as EMOD and prooxidant levels, and appears to enhance the efficiency of PDT. [122, 123] Hyperoxygenation appears to provide effective ways for improving PDT efficiency by oxygenating both preexisting and treatment-induced cell hypoxia. [124]

Relevant General Information

Lest we forget, oxygen and prooxidant EMODs play a central protective role against pathogens, as well as a crucial role in cancer therapy.

Polymorphonuclear cells (PMNs) require oxygen to kill organism by producing prooxidant superoxide, hydrogen peroxide, singlet oxygen and other products via the respiratory burst. [125] The PMN is protected by detoxifying free radicals with superoxide dismutase, catalase and glutathione. It has been shown in numerous studies that the degree of polymorphonuclear cell function in killing of bacteria is directly dependent on oxygen tension. [126, 127]

Scientists at The Ohio State University (OSU) have identified a way to predict very early in the treatment process the outcome

465

of radiation and chemotherapy for cervical cancer patients and it is based on oxygen levels within the tumor. According to Jian Z. Wang, the oxygenation of a tumor is critical for the success of cancer treatment because the amount of oxygen in a cell is directly correlated with the ability of that cell to repair radiation damage. Wang stated that, "Inevitably, those well-oxygenated tumor cells die, tumors are less likely to return, and patient survival rates rise." The research was described in the talk, "When the Oxygen Level Matters Mostly During Radiation Therapy of Cervical Cancer?" presented July 31, 2008 at the 50th annual meeting of the American Association of Physicists in Medicine.

Men with a low oxygen supply to their prostate tumor have a higher chance of the prostate cancer returning, as found by increasing prostate-specific antigen (PSA) levels following treatment, according to Benjamin Movsas, M.D., senior study author and chair of the Department of Radiation Oncology at Henry Ford Hospital. Moreover, recent studies suggest the same finding also appears to apply to patients treated with surgery. Movsas stated that "A tumor's oxygen supply can significantly predict outcome following treatment, independent of tumor stage or Gleason score (a classification of the grade of prostate cancer)." [128]

In short, consideration of oxygen levels in cancer chemotherapy is crucial for successful eradication of neoplasia.

Various cancer chemopreventive agents can induce apoptosis in premalignant and malignant cells *in vivo* and/or *in vitro,* which serve as an anticancer mechanism. Many of these apoptogenic-inducing agents function as prooxidants *in vitro.*

Significant *in vitro* data exists showing that antioxidants can block EMOD-induced apoptosis for a wide variety of cancerous cell types, such as leukemia, lymphoma, retinoblastoma, myeloma, pheochromocytoma and human cancers of the breast, lung, pancreas, liver, colon, rectum and endometrium. This data can not be ignored when considering effective prooxidant cancer therapy. [129]

In 2001, Harvard Medical School investigators observed a dose dependent inhibition of MBT-2 cell (murine bladder cancer) growth after exposure to doxorubicin hydrochloride, which could be enhanced by hydrogen peroxide and inhibited by preincubation with alpha tocopherol. They concluded that hydrogen peroxide may be a relatively inexpensive, nontoxic method of augmenting the cytotoxicity of doxorubicin hydrochloride. [130]

To avoid the confusion with terms of the past, it is suggested that current scientific oxygen related therapies should be referred to as "prooxidant EMOD therapies."

CONCLUSION

The salutary role of EMODs in oncologic therapy has been scientifically substantiated by the use of prooxidant EMODs in currently available anti-cancer therapeutic methods, such as chemotherapy, radiation, photodynamic therapy, etc. Points of confluence exist within the many cancer methods available to treat cancer and many share the interaction of prooxidants. It also suggests potential courses of action clinicians may take when patients express an interest in prooxidant therapies or combinations thereof. Prooxidant EMODs have been proven to exhibit tumoricidal activity in both *in vitro* and *in vivo* studies. We must move forward and beyond the outdated and negative history surrounding so-called "oxidative therapies." Many prooxidant agents suggest selectivity in promoting the death of cancerous cells and avoidance of harm to normal cells. The prooxidant approach to cancer therapy begs for further scientific inquiry and additional validation.

Contrary to the unsupported and irresponsible statements of some major cancer agencies, this review clearly demonstrates that some prooxidant EMODs (a.k.a. oxidative therapies) are currently and have been for decades, integral, effective and safe theoretical and clinical agents in the battle against cancer. To deny the scientific facts supporting prooxidant EMOD therapies is to deny patients significant treatment modalities, which may be crucial to their survival. Various medically related organizations may deny the truth surrounding prooxidant cancer therapy but they can not change the truth, which is exposed to all by a review of the literature.

RMH Note: Hydrogen peroxide is fundamental to the apoptotic process and tumoricidal activity.

CONCLUSION

REFERENCES

1. Harman D, Aging: a theory based on free radical and radiation chemistry. *J Gerontol* 11: 298–300, 1956.

2. Harman D, 1981. The aging process. Proc. Natl Acad. Sci. USA 78, 7124–7128.

3. Beckman KB, Ames, B.N., 1998. The free radical theory of aging matures. Physiol. Rev. 78, 547–581.

4. Finkel T, Holbrook NJ, 2000. Oxidants, oxidative stress and the biology of ageing. Nature 408, 239–247) (Harman D. 1961. Mutation, cancer and aging. Lancet 1: 200-201.

5. Harman D. 1961. Mutation, cancer and aging. Lancet 1: 200-201.

6. Howes RM, The Free Radical Fantasy: A Panoply of Paradoxes. Ann. N.Y. Acad. Sci. 2006;1067:22-26.

7. Aw TY, 1999. Molecular and cellular responses to oxidative stress and changes in oxidation–reduction imbalance in the intestine. Am. J. Clin. Nutr. 70, 557–565.

8. Kwon YW, Masutani H., Nakamura H, Ishii Y, Yodoi J, 2003. Redox regulation of cell growth and cell death. Biol. Chem. 384, 991–996.

9. Duranteau J, Chandel NS, Kulisz A, Shao Z, Schumacker PT, 1998. Intracellular signaling by reactive oxygen species during hypoxia in cardiomyocytes. J. Biol. Chem. 273, 11619–11624.

10. Valko M, et al. Free radicals and antioxidants in normal physiological functions and human disease. Int J Biochem Cell Biol. 2007;39(1):44-84. Epub 2006 Aug 4.

11. White MK. and McCubrey JA. (2001) Suppression of apoptosis: role in cell growth and neoplasia. Leukemia, 15, 1011–10121.

12. Fiers W, Beyaert R, Declercq W,Vandenabeele P. More than one way to die: apoptosis, necrosis and reactive oxygen damage. Oncogene (1999) 18: 7719-30.

13. Howes M.D., PhD., R, (2007). Cancer, Apoptosis and Reactive Oxygen Species: A New Paradigm. *PHILICA.COM Article number 86*. Feb. 26th, 2007.

14. Begin ME, Ells G, Horrobin DF. Polyunsaturated fatty acid induced cytotoxicity against tumor cells and its relationship to lipid peroxidation. J Natl Cancer Inst 1988;80:188–94.

15. Begin ME. Effects of polyunsaturated fatty acids and of their oxidation products on cell survival. Chem Phys Lipids 1987;45:269–313.

16. Das UN, Begin ME, Ells G, Huang YS, Horrobin DF. Polyunsaturated fatty acids augment free radical generation in tumor cells in vitro. Biochem Biophys Res Commun 1987;145:15–24.

17. Lhuillery C, Cognault S, Germain E, Jourdan ML, Bougnoux P. Suppression of the promoter effect of polyunsaturated fatty acids by the absence of dietary vitamin E in experimental mammary carcinoma. Cancer Lett 1997;114:233–4.

18. Block KI, Koch AC, Mead MN, Tothy PK, Newman RA, Gyllenhaal C. Impact of antioxidant supplementation on chemotherapeutic toxicity: a systematic review of the evidence from randomized controlled trials. International journal of cancer. Journal international du cancer 2008;123(6):1227-39.

19. Chabner BA, Collins JM: Cancer Chemotherapy: Principles and Practice, pp 276-297, 314-333. Philadelphia, JB Lippincott, 1990.

20. Enger SM, Longnecker MP, Shikany JM, et al: Questionnaire assessment of intake of specific carotenoids. Cancer Epidemiol Biomarkers Prev 4(3):201-205, 1995.

21. Jarvinen R, Carotenoids, retinoids, tocopherols, and tocotrienols in the diet—the Finnish mobile clinic health examination survey. Int J Vitam Nutr Res 65(1):24-30, 1995.

22. Taylor PR, Wang GQ, Sanford MD, et al: Effect of nutrition intervention on intermediate end points in esophageal and gastric carcinogenesis. Am J Clin Nutr 62(suppl):1420S-1423S, 1995.

23. Frommel TO, Sohrab M, Doria M, et al: Effect of beta-carotene supplementation on indices of colonic cell proliferation. J Natl Cancer Inst 87(23):1781-1787, 1995.

24. Olson RD, Stroo WE, Boerth RC. Influence of N-acetylcysteine on the antitumor activity of doxorubicin. Semin Oncol 1983;10:S29-S34.

25. Roller A, Weller M. Antioxidants specifically inhibit cisplatin cytotoxicity of human malignant glioma cells. Anticancer Res 1998;18:4493-4497.

26. D'Andrea GM. Use of antioxidants during chemotherapy and radiotherapy should be avoided. CA 2005;55:319–21.

27. Parker-Pope T. Cancer and Vitamins: Patients Urged to Avoid Supplements During Treatment; The Wall Street Journal 2005 Sep 20 Sect. D:1.

28. Weijl NI, Cleton FJ, Osanto S. Free radicals and antioxidants in chemotherapy-induced toxicity. *Cancer Treat Rev* 1997. 23:209–40.

29. Judy WV, Hall JH, Dugan W, et al. Coenzyme Q10 reduction of adriamycin cardiotoxicity. In: Folkers K, Yamamura Y, eds. *Biomedical and Clinical Aspects of Coenzyme Q*, Vol. 4, Elsevier, 1984:231–41.

30. Sieja K, Talerczyk M. Selenium as an element in the treatment of ovarian cancer in women receiving chemotherapy. *Gynecol Oncol* 2004;93:320–27.

31. Cascinu S, Cordella L, Del Ferro E, et al. Neuroprotective effect of reduced glutathione on cisplatin-based chemotherapy in advanced gastric cancer: a randomized double-blind placebo-controlled trial. *J Clin Oncol* 1995;13:26–32.

32. Seifried, HE, McDonald, SS, Anderson, DE, Greenwald, P & Milner, JA, (2003) The antioxidant conundrum in cancer. Cancer Res 63:4295-4298.

33. Simone CB 2nd, Simone NL, Simone V, Simone CB. Antioxidants and other nutrients do not interfere with radiation or chemotherapy. Altern Ther Health Med. 2007 Mar-Apr;13(2):40-7.

34. Lawenda BD, Kelly KM, Ladas EJ, Sagar SM, Vickers A, Blumberg J. 2008. Should supplemental antioxidant administration be avoided during chemotherapy and radiation therapy?. Journal of the National Cancer Institute. May 27, 2008. 100(11)773-783.

35. Gray LH, Conger AD, Ebert M, Hornsey S, Scott OC, "The concentration of oxygen dissolved in tissues at the time of irradiation as a factor in radiotherapy". Br J Radiol. (December 1953) 26 (312): 638–48).

36. Dunn T, "Oxygen and cancer". N C Med J. (1997). 58 (2): 140–3.

37. Soengas, MS, Alarcon, RM, Yoshida, H, Giaccia, AJ, Hakem, R and Mak, TW, et al. Apaf-1 and caspace-9 in p53-dependent apoptosis and tumor inhibition. Science 1999; 284: 156-159.

38. Shimizu, S, Eguchi, Y, Kosaka, H, Kamiike, W, Matsuda, H and Tsujimoto, Y, Prevention of hypoxia-induced cell death by Bel-2 and Bel-xL. Nature 1995; 374: 811-813.

39. Giaccia, AJ, Hypoxic stress proteins: Survival of the fittest. Semin Radiat Oncol 1996; 6: 45-58.

40. Howes, RM, *U.T.O.P.I.A. - Unified Theory of Oxygen Participation in Aerobiosis.* © 2004. Free Radical Publishing Co. Kentwood, LA. (available at www.thepundit.com and www.iwillfindthecure.org)

41. Vaupel P and Harrison L, Tumor Hypoxia: Causative Factors, Compensatory Mechanisms, and Cellular Response. Oncologist, November 1, 2004; 9(suppl_5): 4 – 9.

42. Tsang WP., Chau SP., Kong SK., Fung KP. and Kwok TT, (2003) Reactive oxygen species mediate doxorubicin induced p53-independent apoptosis. Life Sci., 73, 2047–2058.

43. Liu L, Trimarchi JR., Navarro P, Blasco MA. and Keefe DL. (2003) Oxidative stress contributes to arsenic-induced telomere attrition, chromosome instability and apoptosis. J. Biol. Chem., 278, 31998–32004.

44. Djavaheri-Mergny M, Wietzerbin J and Besancon F, (2003) 2-Methoxyestradiol induces apoptosis in Ewing sarcoma cells through mitochondrial hydrogen peroxide production. Oncogene, 22, 2558–2567.

45. Gewirtz DA: A critical evaluation of the mechanisms of action proposed for the antitumor effects of the anthracycline antibiotics Adriamycin and daunorubicin. Biochem Pharmacol 1999, 57:727-741.

46. Hasinoff BB, Davey JP. Adriamycin and its iron(III) and copper(III) complexes, glutathione-induced dissociation, cytochrome c oxidase inactivation and protection: binding to cardiolipin. Biochem. Pharmacol., 37: 3663-3669, 1988.

47. Burger RM, Cleavage of nucleic acids by bleomycin. Chem. Rev., 98: 1153-1169, 1998.

48. Byfield JE, Lee YC, Tu L, Kullhanian F, Molecular interactions of the combined effects of bleomycin and X-rays on mammalian cell survival. Cancer Res., 36: 1138-1143, 1976.

49. Ferlini C, Scambia G, Marone M, Distefano M, Gaggini C, Ferrandina G, Fattorossi A, Isola G, Benedetti Panici P, Mancuso S. Tamoxifen induces oxidative stress and apoptosis in estrogen receptor-negative human cancer cell lines. Br J Cancer 1999;79:257–263.

50. Yokomizo A, Ono M, Nanri H, Makino Y, Ohga T, Wada M, Okamoto T, Yodoi J, Kuwano M, Kohno K. Cellular levels of thioredoxin associated with drug sensitivity to cisplatin, mitomycin C, doxorubicin, and etoposide. Cancer Res 1995;55:4293–4296.

51. Erhola M, Kellokumpu-Lehtinen P, Metsa-Ketela T, et al: Effect of anthracycline-based chemotherapy on total plasma antioxidant capacity in small-cell lung cancer patients. Free Radic Biol Med 21(3):383-390, 1996.

52. Halliwell B, Gutteridge JMC: *Free Radicals in Biology and Medicine.* Oxford University Press; 1989.

53. Davies KJ, Doroshow JH: Redox cycling of anthracyclines by cardiac mitochondria. I. Anthracycline radical formation by NADH dehydrogenase. J Biol Chem 1986, 261:3060-3076.

54. Doroshow JH, Davies KJ: Redox cycling of anthracyclines by cardiac mitochondria. II. Formation of superoxide anion, hydrogen peroxide, and hydroxyl radical. J Biol Chem 1986, 261:3068-3074.

55. Nicholson DW, ICE/CED3-like proteases as therapeutic targets for the control of inappropriate apoptosis. Nature Biotechnol., 1996. 14, 297–301.

56. Nicholson DW, (1996) From bench to clinic with apoptosis-based therapeutic agents. Nature, 407, 810–816.

57. Fleury C, Mignotte B, Vayssiere JL, Mitochondrial reactive oxygen species in cell death signaling. Biochimie 2002; 84:131-41.

58. Clement MV, Ponton A, Pervaiz S, Apoptosis induced by hydrogen peroxide is mediated by decreased superoxide anion concentration and reduction of intracellular milieu. FEBS Lett 1998; 440:13-18.

59. Hirpara JL, Clement MV, Pervaiz S, Intracellular acidification triggered by mitochondrial-derived hydrogen peroxide is an effector mechanism for drug-induced apoptosis in tumor cells. J Biol Chem 2001;276:514-521.

60. Simizu S, Umezawa K, Takada M, Arber N, Imoto M, Induction of hydrogen peroxide production and Bax expression by caspase-3(-like) proteases in tyrosine kinase inhibitor-induced apoptosis in human small cell lung carcinoma cells. Exp Cell Res 1998;238:197-203.

61. Mansat-de Mas V, Bezombes C, Quilletary A, et al. Implication of radical oxygen species in ceramide generation, c-Jun N-terminal kinase activation and apoptosis induced by daunorubicin. Mol Pharmacol 1999;56:867-74.

62. Li L, Fattah EA, Cao G, Ren C, Yang G, Goltsov AA, Chinaul ACt, Cai W-W, Timme TL, and Thompson TC. Glioma Pathogenesis-Related Protein 1 Exerts Tumor Suppressor Activities through Proapoptotic Reactive Oxygen Species c-Jun NH_2 Kinase Signaling. Cancer Res 2008;68(2):434–43.

63. Kirshner JR, He S, Balasubramanyam V, Kepros J, Yang C-Y, Zhang M, Du Z, Barsoum J, and Bertin J, Elesclomol induces cancer cell apoptosis through oxidative stress. Mol Cancer Ther 2008;7(8):2319–27.

64. Baker AF, Landowski T, Dorr R, Tate WR, Gard JMC, Tavenner BE, Dragovich T, Coon A, and Powis G. The Antitumor Agent Imexon Activates Antioxidant Gene Expression: Evidence for an Oxidative Stress Response. Clin. Cancer Res., June 1, 2007; 13(11): 3388 – 3394.

65. Isham CR, Tibodeau JD, Jin W, Xu R, Timm MM, and Chaetocin KC: A promising new antimyeloma agent with in vitro and in vivo activity mediated via imposition of oxidative stress. Bible. Blood, March 15, 2007; 109(6): 2579 – 2588.

66. Bhalla S, Balasubramanian S, David K, Sirisawad M, Buggy J, Mauro L, Prachand S, Miller R, Gordon LI and Evens AM. PCI-24781 induces caspase and reactive oxygen species–dependent apoptosis through NF-κB mechanisms and is synergistic with bortezomib in lymphoma cells. Clinical Cancer Research 15, 3354, May 15, 2009.

67. Lecane PS, M. Karaman W, Sirisawad M, Naumovski L, Miller RA, Hacia JG, and Magda D. Motexafin Gadolinium and Zinc Induce

Oxidative Stress Responses and Apoptosis in B-Cell Lymphoma Lines. Cancer Res., December 15, 2005; 65(24): 11676 – 11688.

68. O'Brien PJ. Molecular mechanism of quinone cytotoxicity. Chem Biol Interact 80:1–41, 1991.

69. Little JB. Cellular, molecular, and carcinogenic effects of radiation. Hematol Oncol Clin N Am **7**:337–352, 1993.

70. Borek C, Antioxidants and Radiation Therapy. J. Nutr. 134:3207S-3209S, November 2004.

71. Fang J, Sawa T, Akaike T and Maeda H, Tumor-targeted Delivery of Polyethylene Glycol-conjugated D-Amino Acid Oxidase for Antitumor Therapy via Enzymatic Generation of Hydrogen Peroxide. *Cancer Research* 62, 3138-3143, June 1, 2002.

72. Mallams JT, Balla GA and Finney JW, Regional oxygenation and irradiation in the treatment of malignant tumors. Prog Clin Cancer 1965; 1: 137.

73. Finney JW, Collier RE, Balla GA, Tomme JW, Wakley J, Race GJ, Urschel HC, D'Errico AD and Mallams JT, The preferential localization of radioisotopes in malignant tissue by regional oxygenation. Nature 1961; 202: 1172.

74. Finney JW, Balla GA, Collier RE, Wakely J, Urschel HC and Mallams JT, Differential localization of isotopes in tumors through the use of intra-arterial hydrogen peroxide: Part 1: Basic science. Amer J Roentgen 1965; 94: 783.

75. Schreiner A, Hyperbaric oxygen therapy in bactericides infections. Acta Chir Scand 1974; 140: 73-76.

76. Hampton MB and Orrenius S, Dual regulation of caspase activity by hydrogen peroxide: implications for apoptosis. FEBS Lett (1997) 414: 552-6.

77. Davies KJ, The broad spectrum of responses to oxidants in proliferating cells: a new paradigm for oxidative stress. IUBMB Life. 1999 Jul; 48(1):41-7.

78. Manakata T, Semba U, Shibuya Y, et al. Induction of interferon-gamma production by human natural killer cells stimulated by hydrogen peroxide. J Immunol 985;134(4):2449-2455.

79. Takeuchi T, Matsugo S and Morimoto K, (1997) Mutagenicity of oxidative DNA damage in Chinese hamster V79 cells. *Carcinogenesis*, 18, 2051–2055.

80. Drisko JA, Chapman J, Hunter VJ. The use of antioxidants with first-line chemotherapy in two cases of ovarian cancer. J Am Coll Nutr 2003;22:118–23.

81. Buettner GR. & Jurkiewicz BA, (1996) Catalytic metals, ascorbate and free radicals: combinations to avoid. *Radiat. Res.* 145, 532-541.

82. Halliwell B, (1990) "How to characterize a biological antioxidant", Free Radical Res. Commun. 9, 1-32.

83. Levine M, (1986) New concepts in the biology and biochemistry of ascorbic acid. New Engl. J. Med. 314,892-902.

84. Chen Q, Espey MG, Krishna MC, Mitchell JB, Corpe CP, Buettner GR, Shacter E, and Levine L, Pharmacologic ascorbic acid concentrations selectively kill cancer cells: Action as a pro-drug to deliver hydrogen peroxide to tissues. PNAS. September 20, 2005. Vol. 102. No. 38. pp. 13604-13609.

85. Chen Q, Espey MG, Sun AY, Lee J, Krishna MC, Shacter E, Choyke P, Pooput C, Kirk KL, Buettner GR, and Levine M, Ascorbate in pharmacologic concentrations selectively generates ascorbate radical and hydrogen peroxide in extracellular fluid in vivo. PNAS. May 22, 2007. Vol. 104. No. 21. pp. 8749-8754.

86. Chen Q, Espey MG, Sun AY, Pooput C, Kirk KL, Krishna MC, Khosh DB, Drisko J, Levine M, Pharmacologic doses of ascorbate act as a prooxidant and decrease growth of aggressive tumor xenografts in mice. PNAS. August 12, 2008. Vol. 105. No. 32. pp. 11105-11109.

87. Levine M, Espey MG, and Chen Q, Losing and finding a way at C: New promise for pharmacologic ascorbate in cancer treatment. Free Radical Biology & Medicine. 47 (2008) pp. 27-29.

88. Carr A and Frei B, Does vitamin C act as a pro-oxidant under physiological conditions? The FASEB Journal. 1999;13:1007-1024.

89. Zilberstein, J., Bromberg, A., Frantz, A., Rosenbach-Belkin, V., Kritzman, A. and Pfefermann R, et al. Light-dependent oxygen consumption in bacterio-chlorophyll-serine-treated melanoma tumors: On-line determination using a tissue-inserted oxygen microsensor. Photochem Photobiol 1997; 65: 1012-1019.

90. Al-Waili, NS and Butler, GJ, Phototherapy and malignancy: Possible enhancement by iron administration and hyperbaric oxygen. Med Hypotheses. 2006;67(5):1148-58.

91. Tomaselli F, et al. Photodynamic therapy enhanced by hyperbaric oxygen in acute endoluminal palliation of malignant bronchial stenosis. Eur J Cardiothorac Surg. 2001 May;19(5):549-54.

92. Agarwal ML, Clay ME, Harvey EJ, Evans HH, Antunez AR and Oleinick NL, Photodynamic therapy induces rapid cell death by

apoptosis in L5178Y mouse lymphoma cells. Cancer Res 1991; 51: 5993-5996.

93. Kochevar IE, Lynch MC, Zhuang S, Lambert CR, Singlet oxygen, but not oxidizing radicals, induces apoptosis in HL-60 cells. Photochem Photobiol. 2000 Oct;72(4):548-53.

94. Luna MC, Wong S and Gomer CJ, Photodynamic therapy mediated induction or early response genes. Cancer Res 1994; 14: 315-321.

95. Korbelik M and Dougherty GJ, Photodynamic therapy-mediated immune response against subcutaneous mouse tumors. Cancer Research 1999; 59: 1441-1446.

96. Korbelik M, Induction of tumor immunity by photodynamic therapy. J Clin Laser Med Surg 1996; 14: 315-334.

97. Henderson BW and Dougherty TJ, How does photodynamic therapy work? Photochem Photobiol 1992; 55: 145-157.

98. Moan, J. and Berg, K. The photodegradation of porphyrins in cells can be used to estimate the lifetime of singlet oxygen. Photochem Photobiol 1991; 53: 549-553.

99. Wentworth P Jr, Jones LH, Wentworth AD, Zhu X, Larsen NA, Wilson IA, Xu X, Goddard WA 3rd, Janda KD, Eschenmoser A, Lerner RA, Antibody catalysis of the oxidation of water. Science. 2001 Sep 7;293(5536):1806-11.

100. Wentworth P Jr, McDunn JE, Wentworth AD, Takeuchi C, Nieva J, Jones T, Bautista C, Ruedi JM, Gutierrez A, Janda KD, Babior BM, Eschenmoser A, Lerner RA, Evidence for antibody-catalyzed ozone formation in bacterial killing and inflammation. Science. 2002 Dec 13;298(5601):2195-9.

101. Howes RM, Tumoricidal Activity of An Injectable Singlet Oxygen System Generated From Physiological Agents. (The Howes Singlet Oxygen Cancer Therapy System). In *The Medical and Scientific Significance of Oxygen Free Radical Metabolism.* © 2005. Free Radical Publishing Co. Kentwood, LA. pp. 893-912. (available at www.iwillfindthecure.org)

102. Howes RM and Farber G, Tumoricidal Activity of the Howes Singlet Oxygen Delivery System in Human Basal Cell Carcinoma. In *The Medical and Scientific Significance of Oxygen Free Radical Metabolism.* © 2005. Free Radical Publishing Co. Kentwood, LA. pp. 883-892. (available at www.iwillfindthecure.org)

103. Howes RM and Steele R H, Microsomal chemiluminescence induced by NADPH and its relation to lipid peroxidation. Res. Commun. Chem. Path. Pharmacol., July-Sept. 1971, 2; 4 & 5:619-626.

104. Howes RM and Steele RH, Microsomal chemiluminescence induced by NADPH and its relation to aryl-hydroxylations, Res Commun. Chem. Path. Pharmacol., March 1972, 3; 2:349-357,

105. Yasui, H, Deo K, Ogura Y, Yoshida H, Shiraga T, Kagayama A and Sakurai H, Evidence for singlet oxygen involvement in rat and human cytochrome P450-dependent substrate oxidations, Drug Metab. Pharmacokin. 2002, 17 (5): 416-426.

106. Howes R M, Allen RC, Su CT and Hoopes JE, Altered polymorphonuclear leukocyte bioenergetics in patients with thermal injury, the Surgical Forum, 1976, 27:558-560.

107. Howes RM, Steele RH and Hoopes JE, The role of electronic excitation states in collagen biosynthesis, Persp. In Biol. And Med., Summer 1977, 20; 4:539-544.

108. Howes RM, Steele RH and Hoopes JE, Peroxide induced chemiluminescence in an in vitro proline hydroxylation system, 1976, 8; 1:77-84.

109. Noguchi, N., Nakad, A., Itoh, Y., Watanabe, A. and Niki, E. Formation of active oxygen species and lipid peroxidation induced by hypochlorite. 2002, Arch Biochem Biophys. 397; 2:440-447.

110. Questionable methods of cancer management: hydrogen peroxide and other 'hyperoxygenation' therapies. CA Cancer J Clin. 43 (1): 47–56. 1993.

111. Sweet F, Kao MS, Lee SC, Hagar WL, Sweet WE (August 1980). "Ozone selectively inhibits growth of human cancer cells". Science (journal) 209 (4459): 931–3.

112. Zänker KS, Kroczek R, (1990). "In vitro synergistic activity of 5-fluorouracil with low-dose ozone against a chemoresistant tumor cell line and fresh human tumor cells". Chemotherapy. 36 (2): 147–54.

113. Clavo B, Pérez JL, López L, et al. (June 2004). "Ozone Therapy for Tumor Oxygenation: a Pilot Study". Evid Based Complement Alternat Med 1 (1): 93–98.

114. Kusznieruk K, Tumor Hypoxia and Ozone Therapy". The Stem Cell Patent Journal, October 24th, 2006.

115. Bocci V, Larini A, Micheli V (April 2005). "Restoration of normoxia by ozone therapy may control neoplastic growth: a review and a working hypothesis". J Altern Complement Med 11 (2): 257–65.

116. Clavo B, Ruiz A, Lloret M, et al. (December 2004). "Adjuvant Ozonetherapy in Advanced Head and Neck Tumors: A

Comparative Study". Evid Based Complement Alternat Med 1 (3): 321–325.

117. Borrego A, Zamora ZB, González R, et al. (February 2004). "Protection by ozone preconditioning is mediated by the antioxidant system in cisplatin-induced nephrotoxicity in rats". Mediators Inflamm. 13 (1): 13–9).

118. Borrego A, Zamora ZB, González R, et al. (August 2006)."Ozone/oxygen mixture modifies the subcellular redistribution of Bax protein in renal tissue from rats treated with cisplatin".Arch. Med. Res. 37 (6): 717–22.

119. Potanin et al., Ozonotherapy In The Early Postoperative Period In The Surgical Treatment Of The Lung Cancer. [Written in Russian] Kazanskij Medicinskij Zurnal No. 4, 263-265, 2000.

120. Gretchkanev et al., Role of Ozone Therapy in Prevention and Treatment of Complications of Drug Therapy for Ovarian Cancer. Akusherstvo Ginekologiya No 4, 57-58, 2002.

121. Kontorschikova et al., Ozonetherapy In A Complex Treatment Of Breast Cancer. In Proceedings of the 15th Ozone World Congress, 11-15th Sept 2001, Medical Therapy Conference (IOA 2001, Ed.), Speedprint Macmedia Ltd, Ealing, London, UK, 2001.

122. Tomaselli F, et al. Acute effects of combined photodynamic therapy and hyperbaric oxygenation in lung cancer. Lasers Surg Med. 2001;28(5):399-403.

123. Maier A, et al. Combined photodynamic therapy and hyperbaric oxygenation in carcinoma of the esophagus and the esophago-gastric junction. Eur J Cardiothorac Surg. 2000 Dec;18(6):649-54.

124. Chen Q, et al. Improvement of tumor response by manipulation of tumor oxygenation during photodynamic therapy. <u>Photochem Photobiol.</u> 2002 Aug;76(2):197-203.

125. Babior BM, Oxygen dependent microbial killing by phagocytes. N Engl J Med 1974; 298: 659-668, 721-726.

126. DeChatelet LR, Oxidative bactericidal mechanisms of polymorphonuclear leukocytes. J Infect Dis 1975; 131: 295-303.

127. Hohn DC, Oxygen and leukocyte microbial killing. Davis, J.C., Hunt, T.K. Eds. Hyperbaric Oxygen Therapy, Bethesday, Undersea Med Soc 1977; 101-110.

128. Hypoxic Prostate/Muscle pO2 (P/M pO2) Ratio Predicts for Biochemical Failure in Patients with Localized Prostate Cancer: Long-term Result." Abstract # 5136. ASCO 2009.

129. Howes M.D., PhD., R, (2009). Dangers of Antioxidants in Cancer Patients: A Review. *PHILICA.COM Article number 153.* Published 7th February, 2009.

130. Loughlin KR, Manson K, Cragnale D, Wilson L, Ball RA, Bridges KR, The use of hydrogen peroxide to enhance the efficacy of doxorubicin hydrochloride in a murine bladder tumor cell line. *J Urol.* 2001;165:1300-1304.

Randolph M Howes, PhD, MD

Randolph M Howes, PhD, MD completed residency in general surgery and plastic surgery while doing basic research in oxygen-free radicals at Johns Hopkins University. He invented the triple lumen catheter and, in 2004, published the first selective world review on oxygen metabolism in his book: UTOPIA (Unified Theory of Oxygen Participation in Aerobiosis), which was revised in 2014 and is now available at www.amazon.com.

Pro-oxidant Protection and Oxidative Self-Healing

Dr Howes believes the free radical theory is unfounded and that electronically modified oxygen derivatives (EMOD) are of low toxicity and are essential for energy production, pathogen protection, secondary messenger signaling and as tumoricidal agents. His unified theory states that EMOD deficiency levels allow for the manifestation of diseases, including neoplasia, and is integral in the aging phenomena. Dr Howes recognizes that antioxidants can commonly become pro-oxidants. He points out that antioxidants have failed to control aging and disease and that the scientific literature is increasingly showing that antioxidants can harm biological systems. Please refer to his other companion books also available at www.amazon.com.

www.ingramcontent.com/pod-product-compliance
Lightning Source LLC
Chambersburg PA
CBHW071841200526
45167CB00016B/16